Massa... ...herapists

Massage for Therapists

A guide to soft tissue therapy

Third edition

Margaret Hollis
Edited by Elisabeth Jones

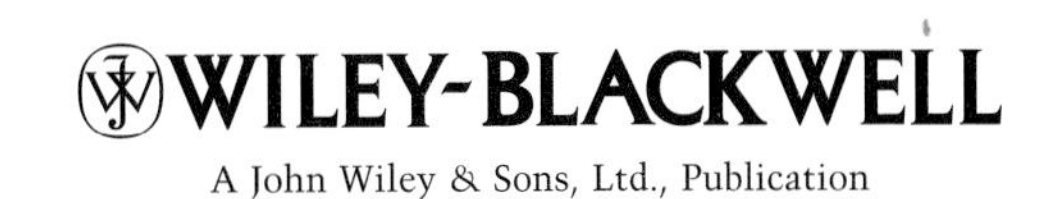

This edition first published 2009

Blackwell Publishing was acquired by John Wiley & Sons in February 2007. Blackwell's publishing programme has been merged with Wiley's global Scientific, Technical, and Medical business to form Wiley-Blackwell.

Registered office
John Wiley & Sons Ltd, The Atrium, Southern Gate, Chichester, West Sussex, PO19 8SQ, United Kingdom

Editorial offices
9600 Garsington Road, Oxford, OX4 2DQ, United Kingdom
2121 State Avenue, Ames, Iowa 50014-8300, USA

For details of our global editorial offices, for customer services and for information about how to apply for permission to reuse the copyright material in this book please see our website at www.wiley.com/wiley-blackwell.

Library of Congress Cataloging-in-Publication Data

Massage for therapists : a guide to soft tissue therapy. – 3rd ed. / edited by Elisabeth Jones.
p. ; cm.
Rev. ed. of: Massage for therapists / Margaret Hollis. 2nd ed. 1998.
Includes bibliographical references and index.
ISBN 978-1-4051-5916-6 (pbk. : alk. paper) 1. Massage therapy. I. Jones, Elisabeth, 1939– II. Hollis, Margaret. Massage for therapists.
[DNLM: 1. Massage–methods. WB 537 M4146 2009]
RM721.H58 2009
615.8′22–dc22

2009005287

A catalogue record for this book is available from the British Library.

Set in 9.5/11.5pt Sabon by SNP Best-set Typesetter Ltd., Hong Kong
Printed and bound in Singapore by Fabulous Printers Pte Ltd

1 2009

Contents

* From the chapter by Janice M. Warriner and the late Alison M. Walker in the second edition of this book (Hollis 1998).

Foreword

Congratulations! You are reading a book which has the potential to educate your hands, improve your massage techniques and increase your understanding of touch and its related therapies.

As someone who has taught massage, I know how immensely useful the book *Massage for Therapists* can be, and I am delighted that this latest edition is going to give a new generation the opportunity to benefit from Margaret Hollis's knowledge and expertise. When Margaret initially wrote this book it was aimed particularly at physiotherapy students, as she had taught many in her capacity as Head of the Bradford School of Physiotherapy, but what she has to say is just as important and relevant to anyone embarking on a career involving massage and soft tissue therapies. It is testament to the appeal of the earlier editions that this book has been translated into many languages, and I well remember Margaret's delight that her book was helping students throughout the world to improve their knowledge of how to massage safely and effectively, and understand the reasons for the treatment.

In this updated version we are indebted to Elisabeth Jones and her eminent band of co-contributors for the excellent additions to Margaret's earlier work. Their contributions provide an updated evidence base for massage, a comprehensive guide to assessing patients, and an insight into the many branches that have 'sprouted' from the massage 'root'. These have led to the numerous soft tissue therapies that are so important in health and well-being today.

My hope for you as a reader of this book is that you will come to understand the three basic principles of massage as a touch therapy. First, as a therapist you will be acquiring, through your hands, an in-depth knowledge of your patients and their tissues. You will then use this knowledge to apply the procedures correctly and in such a way that you help the body to heal. Relief from pain and discomfort through touch is an instinctive human reaction, but it has to be sensitively and thoughtfully administered to achieve its full potential. You use your educated hands!

Second, from the patient's perspective there must be a feeling of trust in the therapist. This stems initially from the two-way exchange of information during the assessment, followed by the receiving of the right depth and presssure of touch, and an explanation of the particular techniques. This then allows the patient to react positively to the treatment.

Third, this book should provide a realisation that this basic knowledge is the ground rock on which all other therapies are based, giving you the key to much greater understanding and ability to improve the human condition.

I wish you good luck in your quest, sensitivity in your fingertips and a focused mind to absorb the knowledge within.

Tessa Campbell MCSP, HPS, MIFPA
Chairman of the Chartered Physiotherapists in Massage and Soft Tissue Therapies (CPMaSTT)

Preface to the third edition

This third edition of *Massage for Therapists* is a follow-up to the first and second editions conceived and written by Margaret Hollis, MBE, MSc, FCSP, who was founding Principal of the Bradford School of Physiotherapy, and published by Blackwell Science, Oxford, in 1987 and 1998 respectively. Sadly Margaret died some years ago and I was invited by Amy Brown, Commissioning Editor, Physiotherapy Professional Division, to edit and write in this edition.

The new, enlarged book is aimed at providing students and therapists in the orthodox, integrated and complementary sectors with a textbook that describes, in detail, techniques that offer models of good practice for the reader to follow.

The chapters are written by different authors because of the need to be scientifically based and also in the interests of accuracy and validity of the techniques. The new chapters expand on, and are relevant to, the practice of massage as follows:

- Chapter 2 outlines the systems of the body that may be affected.
- Chapter 3 further reviews literature on the evidence base in relation to effects achieved, as well as awareness of risk and contraindications.
- Chapter 4 shows how to gather information, vital to the proper application of techniques.
- Chapter 12 revises some of the uses for classical massage techniques.
- Chapter 13 outlines some different techniques.
- Chapters 16 and 17 offer insight into two more specialised techniques.

There has been huge renewed interest in massage, partly due to further evidence-based research into its effectiveness and partly due to public awareness of its therapeutic value and therefore demand for treatment.

The contributors to this book are all health-care professionals and experts in their field. The majority are Members of the Chartered Society of Physiotherapy, UK, (MCSP) and in their curriculum of study one of the core subjects is massage. (Physiotherapists are often termed Physical Therapists in other parts of the world.) I am extremely grateful to them all.

I hope Margaret Hollis would have been proud of this third edition. It is dedicated to her memory.

Elisabeth Jones

Contributors

Andrea Battermann MCSP, HPC, MRSS (T)
Andrea Battermann first qualified with a diploma in social work in Germany in 1985. She is a chartered physiotherapist and a registered practitioner and teacher with the Shiatsu Society UK and qualified in physiotherapy in Germany in 1992. Andrea worked for several years within various specialities in the NHS including neurology rehabilitation, chronic pain management and out-patient clinics. She has built up a successful private practice incorporating physiotherapy, shiatsu, acupuncture, counselling and supervision for colleagues and students. Andrea authored a chapter in *Complementary Therapies for Physical Therapists* (ed. R.A. Charman). Her main interest is to link Oriental and Western medicine with psychology to create a more holistic model of health care.

Ann Childs MSc, MCSP
Ann Childs currently works as a lecturer and practitioner physiotherapist in mental health for the Nottinghamshire NHS Healthcare Trust and the University of Nottingham, Division of Physiotherapy. Her primary interests include touch and movement-based therapies in relation to working with trauma, and moving towards an integrated approach to physical/mental health delivery in the NHS. Ann's lifetime interest and enthusiasm in complementary medicine is expressed in her current role as chairperson for ACPEM, the Association of Physiotherapists in Energy Medicine.

Margaret Hollis MBE, Hon MSc, Hon DSc (Brad), FCSP, DipTP
Margaret Hollis trained as a physiotherapist and teacher of physiotherapy at the Swedish Institute at St Mary's Hospital, London, before teaching in New Zealand from 1946. She returned to the UK in 1950 to become the founding Principal of the Bradford Hospital School of Physiotherapy. The lack of definitive textbooks prompted Margaret to write, and she published several works on massage, exercise therapy, assessment and manual handling. The volume and diversity of her work was acknowledged in 1974 with the award of an MBE, and in 1984 the Chartered Society of Physiotherapy honoured her with a fellowship. Now at peace, we recognise her unique contribution to physiotherapy and to life.

Elisabeth Jones CBE, MCSP, MBABTAC, MIFPA
Elisabeth Jones is a chartered physiotherapist who has lectured and taught massage and aromatherapy worldwide and run a training centre for massage, aromatherapy and reflexology for 25 years. She has worked in the NHS and nursing homes, and currently has her own private practice. She is a

member of two clinical interest groups: Chartered Physiotherapists in Massage and Soft Tissue Therapies (CPMaSTT) and the Association of Physiotherapists in Energy Medicine (ACPEM). Elisabeth is a former Chairman of two organisations: the British Association of Beauty Therapy and Cosmetology (BABTAC) and the Aromatherapy Organisations Council (AOC).

Dr David Lee BSc (Hons), PhD, PGCHEP
Dr David Lee originally trained as a human biologist, qualifying with a BSc in 1999. Thereafter he completed a psychobehavioural PhD in sleep research at the University of Loughborough in 2005, before commencing work as a Research Associate in the Division of Nursing at the University of Bradford, School of Health Studies. David then moved on to lectureships at Bradford in the Division of Rehabilitation and the Graduate School, and is now working as a research fellow at the University of Newcastle-upon-Tyne in the Division of Clinical Psychology. His primary interests include sleep research, NHS service delivery and evaluation, the health and wellbeing of older people and quantitative research methodologies. He is also director of a company offering consultancy for individuals with sleeping problems and companies with shift-working employees whose performance may be affected by sleep disruption.

Stuart Robertson MSc, BSc Physiotherapy, BEd (Hons)
Stuart Robertson is both a qualified teacher and chartered physiotherapist. He has spent over a decade teaching nationally and internationally, predominantly on the integrative role of the fascial system and its importance in dysfunction and disease. This work has acted as an integral bridge between the clinical development and integration of mind–body techniques as well as energy medicine into the teaching of manual therapy skills. His background in physical education has also led him to develop a series of exciting physical exercises linked to the senses, which can be used in the clinical setting for specific injuries or simply for proactive health. His clinical experience has involved him working as a clinical specialist in an NHS chronic pain department through to working with international sportsmen and women. He is currently working towards an MEd, with the aim of introducing his stress reduction programmes into schools.

Ann Thomson FCSP, MSc, M Univ, FMACP, BA, Dip TP
Ann Thomson was a teacher, Vice Principal and Head of School at the Middlesex Hospital School of Physiotherapy until its closure in 1997. She joined the Manipulation Association of Chartered Physiotherapists (MACP) in 1970. In 1998 Ann became Director of Physiotherapy Studies, University College London, to continue the delivery of the MSc programme for physiotherapists. The philosophy of the programme is that quality, highly educated expertise must be developed in physiotherapists who transfer the best scientific and clinical evidence into the treatment and management of patients. Massage and soft tissue therapy have always been an integral part of Ann's teaching. She is a member of the Chartered Physiotherapists in Massage and Soft Tissue Therapy (CPMaSTT) team developing the Fundamentals of Massage and Soft Tissue Therapy course that is piloting an endorsement scheme with the Chartered Society of Physiotherapy (CSP). She has been honoured with a Fellowship award by both the CSP and the MACP.

Joan M. Watt MA, MCSP, MSMA
Joan Watt is a chartered physiotherapist who has worked in private practice since 1981, specialising in musculoskeletal problems, sports medicine and massage. As team physiotherapist and team manager, she has attended many sporting events including Olympic Games, Commonwealth Games and World Championships, and is Honorary Medical Advisor to the Scottish Commonwealth Games. She was lead physiotherapist to GB Athletics from 1984 to 1996 and is currently lead physiotherapist for British Shooting. She was Chair of CPMaSTT, the CSP specific interest group for Massage and Soft Tissue Therapy; she is Honorary President, First Chair person and founder of the Sports Massage Association; and a Member of the United Kingdom Athletics Anti-Doping Panel. In 1999 Joan authored *Massage for Sport*. Joan was President of Scottish athletics from 1999 to 2003, and received the CSP Distinguished Service Award in 2002.

Carol Young MRes, DipRG&RT, Dip Aromatherapy, MCSP
Carol Young qualified as a remedial gymnast and recreational therapist in 1979 and became a chartered physiotherapist in 1985. She worked in clini-

cal posts specialising in older person rehabilitation and stroke rehabilitation in the community. Carol joined the Bradford School of Physiotherapy team in 1990 as a clinical supervisor and made the transition to lecturer in 1993. The School has since become the Division of Rehabilitation within the School of Health Studies at the University of Bradford. Experience in teaching neuromusculoskeletal anatomy and physiotherapy treatment, research and reflective practice has complemented Carol's interest in massage which she is now teaching in the undergraduate physiotherapy programme. She has trained in connective tissue massage and shiatsu and gained a Diploma in Aromatherapy in 1998, continuing to practice in her spare time. Carol is committed to the continuation of massage as a core physiotherapy skill and has a keen interest in the various branches of massage and seeking evidence to support its use.

Acknowledgements

So many people have helped me with this new edition either by help and advice or through personal experience. My grateful thanks to everyone.

For encouragement at an early stage: Bob Chapman FCSP, MCSP, DipTP
For encouragement at later stages: Tessa Campbell MCSP; Ann Thomson FCSP; Joan Watt MCSP
For encouragement throughout: Amy Brown, Commissioning Editor, Professional Division, Wiley-Blackwell, Oxford.

To the authors of the following chapters:

- Chapter 3: Dr David Lee, Carol Young MCSP, Janice M. Warriner MCSP and the late Alison M. Walker MCSP
- Chapter 4: Ann Thomson FCSP
- Chapter 14: Joan Watt MCSP
- Chapter 16: Andrea Battermann MCSP
- Chapter 17: Ann Childs MCSP and Stuart Robertson MCSP

To those who contributed ideas for Chapter 12:

- Robyn Grieg MCSP
- Caroline Griffiths MCSP
- Pauline Melody BA, RGN
- Katy Mitchell MCSP
- Jac Tambellina MSc, RMN

To those who contributed ideas for Chapter 13:

- Bruce Aitkin MCSP
- Andrea Battermann MCSP
- Mary Bromily MCSP
- Ann Childs MCSP
- Suzanne Evans MCSP
- Mark Fairclough MCSP
- Ley Finlayson MCSP
- Donna Gurr MCSP
- Liz Holey MCSP
- Viv Lancey MCSP
- Jill Mintz MCSP
- Penny Nisbet MCSP
- Erica Nix MCSP
- Clare Phillips MCSP
- Stuart Robertson MCSP
- Ann Thomson FCSP
- Joan Watt MCSP

To everyone at the University of Bradford School of Physiotherapy, and in particular:

- Bryan Walkden MCSP who took all the photographs and reproduced the line drawings for this new edition.
- The models, both physiotherapy students at the time: Danielle O'Neill and Laura Robinson.
- Jan Warriner and all the staff, for their hospitality and for the photo-shoot in the precincts of the University of Bradford Physiotherapy School – where Margaret Hollis first set up

photographic pictures to illustrate her original edition of *Massage for Therapists*, of which Chapters 5–11 are the central core.

To the International Federation of Aromatherapists and the International Federation of Professional Aromatherapists.

To the indefatigable work of John Perrott AFC who set up and who copied all the contributions in this book, and without whom this edition could not have been put together.

To the students and patients I have had the good fortune to be involved with and from whom I have learnt so much about the therapeutic value of massage and soft tissue therapies.

Finally to my daughters, Felicity and Lucy, who have listened to and supported me throughout the editing of this book.

The basis for massage

1 Introduction to massage

Elisabeth Jones

Massage is an ancient art and modern clinical research has provided increasing scientific evidence for its therapeutic use. Since time immemorial 'the laying on of hands' has been known to have beneficial effects, not only on the body but also on the mind.

Think of a small child who has just had a tumble. The reaction of the worried parent is to hold her/him with a loving touch. Similarly, if we hurt ourselves, our instinct, more often than not, is to press and/or rub the affected part. Such gestures seem to be rooted deep in the psyche. The comfort that may be gained by such touch brings with it one of the fundamentals of healing, namely transference of caring energy to the traumatised person, wholly or in part.

The word 'massage' comes from 'mass' the Arabic term denoting 'to press'. There are many definitions of massage. Early in the twentieth century, Araminta Ross, Principal of the Dublin School of Massage, wrote in her book *The Masseuse's Pocketbook* (1907) the following:

> 'Massage is the term used to express certain scientific manipulations, which are performed by the hands of the operator upon the body of the patient. It is a means used for creating energy, where such has become exhausted, from whatsoever cause and is a natural method of restoring the part either locally or generally injured, to its normal condition'.

Prosser in 1941 gave another: 'The scientific manipulation of the soft tissues of the body as apart from mere rubbing'. Vickers in 1996 offered: 'Technically it can be described as the therapeutic manipulation of soft tissue'.

Its value as a therapy has been utilised throughout history by primitive peoples and by many civilizations, from the Chinese almost 5000 years ago to the Hindus of India, the Japanese, the Thai and the ancient Egyptians, some time later. The Greeks and the Romans were also proponents of massage. Hippocrates (460–377 BC) described its medical uses. The Roman Bath concept, where massage played an important part, was preserved in Turkey long after the fall of the Roman Empire. Not much documentary evidence is available on the use of massage in the Middle Ages. It was not until French missionaries returned in the early nineteenth century from China, carrying information from ancient Chinese manuscripts on massage, that its use as a therapy became popular in Europe and in the USA.

Western forms of massage

Per Henrik Ling (1776–1839) of Sweden founded an Institute in Stockholm in 1813 and promoted the therapeutic use of techniques termed 'Swedish massage and gymnastics'. In 1856 the Taylor brothers (Charles and George) brought Swedish Massage to the USA. In 1894 the Society of Trained Masseuses was formed (later incorporated into the Chartered Society of Physiotherapy) in the UK.

In 1932 Mary McMillan of Harvard Medical School, USA, was responsible for more advanced techniques in massage. In 1943 the American Association of Masseurs and Masseuses was formed and in the 1950s Gertrude Beard of North Western University, Evanston, Illinois, together with Francis Tappen, wrote a number of influential books on massage. Also in the 1940s and 1950s James Cyriax of St Thomas's Hospital, London, UK, developed transverse friction massage techniques.

Many other practitioners offered their ideas, too numerous to mention here.

Eastern forms of massage

As mentioned above, the Chinese, the Japanese, the Hindus of India and the Thais had developed their own types of massage centuries ago. *The Yellow Emperor's Classic of Internal Medicine* (*c.* 500 BC) was a book on Chinese medicine that provided a foundation for traditional medicine, practised in many Asian countries. Tui-na – a form of acupressure – originated in China. Anma (amma), a type of Japanese massage, came from China, whilst Shiatsu, a modern form of acupressure, was developed in the twentieth century AD. In India the 'Ayurvedic' massage techniques were based on the 'Vedas' which were ancient books written centuries before the birth of Christ, defining spiritual and philosophical beliefs.

Globalisation

With 'globalisation', many techniques are being incorporated within the modern practitioner's portfolio. Public awareness of the benefits of massage has grown and with it an ever-increasing demand for safe and effective treatment. It is therefore very important to have a knowledge of human anatomy and physiology, and the next chapter is written with the intention of providing an outline of the body systems relevant to the practice of massage.

Further reading

Beard, G. and Wood, E.C. (1965) *Massage Principles and Techniques*. W.B. Saunders, Philadelphia.

Benjamin, P.J. and Tappan, F.M. (2005) *Tappan's Handbook of Healing Massage Techniques: Classic, Holistic and Emerging Methods*. Pearson Prentice Hall, Upper Saddle River, New Jersey.

Cyriax, J.H. and Cyriax, P.J. (1993) *Illustrated Manual of Orthopaedic Medicine*, 2nd edn. Butterworth Heinemann, Oxford.

Fritz, S. (2004) *Fundamentals of Therapeutic Massage*, 3rd edn. Mosby, St Louis.

Holey, E. and Cook, E. (2003) *Evidence Based Massage, a Practical Guide for Therapists*. Churchill Livingstone, Edinburgh.

Hollis, M. (1998) *Massage for Therapists*, 2nd edn. Blackwell Science, Oxford.

Prosser, E.M. (1941) *A Manual of Massage and Movements*, 2nd edn. Faber and Faber, London.

Ross, A. (1907) *The Masseuse's Pocketbook*. Scientific Press, London.

Vickers, A. (1996) *Massage and Aromatherapy, a Guide for Health Professionals*. Chapman and Hall, London.

2 Relevant anatomy and physiology: an overview

Elisabeth Jones

This chapter gives an overview of the anatomy and physiology that is relevant, in this book, for the practice of massage, in particular classical massage.

THE SKIN

The skin is the outer covering of the body (Fig. 2.1).

Function

Protection: due to its structure it is a strong tensile barrier which protects the underlying tissues:

- From dehydration and from externally applied entry of fluids.
- From most chemicals and micro-organisms.
- From ultraviolet (UV) rays.
- From trauma.

Regulation of temperature: through conduction, convection, radiation and evaporation, the skin:

- Helps to remove excess heat in the body, via regulation of the circulation and thence the capillary network in its tissues, together with the evaporation of sweat.
- Maintains heat levels in the body, via regulation of circulation and therefore its capillary network, by virtue of the insulating effect of the adipose tissue below the skin and by the hair on the surface of the skin.

Sensation: the skin provides sensory nerve endings which conduct pain, touch, vibration, pressure, cold and heat. Some areas of the body have more neural receptors than others, e.g. the fingers have more than the back. Examples are as follows:

- Nociceptors: pain, temperature, itch, stretch, discriminatory touch, mechanical stimuli.
- Ruffini's corpuscles: tactile (crude pressure).
- Pacini's corpuscles: deep pressure, stretch, vibratory sensation, mechanical stimuli.
- Merkel's discs: light pressure, shear forces, vertical pressures, discriminatory touch.
- Meissner's discs: tactile, discriminatory touch, mechanical stimuli, vibration.

Excretion: excess fluid as well as waste products are excreted through the sweat glands.

Production of vitamin D: when UV rays are absorbed by the skin, they act on a chemical called 7-dehydrocholesterol, which is converted ultimately into vitamin D.

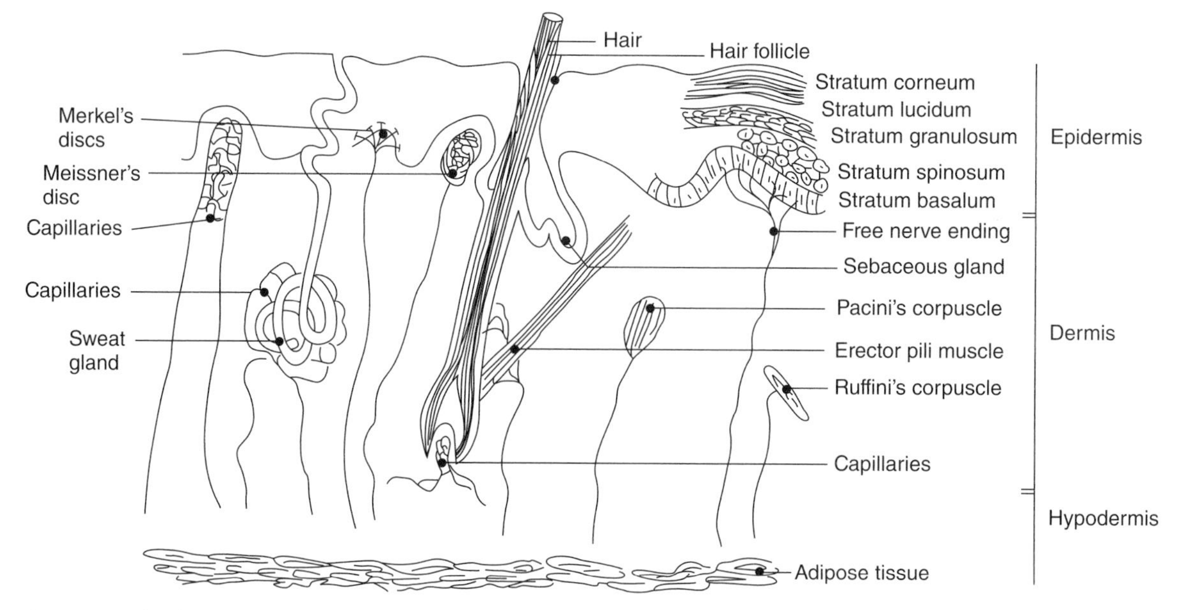

Figure 2.1 The skin.

Absorption: drugs and some other substances, such as essential oils, can be absorbed through the skin.

Immunity: specialised cells destroy pathogenic organisms, and Langerhans' cells function with T cells to provide immune reactions to some diseases.

To convey emotions: reddening of the skin may convey anger or embarrassment. Blanching of the skin can show anger or fear. Even tiny hairs may become erect in frightening situations.

Structure

Epidermis

This is made up of five layers or strata. The cells are mitotically active (i.e. they reproduce by splitting in two) in the lowest zone. As they work through the layers, they change, gradually hardening and drying until they become keratinised dried cells in the topmost layer, the stratum corneum. Here they desquamate (fall off). This process takes about 35 days under normal circumstances, which maintains the constant thickness of the epidermis. 'Thin' skin covers most of the body surfaces, 'thick' skin being found where there is a likelihood of much friction, e.g. soles of the feet and palms of the hands.

- Stratum basalum: the deepest layer of the epidermis. It consists of a layer of column-shaped, hydrated cells that contain nuclei and are mitotically active. This layer also contains melanocytes (melanin pigment cells), the number of which account for variations in skin colour as well as helping to protect from excessive UV rays.
- Stratum spinosum: this layer of irregularly shaped cells lies on top of the stratum basalum. There are intercellular bridges between the cells, giving a prickly or spiny appearance. Ribonucleic acid (RNA) is present and initiates the production of keratin, a water-repellent protein. The stratum basalum together with the stratum spinosum form the germinativum layer.
- Stratum granulosum: this layer lies on top of the stratum spinosum and has spindle-shaped cells. The nuclei of the cells are missing or disintegrating. This layer together with the stratum lucidum, the next layer above, may be missing in 'thin' skin. The process of keratinisation starts here due to the presence of kerato-hyaline.

- Stratum lucidum: this appears as a clear layer of closely packed cells with no nuclei. The cells have a soft substance called eleidin, which is gradually being turned into keratin.
- Stratum corneum: this is the most superficial layer and acts as a barrier and a protection against trauma to the skin due to its many layers of horny epithelial scales, containing keratin, in which no nuclei are discernible. This is particularly evident in 'thick' skin. It is the only completely keratinised layer, and is where desquamation continually takes place.

Dermal–epidermal junction

This cements the epidermis and dermis together, provides support for the epidermis and acts as a partial barrier to certain cells and large molecules.

Dermis (corium)

The dermis lies below the epidermis and the dermal–epidermal junction. It consists of two parts:

- Papillary layer: this is the upper layer. It has fibrous and connective material which forms 'convex humps' into the epidermis called papillae. Sensory nerve endings and capillary and lymphatic vessels project into the papillae.
- Reticular layer: this has a much more dense network of fibres than in the papillary layer. Collagen and elastic fibres are present, helping to give structure, support and elasticity to the skin.

Sensory nerve fibres and receptors, capillaries and lymph vessels as well as sweat glands and hair follicles are to be found in the dermis. Voluntary muscles such as the facial and scalp muscles are attached to the dermis, and involuntary muscles such as the erector pili, which cause the hair to become erect, are also attached to the dermis.

Subcutaneous adipose layer (superficial fascia) (hypodermis)

Below the skin proper lies the subcutaneous adipose layer. This is made up of areolar tissue (loose connective cells, rather like bubble wrap) and adipose tissue (fat cells) with capillaries and lymphatic and nerve fibres passing through.

Function

- To pack and support blood vessels, lymphatic and nerve fibres and some organs.
- To bind the skin to underlying layers.
- To store fat in the body, act as an insulator and play a part in heat regulation.
- To protect the organs.
- To give mobility to the skin.

Skin thickness varies. It is 5 mm in some places, such as the back, and 0.5 mm in others, such as in the eyelids.

Appendages of the skin

Nails

These are formed by cells, which originally developed in the stratum basalum and have become keratinised. Although nails do not have sensory nerve endings, pressure on them can cause sensation in surrounding tissues, and can help with the sense of touch.

Hair

Hair grows on most parts of the body, but not on the palms or the soles of the feet, lips and some genitalia. The hair is a keratinised structure with no sensory endings and arises from the base of the hair follicle, which is a deep indentation in the skin. The erector pili muscle is attached to the follicle and, when required, it makes the hair erect, e.g. in cold or in fear.

Sweat glands (sudoriferous glands)

There are two types:

- Eccrine: these are the most numerous, to be found over almost all the body surface other than the lips, nails, ears and glans penis. They arise from the subcutaneous tissue and are simple tubes, coiled at the base, secreting sweat which contains salts and waste products. As a result they help to regulate temperature and waste excretion.
- Apocrine: these are found in the axilla (armpit), the areola of the breast and around the anus. They arise from the subcutaneous tissue and are larger than the eccrine glands. They are associated with hair follicles and are simple

branching tubes. They have a viscous secretion, begin to function at puberty and appear to have a sexual function, possibly exuding a subliminal scent.

Sebaceous glands

These are usually associated with hair follicles. They are simple branching structures, situated in the dermis, other than on the palms and the soles of the feet. Some glands open directly onto the skin, namely those around the glans penis, eyelids and lips. They secrete sebum, an oily fluid which maintains the suppleness of skin and hair and has antifungal properties. In adolescence they can be overactive.

Ceruminous glands

These are a special type of apocrine gland, which are simple coiled tubes, opening into the ear and secreting a waxy substance.

Connective tissues

Connective tissue is composed of fibres, cells and sometimes fluids, in varying amounts, according to its purpose, together with a ground substance. Collagen and reticulin fibres give support, and elastin fibres offer elasticity. Among some of the cells are fibroblasts which help repair tissue, mast cells which are involved in inflammatory changes, and plasma cells which produce antibodies. The skin is a major connective tissue; others include bone, cartilage, ligaments and tendons, as well as blood.

Function

Connective tissue supports, transports, connects and protects the body. Damaged tissue requires healing by the formation of connective tissue. Adhesions occur when fibrous tissue becomes adhered to structures that have been traumatised. Overuse in a structure may cause extra fibrous tissue to be laid down in the musculoskeletal framework and it may become fibrosed, causing dysfunction.

Piezo-electricity

Physicists have found that electric fields are generated when pressure or stretch is applied to certain crystals (piezo-electric effect). Living crystals are soft and flexible, and crystalline arrangements are the rule, not the exception, in living systems. Connective tissue is considered by many to be piezo-electric. When bone and cartilage is compressed or when tendons, ligaments or skin are stretched, minute electrical pulsations are set up (Oschman 2000). This has led to the possibility that connective tissue may have energy-related properties which can be used in certain forms of therapy such as massage.

Fluid balances of the skin

The fluid within the systemic circulatory system is a transport mechanism which carries oxygen, carbon dioxide, nutrients, electrolytes, hormones, chemicals and many other substances, including waste products, to and from all parts of the body via arteries, arterioles, capillaries, venules and veins.

The lymphatic system primarily carries away excess fluids and waste products from different parts of the body. It produces antibodies in the lymph nodes to fight infection. There are capillary loops and lymphatic vessels passing up through the dermis into the papillary layer and it is vital that they function normally, so as to maintain the correct fluid balance not only in the skin but also in the body.

THE MUSCULOSKELETAL SYSTEM

The skeleton

The skeleton (Fig. 2.2) is the framework of the body and is composed of two types of tissue:

- Bone proper
- Cartilage

Both these are forms of connective tissue. Bone is a rigid non-elastic tissue. There are 206 separate bones. Movement of the body is possible because

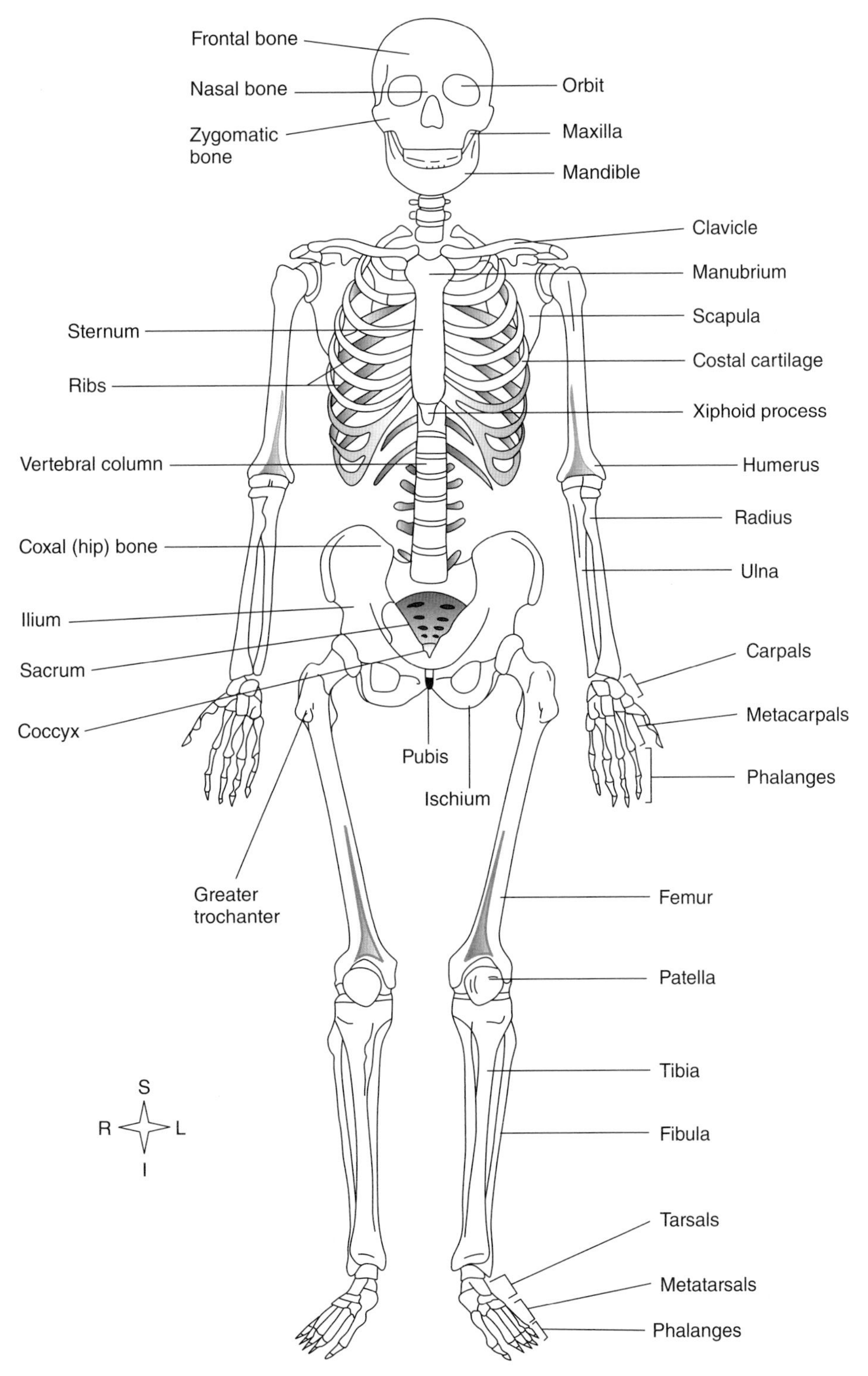

Figure 2.2 The skeleton. Reproduced from Thibodeau, G.A. and Patton, K.T. (2003) *Anatomy and Physiology*, 5th edn. Mosby, St Louis, copyright 2003 with permission of Elsevier.

when bones come together at joints, the skeletal muscles attached to the bones either side can by virtue of contraction and relaxation move them. Stimulation of the nerve endings in the muscles allows this to take place.

Cartilage is softer than bone, slightly elastic and less rigid. It forms the temporary skeleton in the developing fetus but is gradually almost entirely replaced by bone. It remains on most bone ends forming part of the joint and also in part of the rib cage and the respiratory tract.

Function

- **Support:** it provides the framework, position and shape of the body.
- **Protection:** it provides a protecting environment for the structures within, e.g. ribs for the lungs and skull for the brain.
- **Movement:** the muscles attached to bone at joints, by virtue of their contraction and relaxation, provide movement for the body.
- **Storage:** bones provide storage for minerals such as calcium and phosphorus.
- **Blood cell formation:** red bone marrow inside the ends of long bones such as the humerus and the femur, and flat bones of the skull, etc., provide blood cells.

Muscles

The muscles are soft tissue structures responsible for movement (see Figs. 2.3 and 2.4).

Function

Contraction: muscles have contractile tissue, which when activated facilitate movement, produce heat and maintain posture.

Structure

The muscular system is under the control of the nervous system. It can be divided into the following muscle types:

- Voluntary muscles (skeletal)
  These are under the control of the will and the central nervous system (CNS). The fibres are long and striped. They are attached to the skeleton and are responsible for body movement.
- Involuntary muscles (visceral)
  These are not under the control of the will but under the autonomic nervous system (ANS). The fibres are short and unstriped, lie in the visceral walls and move on the contents.
- Cardiac muscle
  This is a form of involuntary muscle, found only in the heart, not being under the control of the will but under the ANS. It also has its own nerve supply, and the fibres are short and striped. They create a wave of contraction which pumps the blood onwards through the heart, to the blood vessels.

There are over 600 voluntary muscles. The contraction of these muscles creates purposeful movement. Each muscle cell or fibre is roughly cylindrical in shape and consists of tiny parallel subunits called myofibrils. Different structures help protect the individual elements that compose muscle and are as follows:

- Endomysium: this is a delicate membrane of connective tissue covering the muscle fibres.
- Perimysium: this is a stronger connective tissue membrane which covers the groups of fibres.
- Epimysium: this is the coarser connective membrane sheath which covers the whole muscle formed by a collection of the groups of fibres.

Associated with muscles are the following: tendons, aponeurosis, ligaments and fascia.

Tendons

The fibrous tissues that attach muscles to bone are called tendons.

Aponeurosis

This is a flat band of connective tissue which connects one muscle to others by merging with the sheaths of these other muscles.

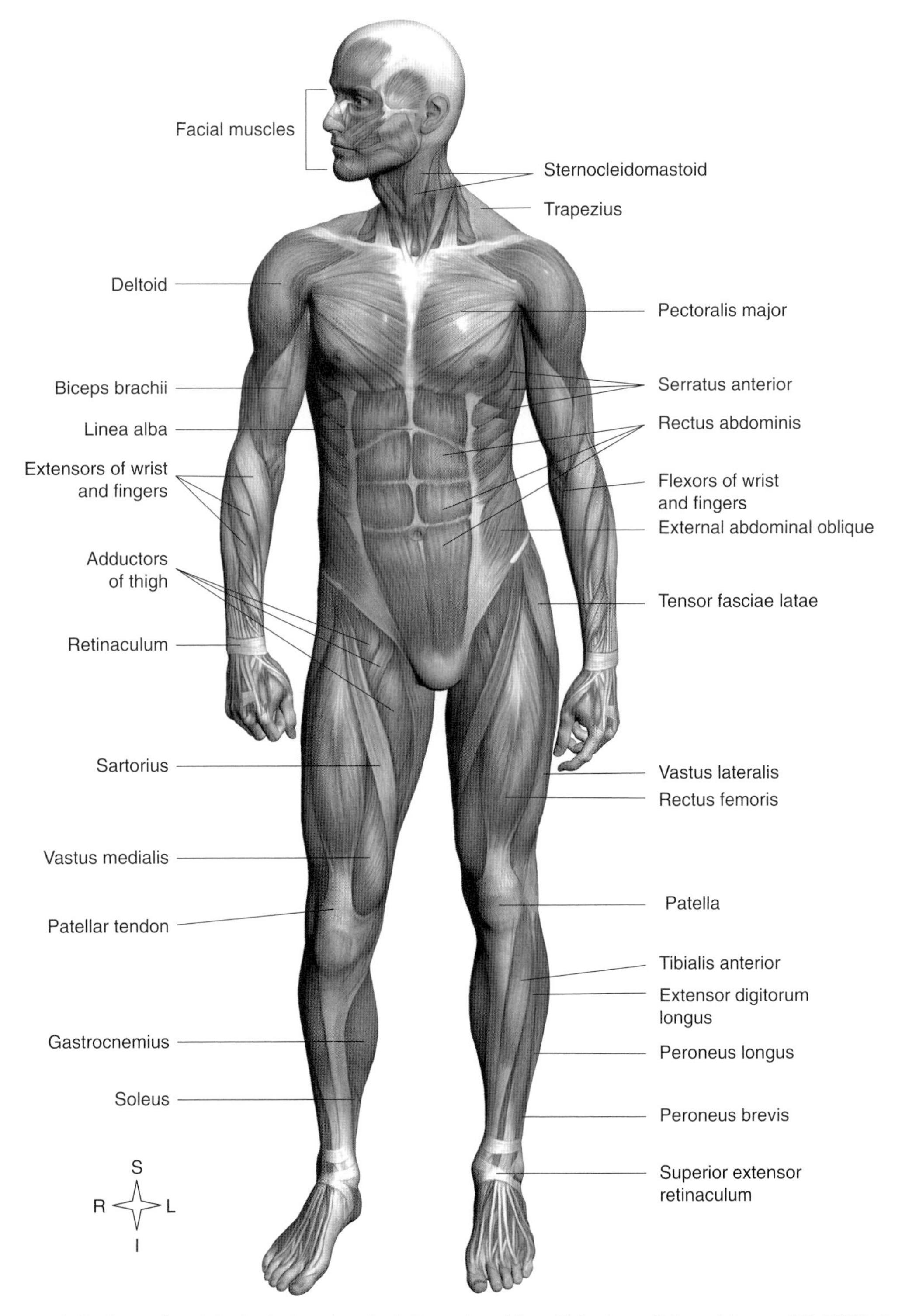

Figure 2.3 Skeletal muscles of the body (anterior view). Reproduced from Thibodeau, G.A. and Patton, K.T. (2003) *Anatomy and Physiology*, 5th edn. Mosby, St Louis, copyright 2003 with permission of Elsevier.

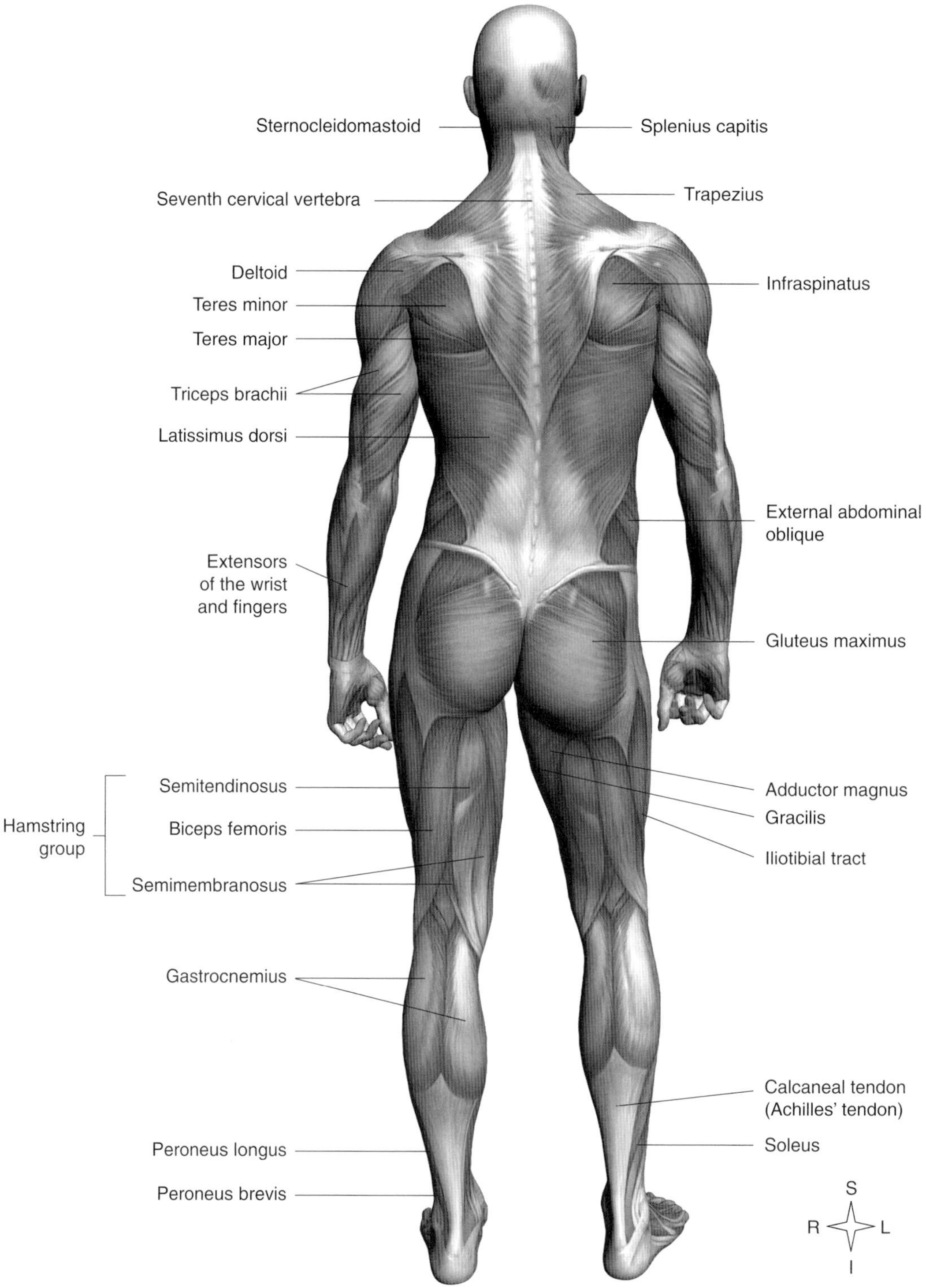

Figure 2.4 Skeletal muscles of the body (posterior view). Reproduced from Thibodeau, G.A. and Patton, K.T. (2003) *Anatomy and Physiology*, 5th edn. Mosby, St Louis, copyright 2003 with permission of Elsevier.

Ligaments

These are strong bands of fibrous connective tissue which hold bones together at a joint and also protect it.

Fascia

This is a structure that covers the whole body, lies below the skin and is made up of two layers of connective tissue.

- Deep: this surrounds the muscles, bone and deep organs.
- Superficial: this is the layer just under the skin.

Definitions associated with muscle action

'Neuro' refers to 'nerves' and 'muscular' refers to 'muscles'.

- Motor unit: a muscle and the nerve supplying it make up a 'motor unit'.
- Motor neuron: a muscle cannot contract unless it is stimulated by a nerve (motor neuron).
- Neuromuscular junction: a motor nerve (action nerve) stimulates a muscle through a motor end-plate at the 'neuromuscular junction'.
- Neurotransmitter: a chemical such as acetylcholine, which transmits signals across a gap (between two neurons) called a synapse.
- All-or-none law: muscle fibres obey the 'all or none law', i.e. each muscle fibre contracts maximally.
- Aerobic respiration: muscles get their potential energy from reactions between glucose molecules and adenosine triphosphate (ATP) in the presence of oxygen.
- Anaerobic respiration: if the oxygen supply to a muscle is reduced, as in high-intensity exercise, then the ATP is provided by 'glycolysis', a process that can proceed in the absence of oxygen, using glycogen stores in the muscle. Lactic acid is an end product of this process and causes temporary aches in muscle.
- Proprioceptors (mechanoreceptors): these are specialised nerve receptors which receive and transmit information about joint position, muscle tension, muscle tone, stretch, speed, direction of movement and body position.

Reflexes

Reflexes are automatic motor responses to sensory stimuli. Nervous system receptors when stimulated are interpreted and conducted through 'somatic' reflex arcs in the spinal cord.

- Stretch reflex: this is a 'feedback' mechanism controlling muscle length by causing contraction of muscle. The sensitivity of the muscle spindles to stretch has an effect on muscle tone throughout the body. Hyperactivity of these stretch reflexes causes increased tensions in muscle.
- Tendon reflex (Golgi receptors): this is a feedback mechanism whereby tendons react to the pull of a muscle contraction and respond by setting up muscle relaxation, to protect the muscle from excessive tension which might tear it from the tendon.
- Flexor and crossed extensor reflexes: the flexor reflex is elicited when an unpleasant sensation is received in one part of the body and other parts of the body go into action with the intention of withdrawing from the pain or noxious stimuli, (e.g. if the right foot stands on a drawing pin, the reflex action withdraws the foot and the individual rebalances, and possibly shouts).

Reciprocal innervation

This occurs when one muscle contracts and its opposite muscle relaxes, e.g. when the biceps contracts, the triceps reciprocally relaxes.

Common terms

Origin: this is the point from which a muscle arises.

Insertion: this is the point at which the muscle is finally attached. The origin is usually the 'fixed' point and the insertion is the 'moveable' point. Sometimes muscles do work from a reversed origin.

Action: this is the movement that occurs as a result of muscle contraction.

Tone: continuous partial contraction of some of the muscle fibres causes tautness in a muscle but not movement. For example, the postural muscles that keep us upright in standing or sitting are constantly finely adjusting their contractions to counteract gravity.

Anatomical position

Fig. 2.5 shows what is termed the anatomical position of the human body. Movement of the head, trunk and limbs, and position of these parts, is given particular terminology in relation to the anatomical position (Fig. 2.6).

Common terms

Anterior: to the front.
Posterior: to the back.
Medial: nearest to the midline.
Lateral: furthest from the midline.
Proximal: nearest to the trunk.
Distal: furthest from the trunk.
Abduction: away from midline.
Adduction: towards midline.
Flexion: bending.
Extension: straightening.
Lateral rotation: turn outwards.
Medial rotation: turn inwards.
Circumduction: abduct, adduct, flex, extend, rotate outwardly and rotate inwardly, all in one full movement.
Pronation: to place the anterior aspect face down.
Supination: to place the anterior aspect face upwards.
Opposition: to pull across (the thumb across the palm).
Dorsum: anterior aspect of the foot or hand.
Plantar: underside of the foot (sole).
Palmar: palm aspect of the hand.

Trigger points

These are small areas of tension or micro spasms in muscle or connective tissue (also known as myofascial trigger points, or MTPs). MTPs are sensitive to pressure and can feel tight (taut bands) and very tender. Pain is often referred from these points elsewhere. The local circulation is altered due to many different factors (metabolic, stress, nutrition, mechanical, posture, etc.). A 'twitch' response may occur when points are palpated. The painful points and areas are often found in similar zones in different individuals.

Nerve impingement

Soft tissues may cause compression or entrapment of a nerve, causing altered sensation or pain.

THE NERVOUS SYSTEM

The nervous system is divided into the central nervous system (CNS) and the peripheral nervous system (PNS).

The CNS

The CNS is composed of the brain within the skull, i.e. the cerebrum, the cerebellum, the midbrain, the pons, the medulla oblongata, the hypothalamus, the ventricles, the pineal body, the thalamus and the basal ganglia. Covering the brain are the meninges and the cerebrospinal fluid (CSF). The spinal cord within the vertebrae, and its coverings, the meninges and the CSF are also part of the CNS.

The PNS

The PNS is composed of nerves and ganglia:

- Cranial nerves (12 pairs) originate in the brain but go beyond the anatomical boundaries of the brain and the spinal cord.

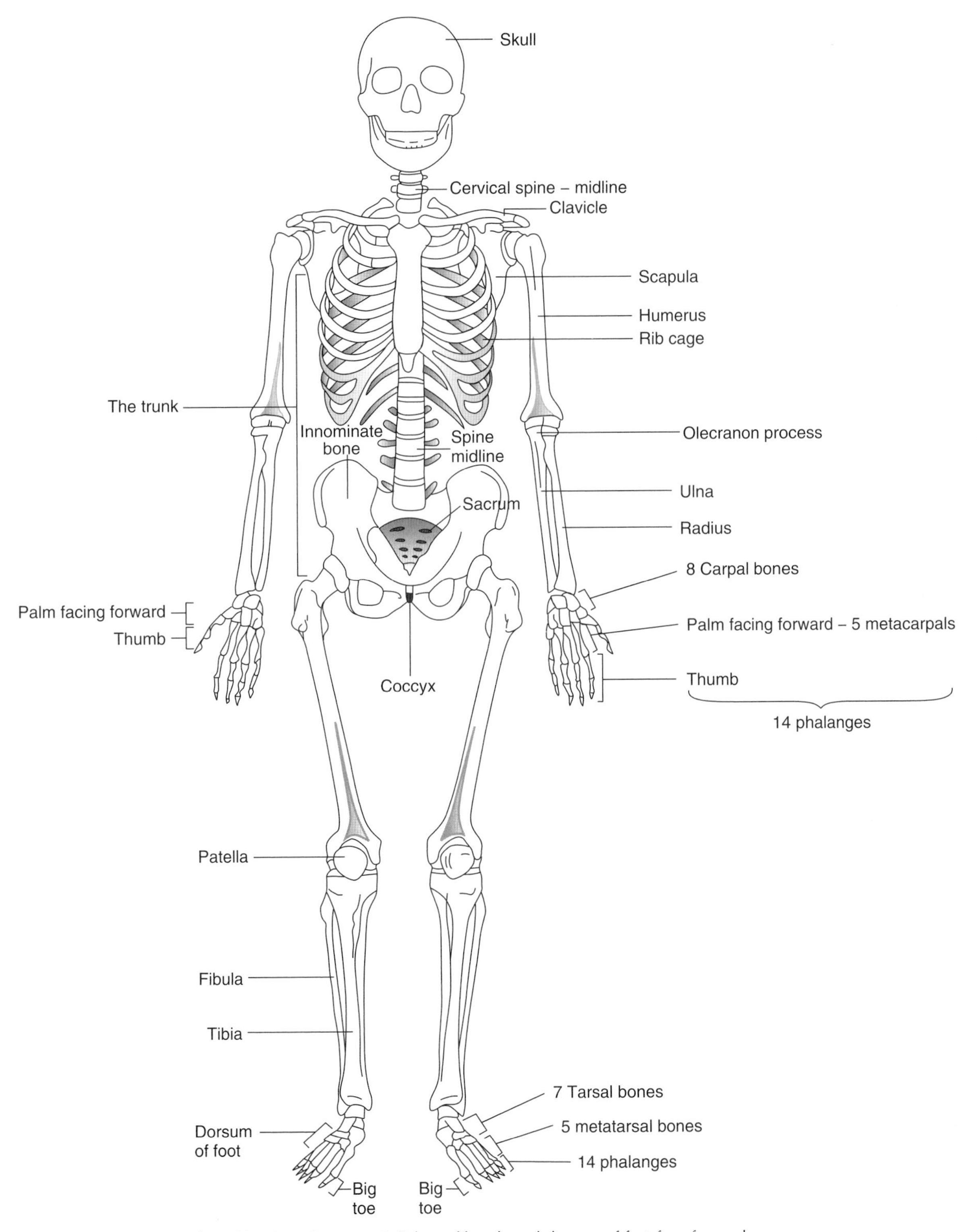

Figure 2.5 Anatomical position (anterior aspect). Palms of hands and dorsum of feet face forward.

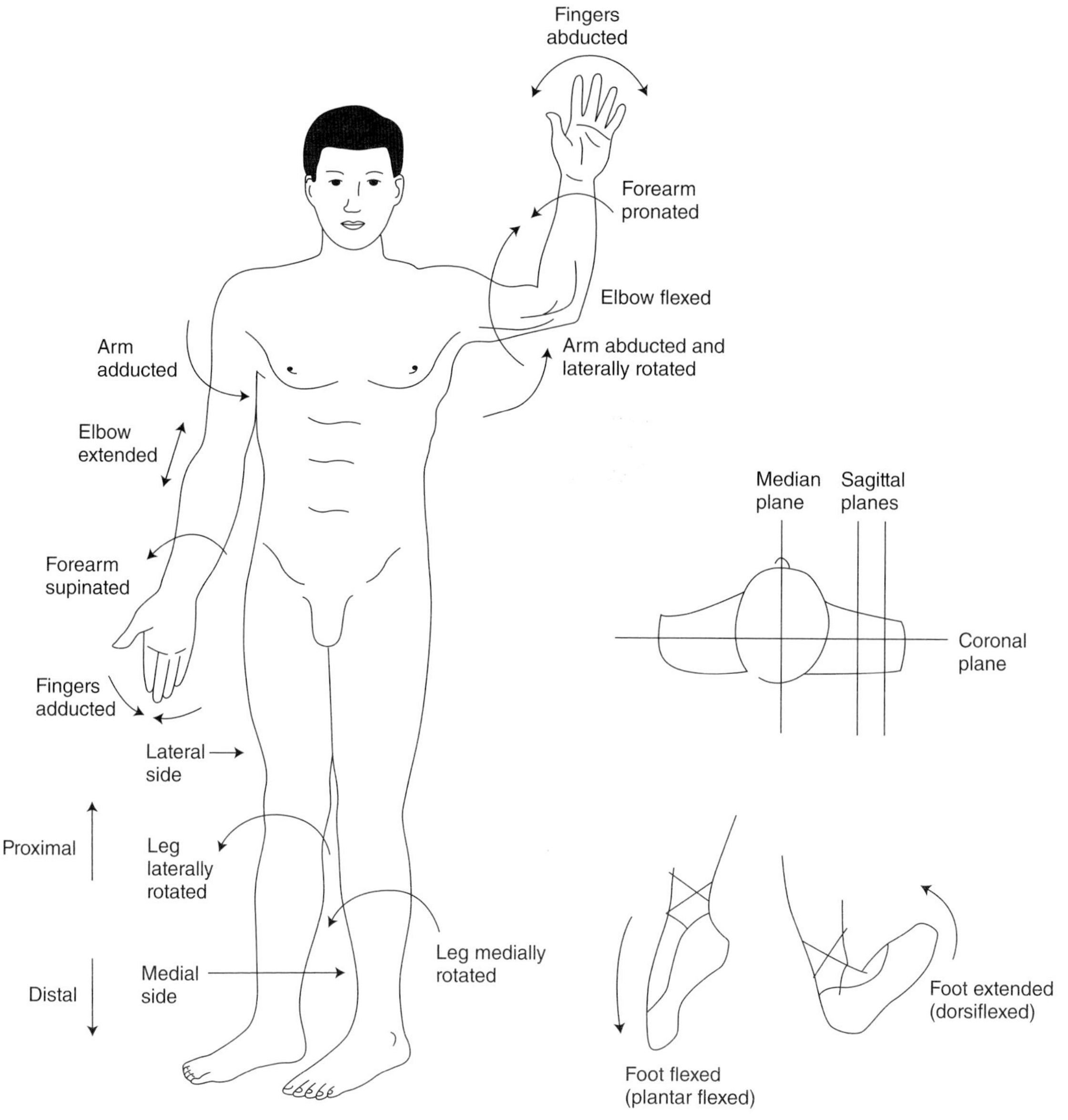

Figure 2.6 Some anatomical terminology. Reproduced from Faiz O. and Moffat D. (2006) *Anatomy at a Glance*, 2nd edn., copyright 2006 with permission of Blackwell Publishing Ltd.

- Spinal nerves (31 pairs) pass from the spinal cord to its periphery (anterior motor roots) and from its periphery back to the spinal cord (posterior sensory roots).

There are two types of spinal nerves:

- Spinal nerves which innervate muscles, joints and other structures, namely motor (action) efferent nerves and sensory (sensation) afferent nerves and a combination of these called mixed nerves.
- Autonomic spinal nerves (ANS) which innervate the viscera. There are two types of autonomic nerves:
  - Sympathetic nerves which have an excitory stimulating role (fight or flight syndrome).

- Parasympathetic nerves which have an inhibitory role (rest and repair syndrome).

Basic structure of the nervous system

- Neurons: a neuron is made up of a nerve cell, with its receiving processes, the dendrites, and its transmitting processes, the axon fibre and its nerve endings. White nerve fibres are medullated (covered in a fatty sheath called myelin). Grey fibres have no such myelin sheath.
- Neuroglia (glia): this is the supporting structure around the neurons.

The neuro-endocrine mechanism

Many cells have receptors for neurotransmitters and hormones and can therefore be influenced by both types of chemicals. The endocrine system influences the nervous system and likewise the nervous system influences the endocrine system – a feedback loop.

The neuro-endocrine content regulates physiological function. In an ever-changing chemical mixture there are fluctuations depending on body demands. Mood and perceptions of pain and stress can be affected by the variations in proportion of these chemicals.

For example, Dr Candace Pert and others discovered endorphin and non-endorphin pain-inhibiting hormones associated with activity of the CNS (Fritz 2004). Moreover, the body produces several opiate-like compounds such as enkephalin and beta endorphins. These help to relieve particularly chronic pain and produce euphoria. The body also produces cortisol hormone, which is at high levels when the nervous system is under stress.

Entrainment

This is an important reflex action which appears to be processed through the ANS and is the co-ordination of a synchronisation of various system rhythms. In the body, biological oscillators such as the thalamus of the brain and the heart set this pattern of rhythm. Research at the Institute of HeartMath in California, USA, indicates that the heart rhythm is the guide for other rhythms (McCraty *et al.* 1995). The synchronisation of the rhythms of the heart, respiration and digestion promotes body balance or homeostasis to create a healthy body.

THE CIRCULATORY SYSTEM

This is composed of two main parts, the cardiovascular system and the lymphatic system.

The cardiovascular system

This consists of the heart, the arteries, the arterioles, the capillary network, venules and veins, which form a closed system (Fig. 2.7).

Function

Transport: it carries oxygen, nutrients, salts, hormones, leucocytes to fight infection, clotting factors and other substances to the tissues, and returns waste products, carbon dioxide, water, dead cells, etc. back to the excretory organs of the body, as well as regulating temperature by movement of fluids.

Structure

The heart is the centre of this system, being a muscular organ which pumps blood out through the arteries and arterioles into a capillary network surrounding tissue cells, and back through venules and veins (which have valves to prevent backflow) to the heart (which also has valves to prevent backflow). The contracting period of the heart is called 'systole' and the resting period is called 'diastole'. The blood itself is an alkaline fluid, total volume approximately 5–6 litres (10 pints) and consists of plasma and blood cells.

Plasma

Plasma is the liquid part, clear and straw coloured, containing various substances including salts, hormones, plasma proteins, sugars, urea and amino acids.

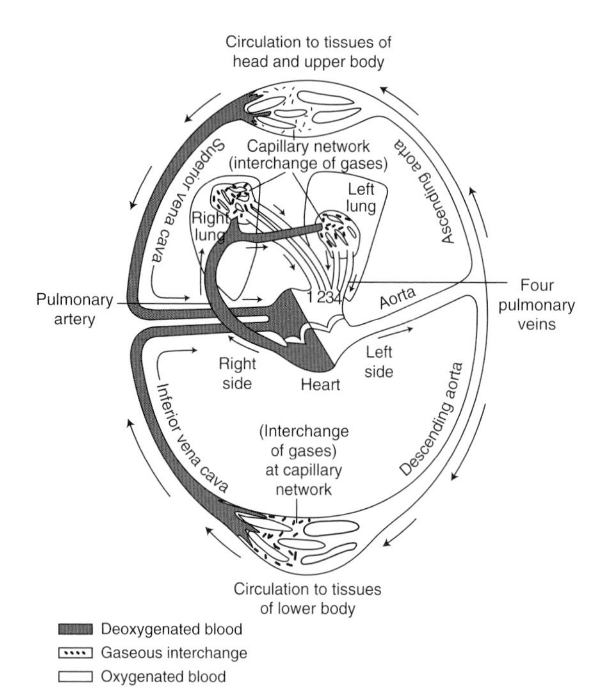

Figure 2.7 The cardiovascular system. Adapted from Thibodeau, G.A. and Patton, K.T. (2003) *Anatomy and Physiology*, 5th edn. Mosby, St Louis, copyright 2003 with permission of Elsevier.

Blood cells

- Red cells or corpuscles (erythrocytes) (RBCs). There are approximately 5 million per cubic millimetre (mm) of blood, and they are bi-concave with no nucleus. They are very small and so can pass through a capillary wall. They contain a substance called haemoglobin which carries oxygen to all parts and takes away carbon dioxide. They are manufactured in the red bone marrow.
- White cells or corpuscles (leucocytes or phagocytes) (WBCs). There are approximately 8000 per cubic mm of blood, and there are different types. Larger than RBCs, they have a nucleus generally irregular in shape. They are produced in bone marrow. They help with the defence of the body, being part of the immune system.
- Platelets (thrombocytes). There are approximately 250,000 per cubic mm of blood. They are minute spherical structures produced in red bone marrow. They are essential for clotting.

Blood pressure

This is the force or pressure exerted on the walls of an artery by the blood contained within it. It is influenced by age, exercise, rest, emotion, haemorrhage, arteriosclerosis (or hardening of the arteries by deposits of certain salts) and atherosclerosis (furring up of the arteries by certain types of cholesterol deposits).

Variations in blood pressure are considerable, but approximate readings in normo-tensive individuals should be, at rest, below 140 mm of mercury (or electric reading) for systole and below 90 mm of mercury (or electric reading) for diastole.

The lymphatic system

The lymphatic system is shown in Fig. 2.8.

Function

Drainage: of excess tissue fluids, maintaining fluid balances via lymph and blood capillary vessels.

Immunity responsibility: via lymphocytes manufactured in the lymph nodes.

Absorption: of fats and other nutrients via the lacteals which carry 'chyle', a specialised type of lymph, from the villi projections of the small intestine into the cisterna chyli, a chamber at the base of the thoracic duct in the thorax. Ultimately the contents of the duct flow into the cardiovascular system, where the duct joins the left subclavian vein.

Structure

The lymphatic system is not a closed circulatory system like the cardiovascular system. It consists of lymph capillaries (starting with blind-ended ducts in the tissues), lymph vessels, lymph nodes and two ducts, the right lymphatic duct and the thoracic duct, both found in the trunk. Tonsils, Peyer's patches, the spleen and the thymus gland are also part of the lymphatic system.

Lymph

Lymph (which closely resembles blood plasma and intercellular fluids) is the liquid that is absorbed by the lymph capillaries and is then carried through

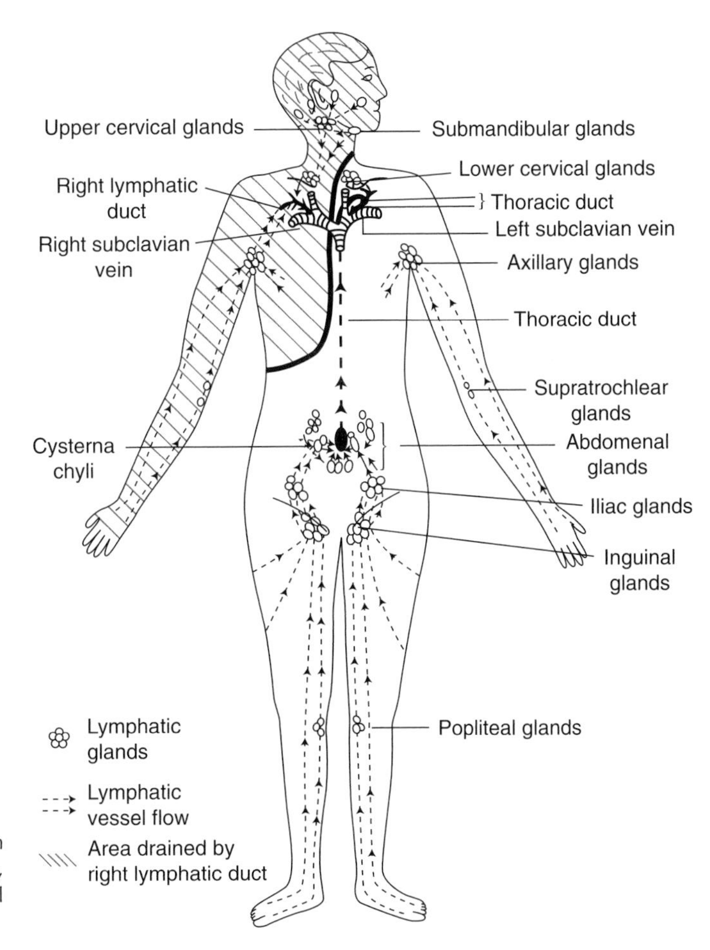

Figure 2.8 The lymphatic system. Adapted from Faiz O. and Moffat D., *Anatomy at a Glance*, copyright 2006 with permission of Blackwell Publishing Ltd.

lymph vessels and nodes, to be drained via the two ducts into the cardiovascular system at their junction with the right and left subclavian veins.

Lymphatic pump

The lymph flows steadily through the lymphatic system to the right lymphatic duct and the thoracic duct and thence into the two subclavian veins. The pumping action of contracting muscles and respiration aids this, together with the valves in the vessels which prevent backflow of the liquid.

THE CEREBROSPINAL FLUID SYSTEM

Function

Cerebrospinal fluid (CSF) nourishes, cools and protects the brain and spinal cord and influences breathing through its carbon dioxide levels. The movement of CSF has a pumping rhythm that some contend can be palpated. This rhythm seems to affect the phenomenon of fascial movement and is independent of other body rhythms.

Structure

The brain and spinal cord have three coverings, and a cushion of fluid. The coverings are:

- The **outer dura mater**
- The **middle arachnoid mater**
- The **inner pia mater**

The fluid is:

- The **cerebrospinal fluid (CSF)**

In the subarachnoid space around the brain and the spinal cord, and within the canals and cavities of the brain and spinal cord, there is CSF. It is separated from the blood in the choroid plexuses which are networks of capillaries in the brain. It circulates in the subarachnoid space and is reabsorbed into the venous blood through fingerlike projections (villi) of the arachnoid membrane.

Fluid balances

If we did not maintain the chemical nature and other characteristics of our internal body environment, we could not survive. Circulatory fluid in the cardiovascular system, the lymphatic system and indeed the CSF system shifts chemical products from place to place, and redistributes heat, pressure, nutrition and waste, etc. and helps to keep this environment normal.

This balance of fluids is a vital part of homeostasis balance which keeps the body healthy.

THE ENDOCRINE/HORMONAL SYSTEM (DUCTLESS GLANDS)

Function

The nervous system and the endocrine system work on their own or together as the neuro-endocrine system, to help maintain communication, integration and control. Both perform their function via chemical messages sent to specific cells.

Structure

There are glands in different parts of the body which perform specific functions via 'hormones', types of chemical messenger secreted by each gland and sent not through an opening (duct) but directly into the bloodstream.

The following constitute the main glands:

- **Pituitary** (**anterior** and **posterior**)
- **Pineal**
- **Thyroid**
- **Parathyroids**
- **Adrenals** (**cortex** and **medulla**)
- **Pancreas**
- **Gonads** (**ovaries** in the female and **testes** in the male)

The effects of stress on the endocrine system

Although difficult to define, stress can be anything to disturb a person's sense of wellbeing. What may for one person be an enjoyable challenge, to another may be a stressful situation. In particular will be those times when there are major life changes. There are obvious events that are considered to be stressful for nearly everyone: divorce, separation, bereavement, moving house, injury or illness, and job loss are examples.

The body's natural response to stress is to produce extra adrenaline, noradrenaline and corticosteroids. These increase heart rate and respiration as well as blood flow to muscles, so we are better equipped to run away from the event or stay and fight it. Selye researched these phenomena and termed it the 'fight or flight' reaction to stress (Antony and Thibodeau 1979).

Over a period of time, if unrelieved, stress may lead to conditions such as undue anxiety, insomnia and depression, as well as symptoms such as headaches, fatigue and digestive upsets.

Chronic stress where pressures are relentless, unmanageable or overwhelming is acknowledged as a risk for serious illness, hypertension, heart disease and mental illness.

THE RESPIRATORY SYSTEM

Function

Inspiration: the respiratory system is responsible for taking in oxygen, which is vital for all living cells as they require a constant supply in order to carry out their energy processes (metabolism). This is called inspiration.

Expiration: the respiratory system also gives up carbon dioxide and water vapour, which occurs as a waste product of the metabolism. This is called expiration.

Structure

The organs of respiration are:

- The **upper respiratory tract**: which comprises the nose, the mouth, the throat, the larynx, the sinus cavities and the Eustachian tubes.
- The **lower respiratory tract**: which comprises the trachea (windpipe), the bronchi, and bronchioles and alveoli (air cells) of the two lungs. The two lungs (right and left) lie in the thorax (chest) and either side of the heart. They are inert organs, meaning they work by a variation in the atmospheric pressure, caused by the work of the intercostal muscles and diaphragm muscle, to which they are attached. These muscles are themselves attached to the ribs (intercostals) and the vertebrae behind (diaphragm).

External respiration

Inspiration occurs when these muscles contract and expand the thorax, sucking air through the upper and lower respiratory tracts into the alveoli of the lungs. Expiration occurs when these muscles relax, the ribs revert to their original position and the lungs recoil, driving air out through the lower and the upper respiratory tracts and expelling it through the mouth.

Internal respiration

The inspired air containing oxygen passes through millions of air cells (alveoli) which have very thin walls. Oxygen is absorbed through these walls into the blood capillary networks surrounding the alveoli and travels via the cardiovascular system to all the tissues of the body. Carbon dioxide and water vapour pass out from the blood capillaries back into the alveoli during expiration.

Nervous and chemical control of respiration

The carbon dioxide and hydrogen ion content of arterial blood influences respiration by stimulation of chemo-receptors within the brain (medulla oblongata). Above-normal levels of these chemicals will promote faster breathing and a greater volume of air passing out in expiration.

THE DIGESTIVE SYSTEM

Function

Absorption of nutrition: the main function of the digestive system is to change nutrition taken via the mouth into a suitable form so that it can be easily absorbed into the body and utilised for growth, repair, heat and energy, with the waste products of these metabolic processes excreted at the anus, and by the urinary system, and sweat glands.

Structure

The digestive system proper is in essence a long tube stretching from mouth to anus with vital digestive structures incorporated along its route. These are the **mouth, oesophagus, stomach, small intestine** and **large intestine** (Fig. 2.9).

The digestive contents, once they leave the mouth and upper part of the oesophagus, are moved by the action of the involuntary muscles of the digestive tract, by a wave-like phenomenon called 'peristalsis'.

Accessory organs of digestion

Liver: which produces bile to emulsify fats in the digestive tract and stores products of digestion, among other important functions.

Gallbladder: which stores bile from the liver, to be used when there is more fat than usual in the digestive tract.

Pancreas: which produces enzymes used to act on fats, carbohydrates and proteins in the digestive tract, as well as producing insulin for sugar metabolism.

THE ENERGY SYSTEM

Technology is beginning to enable researchers to measure this subtle body system, to show that these electrical fields exist. Animal studies show, for example, that the platypus detects its living food source by sensing the electrical field around its prey

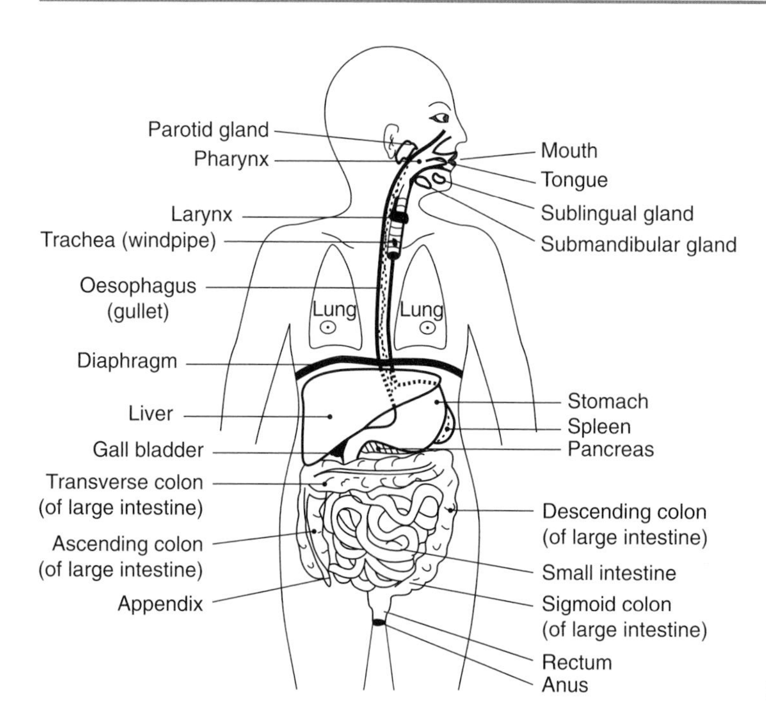

Figure 2.9 The digestive organs.

(Alcock 1989). There is considerable scientific debate, however, on the truth of the effectiveness of therapies based on such piezo-electric components of the body. Connective tissue, as already noted, is piezo-electric, and it extends throughout the body even to the innermost parts of each cell (Oschman 2000). Stimulation of a piezo-material causes either generation of an electric current or a vibration. Kirlian photography demonstrates the electromagnetic aura of energy which emanates from the body.

Dr Candace Pert theorises that energy healers may use their own energy fields to enhance the energy in their patients (Pert 1999). Massage by application of pressure has an effect on connective tissue which may enable it to conduct piezo-electricity.

References

Alcock, J. (1989) *Animal Behaviour: An Evaluatory Approach*. Sinawar, Sunderland, Massachusetts.

Antony, C.P. and Thibodeau, G.A. (1979) Anatomy and physiology. In: *Selye's Concept of Stress* (ed. H. Selye), p. 664. Mosby, St. Louis.

Faiz, O. and Moffat, D. (2006) *Anatomy at a Glance*, 2nd edn. Blackwell, Oxford.

Fritz, S. (2004) *Fundamentals of Therapeutic Massage*, 3rd edn. Mosby, St Louis.

McCraty, R., Tiller, W.A. and Atkinson, M. (1995) *Head–Heart Entrainment – A Preliminary Survey*. Institute of HeartMath, Boulders Creek.

Oschman, J.L. (2000) Energy medicine – the new paradigm. In: *Complementary Therapies for Physical Therapists* (ed. R.A. Chapman), Part 1, pp 3–36. Butterworth-Heinemann, Oxford.

Pert, C.B. (1999) *Molecules of Emotion; Why You Feel the Way You Feel*. Simon & Schuster, London.

Further reading

Field, T. (2006) *Massage Therapy Research*. Churchill Livingstone, Edinburgh.

Guyton, A.C. (1991) *Textbook of Medical Physiology*. W.B. Saunders, Philadelphia.

Rowett, H.G.Q. (1999) *Basic Anatomy and Physiology*, 4th edn. John Murray, London.

Thibodeau, G.A. and Patton, K.T. (2002) *Anatomy and Physiology*, 5th edn. Mosby, St Louis.

Thomson, A., Skinner, A. and Piercey, J. (1991) *Tidy's Physiotherapy*, 12th edn. Butterworth-Heinemann, Oxford.

3 Evidence-based effects, risk awareness and contraindications for massage

Dr David Lee and Carol Young*

Observation of the animal kingdom suggests that 'rubbing' of different types is useful to deal with the various discomforts of living. We have all observed domesticated animals 'licking' and 'stroking' wounded areas. Puppies and kittens are licked to facilitate digestive functions. Some primates rub each other to assist toleration of or to relieve a disorder. Every one of us has been rubbed or patted in infancy to assist voiding of wind and also to comfort and induce sleep in the fretful. Most of us will have held and then rubbed our bumps and painful areas such as disordered joints and muscles. These are subjective glimpses of some of the perceived benefits that massage may provide.

Massage has been regarded for a long time as having a variety of physiological and psychological effects (if from a largely empirical base). In recent years the therapeutic trend is ever more towards evidence-based practice and this has led to an ever-growing body of research seeking to establish scientifically the effects of massage. The research investigating the effects of massage, as with many areas of medicine, has produced evidence that is incomplete and often contradictory.

The potential effects of massage are many and variations in technique introduce yet another array of variables. Replication of studies is hindered by such subtleties as changes in rhythm or depth of technique and the length of application of massage. Many studies report misleading findings due to methodological inadequacy and inconsistency between studies.

Despite the problems with some of the research into the effects of massage, there would seem to be reasonable consensus with subjectively claimed benefits as to the systems and areas of the body affected by massage. Massage has effects that have been described traditionally under the following main headings:

- Mechanical
- Physiological
  - on the circulatory system
  - on the nervous system
  - on the musculoskeletal system
- Psychological

There is some difficulty in completely separating the effects under these individual headings as it would seem some effects could have appeared under at least two headings; for example, circulatory effects on the skin may be viewed as both mechanical and physiological. Part of the problem arises from the fact that massage is a system of mechanical techniques and when applied to living tissues

* From the chapter by Janice M. Warriner and the late Alison M. Walker in the second edition of this book (Hollis 1998).

subsequent effects are usually physiological – if at times bordering on the pathophysiological. Few effects would seem to be mechanical only. Subdivision of physiological effects into circulatory and neurological may also be problematic as not all of the reported effects fit neatly into these subheadings.

The effects of massage will be discussed under these main headings, while acknowledging semantic variations. Following this description of the effects of massage under these broad headings an examination of the issues surrounding the efficacy of massage therapy in vulnerable groups will be presented along with situations where massage therapy might be contraindicated or even ill advised.

Mechanical effects

Massage may have a number of effects on the skin. The constant passage of the hands over the skin will remove dead surface cells and allow the sweat glands, the hair follicles and the sebaceous glands to be free of obstruction and to function better. The increased lubricant effect is seen especially when desquamation is a problem. The circulatory effects on the skin are exhibited in some subjects by obvious reddening and by an increase in warmth often commented on by the patient.

Mobilisation of the skin and tissues at deeper levels is possible through the mechanical influence of the massage. The lightest massage will cause movement of the epidermis by the movement of the hand over the skin. In turn the epidermis moves on the underlying tissues and the dermis on deeper tissues.

Therapeutically, massage has been used widely in the management of scar tissue, the benefits of which can be observed most readily when healing of the skin is involved. Approximately 5 days after any damage has been sustained the weaker type III collagen is laid down as part of the repair process and begins to be converted to the stronger type I collagen (Lakhani *et al.* 1993). Massage may provide externally applied stresses that can influence the conversion of one type of collagen to another as well as the alignment of fibres which tends to be along lines of stress.

The stretching effects of carefully selected massage manipulations can help in promoting or retaining mobility of new 'skin' tissue relative to underlying tissue layers. The mechanical stresses of massage are useful to attempt to counter the tendency for repair scar tissue to shrink and shorten. Massage is often very successful in maintaining scar length while contributing to the strength of the repair and maybe assisting with other changes in the surrounding area, even if they are more through circulatory effects.

There is good reason to believe these positive influences on superficial scar tissue can be repeated at deeper tissue levels. Mobility between tissue interfaces occurs normally unless fibrous adhesions are present, when massage may stretch the tissues on one another. Appropriately timed massage intervention to encourage strength and alignment of repair fibres can enhance the natural process of healing in the tissues.

The percussive manipulations performed over the lungs have the mechanical effect of jerking adherent mucus free from the bronchial tree and, aided by gravity, assisting the removal of sputum towards the upper respiratory passages. The jarring effect and the vibratory effect probably cause some mixing of respiratory gases, while vibrations performed on the distended, wind-laden abdomen cause movement of the wind and relief of discomfort, whether in the infant after a feed or patients in the post-operative abdominal recovery stage. The mechanical effects of massage have for a long time been reported to be effective in terms of encouraging hyperaemia (resulting from histamine release), increasing the suppleness of tissues and parasympathetic activity, relaxing muscle tone, reducing oedema, activating mast cells and relieving subcutaneous scar tissue (Ironson *et al.* 1996; Duimel-Peeters *et al.* 2005).

Physiological effects

Physiological effects on the circulatory system

When massage is applied to the skin there is quite often an observable change of colour in the area. This change has been attributed most usually to the massage having an effect on the circulatory system. It has been reasonable to consider that massage applied to deeper structures would have similar effects on the blood vessels within such structures. Research papers have attempted to explore many aspects of the circulatory effects achieved by massage. Circulatory flow (venous, lymphatic, arterial), blood velocity and blood viscosity have all been areas of investigation during the last 50 years.

The squeezing, compressive and pushing elements of the massage manipulation carried out with centripetal pressure are widely considered to bring about drainage of venous blood and lymph. This was a view held by Scull (1945) who considered that venous and lymphatic flow could be mechanically enhanced in this way by 'displacement of their contents into regions subjected to lesser pressure'. Scull hypothesised further that such changes in circulatory flow may have occurred due to neurovascular adjustments.

A more recent study by Mortimer *et al.* (1990) looked at skin lymph flow in anaesthetised pigs using a 'hand-held' massager. The researchers found significantly increased ($p < 0.005$) isotope clearance rates in the massaged leg compared with the contralateral leg.

It is difficult to relate these findings directly to the effects of manual massage on the conscious human, but it does encourage speculation as to how changes in venous and lymphatic flow may be achieved.

The drainage of venous blood can be observed if a dependent hand in which the superficial veins are easily observed is stroked firmly. The soft-walled veins are compressed and the blood within them flows onward or centripetally. Its return is stopped by the presence of valves, which prevent backflow, and by the blood behind waiting to take its place. Lymph vessels are also thin walled and affected in the same way. All the minute drainage vessels must be equally affected so that as blood and lymph flows onwards more rapidly due to the massage, the replacing blood moves more quickly. In this way the drainage of treated tissues is enhanced, allowing fresh blood an unimpeded flow.

A number of studies have attempted to investigate changes in blood flow and have produced variable findings. Wakim *et al.* (1949) examined blood flow using venous occlusion plethysmography, a technique whereby the arterial flow is calculated from increased limb volume following venous occlusion. Following the application of vigorous, stimulating massage to normal subjects, average increases in blood flow of 57% and 42% for upper ($n = 12$) and lower ($n = 14$) extremities respectively were found. Even greater increases averaging 103% were shown following massage of limbs ($n = 7$) that were flaccidly paralysed following poliomyelitis. However, Wakim states that this massage is more forceful than that normally used by therapists and suggests that such pressure could be damaging to flaccid limbs. No evidence is provided for these assumptions and the sample sizes reported in this study are obviously small, limiting the generalisability of these findings.

In the same paper Wakim also reports findings on blood flow alterations using a less vigorous 'modified Hoffa type of deep stroking and kneading'. In one 'normal' subject no significant increases in blood flow were found. Taking a 15% or above increase as clinically significant Wakim reported significant increases in four out of six observations of massage to flaccidly paralysed limbs, with an average increase of 22% over the six readings.

Similarly, Severini and Venerando (1967) found significant increases in blood flow with deep massage. Only insignificant changes were noted with superficial massage.

In 1952 Ebel and Wisham, using sodium radioisotope clearance procedures, found no increase in calf muscle blood flow after 10 minutes' massage in comparison with a control test the previous day ($n = 7$). Hansen and Kristensen (1973), using 133 xenon isotope clearance, found a significant increase ($p < 0.01$) in muscle blood flow during 5 minutes' effleurage. This was followed by a significant decrease ($p < 0.05$) for 2 minutes post massage before returning to baseline values. The authors hypothesise that increases in blood flow during massage may be due to emptying of the capillary bed, leading to a decrease in blood flow post massage as the capillary bed refills. The authors also comment that the increases are relatively small, even less than in light exercise.

Also using 133 xenon clearance as an indicator of muscle blood flow, Hovind and Nielsen (1974) compared the effects of 2 minutes' petrissage to the thigh and forearm with 2 minutes' tapotement to the contralateral thigh and forearm ($n = 9$). Resting values were recorded prior to the intervention. Blood flow significantly increased ($p < 0.01$) following tapotement, but no significant change was noted following petrissage. The researchers suggest that tapotement might cause repeated muscular contractions, precipitating increased blood flow.

In a more recent study Tiidus and Shoemaker (1995) measured muscle blood velocity using ultrasound velocimetry ($n = 9$). Arterial blood velocity was measured before and during a 10-minute massage comprising deep and superficial effleurage, at 1 hour and 72 hours post treatment. Venous blood velocity was measured at 72 hours post treatment. No significant differences were noted between the rest and massage conditions for either arterial or venous velocities. Further investigation using Doppler ultrasound to assess blood flow in the lower limbs was conducted by Shoemaker *et al.* (1997). These authors reported that manual massage did not elevate muscle blood flow in any of the muscle groups massaged, nor did the type of massage used impact on muscle blood flow. They concluded that if increased blood flow is the desired therapeutic outcome, then light exercise would be beneficial, whereas massage would not (Shoemaker *et al.* 1997). These findings contradict those described by Hovind and Nielsen (1974) who reported a 35% increase in blood flow in skeletal muscle following massage using the tapotement technique. However, these authors report that the technique is rather painful and contraindicated for older people with thin skin/underlying tissue damage.

All these studies are hampered by small sample sizes and the gross nature of the measurements. Studies of the minute circulation to specific areas where the blood flow was compromised by trauma or disease might prove a more useful source of information. Comparison of these findings is difficult due to variations in massage applications and study designs.

Ernst *et al.* (1987) explored the effects of massage on blood viscosity. Using 12 healthy adults, blood viscosities were measured before and after a 20-minute whole body massage. A significant fall ($p < 0.05$) in native blood viscosity, haematocrit and plasma viscosity was noted. The researchers concluded that such viscosity changes suggest an inflow into the general circulation of low viscosity fluid derived either from stagnant microvessels or from interstitial fluid. Either of these could have therapeutic benefits. However, no control group was included in this study to compare the effects of rest and postural changes alone. The authors do state that they had studied these effects previously and found only small, insignificant falls in viscosity. In opposition to the findings of Ernst, Arkko *et al.* (1983) had previously found no change in haematocrit values following a 1-hour whole body massage.

On a cautionary note, when studying both humans ($n = 6$) and dogs ($n = 8$), Eliska and Eliskova (1995) found that massage applied at pressures of 70–100 mmHg caused damage to lymphatic vessels. The damage was greater if oedema was present.

Blood pressure, heart rate, skin temperature and conductivity, and oxygen consumption are among the factors researched. The findings of these studies into the effects of massage on these parameters are inconsistent. Comparison of studies is fraught with difficulties: study groups vary from the healthy to the critically ill, and the massage applied varies from a 1-minute back rub to a 1-hour whole body massage.

A number of well-designed studies failed to find significant differences in a variety of physiological measures as a result of massage. However, many of these studies had very small sample sizes. Some studies found significant increases while others found significant decreases as a result of massage. A number of studies continued measurements for some minutes after massage with variable findings as to the persistence of the effect. Until large-scale well-controlled studies using similar massage intervention have been conducted the picture will remain unclear.

However, it appears unlikely that the changes in blood pressure or heart rate will be great enough to be of danger to patients. The benefits of any decrease in blood pressure would only be of clinical usefulness if any carryover effects persist. Further studies into this aspect are required.

The observable effects in the human are cutaneous circulatory responses occurring in the following order:

- A transient white line appears in response to light pressure and is the result of an initial capillary constriction.
- Because the tissues are slightly traumatised by most massage manipulations and more so by those such as skin rolling and percussive manipulations, a histamine-related substance is released.

Histamine is stored in mast cells in the connective tissues, and in the basophil cells and platelets of blood, all of which may be disturbed or traumatised by the various massage manipulations. The release of this substance initiates the following triple response involving three reactions which follow each other rapidly. A red line appears and is caused by dilatation of the minute blood vessels independent of the somatic supply of the skin area. A flare of redness often described as a 'flush' then appears around the area and is due to a widespread dilatation of skin arterioles. This is brought about by the axon reflex. The third feature of the triple response is slight swelling, usually described as a wheal. The increased permeability of the capillary walls allows escape of more tissue fluid so that the area becomes slightly swollen. This fluid is almost identical to lymph.

Physiological effects on the nervous system

Massage is recognised as having an effect on the nervous system. Different methods of application will provide subtle variations of afferent input which, in turn, may cause a number of possible effects. Practice suggests that manipulations need to be selected for the specific effects that they may cause. It is believed that the diametrically opposite effects of sedation or stimulation of a patient may be achieved by selection of appropriate tempo, degree of pressure and length of continuity of each manipulation and the massage as a whole. It is noticeable that the sedative effect appears to require longer to achieve than the stimulatory effect, whether applied to the patient as a whole or to individual parts of the body.

In recent years researchers have begun to turn their attention to proving some of the claimed effects. An ever-increasing knowledge of the mechanisms operating within the nervous system has encouraged this research, along with a revival of interest in massage as a therapy and the development of suitable means of measurement.

Alpha motoneuron excitability

A team of researchers from Montreal conducted a series of studies on the effect of massage on the 'Hoffman' or 'H-reflex' excitability. The 'H-reflex' represents an indirect measure of spinal motor neurone excitability and therefore the excitability of the spinal reflex pathway. All these studies, published between 1990 and 1994, have consistently shown a decrease in the H-reflex amplitudes during massage. This denoted a decrease or inhibitory influence on alpha motoneuron excitability. A similar experimental design was used for all the studies: pre-treatment, baseline control readings followed by a few minutes' massage with readings (individual studies used 3-, 4- and 6-minute timings), terminating with post-treatment readings. The triceps surae muscle group was used on each occasion.

Morelli *et al.* (1990), by studying nine healthy subjects, were able to demonstrate a 71% decrease in H-reflex amplitude during a 3-minute application of petrissage to the ipsilateral triceps surae, but this amplitude reverted to normal levels when the massage was terminated. This suggests that reduced motoneuron excitability occurs only when the massage is being applied and there is no apparent carryover effect. A further study demonstrated that this inhibitory effect is only achieved in the muscle group receiving the petrissage and not in other muscle groups (Sullivan *et al.* 1991).

The study by Morelli *et al.* (1991) using more subjects ($n = 20$) and a 6-minute period of petrissage confirmed the decreased amplitude of the H-reflex in the triceps surae with still no carryover effects noticeable in the post-massage period. However, these authors went on to exclude factors such as changes in skin temperature, nerve conduction velocity and antagonist activity as being responsible for the decrease in H-reflex excitability. Rapidly adapting cutaneous and/or muscle receptors along with inhibitory polysynaptic, non-segmental pathways were proposed by the authors as possible mediators of these change(s) because of the immediacy of the noted response(s).

In 1992 Goldberg *et al.* reported that reduction of H-reflex excitability occurred with both light petrissage (pressure = 1.25 kPa) and deep petrissage (pressure = 2.5 kPa). A greater effect was noted with deep massage and this research team suggested that pressure-sensitive receptors must be implicated in the mechanisms bringing about the inhibition. Sullivan *et al.* (1993) went on to report that H-reflex excitability could also be decreased during effleurage.

Goldberg *et al.* (1994) reported a similar reduction in H-reflex amplitude during petrissage of the triceps surae in eight out of ten subjects with spinal cord injuries. The sample included both complete and incomplete lesions. One patient with complete and one patient with incomplete lesions failed to show the reduced H-reflex amplitude. Despite this the main effects of the massage treatment were statistically significant ($p = 0.008$). The decrease in H-reflex amplitude was not as great and was considered to be less uniform than noted in the participants of previous studies. This study did indicate a tendency to some carry-over effects post massage. Although the sample population was small and this might detract from the potency of the reported findings, it was felt to be 'encouraging' with possible clinical implications if future research could further delineate the potential effects of massage therapy on H-reflex amplitude. Sustained decrease in H-reflex amplitude was not noticed in this particular study (Goldberg *et al.* 1994).

Pain

Pain is a complex phenomenon of many components and at the very least encompasses physical and emotional elements. There are different types of pain: acute, sharp, fast pain, which is carried to the central nervous system (CNS) along 'A delta' nerve fibres; and chronic, aching, slow pain, which is served by the so-called C fibres. Sensitivity to pain is perceived individually and perception thresholds seem to be variable. This variability appears to be demonstrable both between individuals and even within a given individual at different times. Pain perception is thought to be influenced by many factors, one of these being afferent input to the CNS, and this may be where massage is able to exert its effects.

Control or suppression of pain is deemed to occur at different levels within the nervous system, although these mechanisms are still more hypothetical than fully proven (Carreck 1994). Critical key sites for influencing pain are: (1) peripheral areas where there is presence of tissue damage; and (2), chemical substances such as bradykinin, serotonin and substance P which are released and stimulate the free pain receptors (nociceptors) commonly producing the characteristics of slow pain previously described (Guyton 1992). Hernandez-Reif *et al.* (2001) reported significantly increased serotonin levels in their massage treatment group after intervention ($p = 0.05$) and describe this finding as important as chronic pain patients have been shown to have depleted serotonin levels.

The spinal cord is taken to be the next point at which pain may be blocked before signals ascend to the cerebrum for conscious appreciation of the sensation. Since the presentation of the pain gate theory of Melzack and Wall in 1965 and subsequent modifications to this, there has been a basis for believing that sensory traffic, into the dorsal grey areas of spinal cord segments, is sifted and sorted. This is performed by complex neuronal circuitry including that within the substantia gelatinosa. Signals from different sources are carried along fibres of different diameters and compete across the synapses of the circuitry for which signals will have the right to further transmission. Input of signals along large-diameter fibre pathways competes with pain signals along smaller diameter fibre pathways and can close the 'pain' gate. This occurs via various influences on synapses – preventing pain signals from further transmission to conscious level. Higher levels of the CNS are considered to be involved in pain control, most probably involving descending pathways and release of endogenous opiate substances (endorphins).

Some of the descending fibres are thought to emanate from areas such as the reticular formation of the brainstem and are triggered by certain pain signals reaching that level within the CNS. Some of the subsequent endogenous opiate release will be at the reticular formation and at higher levels, but also at the spinal cord level. It has been suggested that this will result in the suppression of pain signals entering at these sites (Holey and Cook 1997).

It has been put forward that the setting of the pain gate is controlled by higher centres and this can dominate neural activity at the spinal cord level (Melzack and Wall 1988, cited in Carreck 1994). It is difficult to define with certainty exactly which higher centres may be involved, but parts of the cerebral cortex and limbic system have been implicated (Holey and Cook 1997).

Massage may contribute in some way to pain control at all the indicated levels and therefore may influence pain perception and its threshold. Pain receptors are not readily adaptive (Guyton 1992) so if harmful chemicals are present as a result of injury, pain signals are likely to be triggered and carried to the CNS. Massage, used appropriately in accessible peripheral areas of damage, has been observed as having a positive effect in reducing pain. It is speculated that under these circumstances the massage may have altered the local circulation in such a way as to reduce or remove noxious substances, thereby reducing or removing stimuli, reflected in a corresponding reduction of response by the pain receptors.

Massage can provide the CNS with afferent inputs, some along the larger diameter 'A beta' fibres, that will compete with incoming pain signals to the spinal cord. This input (if of adequate level) may block pain signals by a process of presynaptic inhibition and may reduce or prevent transmission to conscious level.

Massage input, relative to the higher centres and the release of endorphins, is a somewhat hypothetical area. It may be possible that sensory signals triggered by certain massage techniques stimulate higher levels of the CNS. These areas may be those capable of sending descending signals and this may result in opiate release; some in turn afford pain control through post-synaptic inhibition at spinal level. Quite how the highest levels of the CNS are involved is hard to assess. Can they influence brainstem areas or other areas within the cerebrum? How is this influence exerted via opiate release? Can these areas be affected by sensory input from massage, and is this the cross-over point with what has been labelled the 'psychological effect' in times past?

Research studies into the relationship between massage and pain control have produced some very mixed results. Some of the studies have examined normals, i.e. subjects without pain, and lead one to wonder if responses are inclined to be different in normals compared with those found in subjects already experiencing pain.

Day *et al.* (1987) chose to investigate the effect of massage on endogenous opiates within the peripheral venous blood. The study consisted of 21 healthy adult volunteers. One group rested for 40 minutes and the other group received 30 minutes' back massage using mineral oil. Venous beta endorphin and beta lipotropin were measured pre and post treatment. Massage in this set of circumstances did not change the levels of the endogenous opiates. The researchers recommended that a follow-up study using subjects with acute and chronic back pain might give different results. Massage and endogenous opiate release was still considered as the possible mechanism of pain relief.

Weinrich and Weinrich (1990) investigated the effect of massage on patients with cancer pain. The main significant positive finding was a decrease of pain immediately post massage, but only for the male subjects. There were a number of problems with this study. Only 10 minutes' back massage was performed by student nurses after a minimal training period of 1 hour. The control group subjects were simply visited by the data collector for 10 minutes. The researchers felt that where there was significant pain reduction this had tended to occur in male subjects already experiencing higher levels of pain than the female subjects, and males within the control group. Pain levels were self reported. This pilot study posed many questions, which have largely remained unanswered. It was considered that massage may be a useful option for short-term pain relief.

Puustjarvi *et al.* (1990) investigated 21 female subjects with chronic tension headaches. Each subject received 10 sessions of upper body massage – kneading and stroking, with prolonged work over trigger points. Pain measured by questionnaire and visual analogue scale decreased and the number of days with neck pain decreased in the follow-up period at 3 and 6 months. Additionally cervical movements improved, and reduced electromyogram (EMG) activity was shown in the frontalis muscle. The researchers felt the study confirmed positive clinical and physiological effects of massage.

Carreck (1994) explored the pain perception threshold of 40 healthy subjects, using 15 minutes' lower limb massage with 20 subjects and 15 minutes' rest with the other 20 subjects. Transcutaneous electrical stimulation was used to elicit the point at which the participants first perceived pain. The results showed increased pain perception thresholds in the group who had received massage and it was concluded that massage is a valuable option in the management of pain.

Mancinelli *et al.* (2006) described a significant decrease in perceived muscle soreness after 17 minutes' massage (including effleurage, petrissage and vibration techniques) applied to the thighs of 11 sportswomen ($p < 0.0011$). However, the reported findings were derived from a small sample size and only from fit and healthy women, and how these findings may extend into other populations is not known.

Hasson *et al.* (2004) reported a large, randomised, 3-month follow-up design study into the effectiveness of massage on diffuse chronic pain patients ($n = 129$). They described an initial effectiveness of massage therapy ($n = 62$) in the chronic pain patients compared with a relaxation control group ($n = 55$) on functional pain outcomes assessed using a questionnaire at baseline, immediately following intervention and at 3 months follow-up. These authors described a significant improvement in muscle pain immediately post intervention in their treatment group (Fischer's F ratio (F) (48.2) = 5.8; $p < 0.01$), with no such improvements described by the control participants. However, these positive effects of massage were not noticed at the 3-month follow-up; some of the treated patients even described more pain at 3-months than at baseline, and the authors commented that the reasons for this deterioration were not known (Hasson *et al.* 2004).

A randomised controlled trial of massage therapy for low back pain reported by Preyde (2000) described improvements in pain outcomes in a treatment group (comprehensive massage $n = 25$ and soft-tissue manipulation n = 25] compared to exercise ($n = 22$) and sham laser ($n = 26$) control groups after 1 month of intervention and at 1 month subsequent follow-up. Significant improvements were also reported in the comprehensive massage group compared to the soft-tissue manipulation group in measurements of function ($p < 0.00$ 1), pain intensity ($p < 0.001$) and pain quality ($p = 0.001$), although the author stated that these improvements were modest (Preyde 2000).

Hernandez-Reif *et al.* (2001) reported improved pain outcome measurements as assessed using the Short-Form McGill Pain Questionnaire (Melzack 1987). Group by time analyses identified reduced pain in both groups, but effects only persevered in the massage treatment group and not in the relaxation group at 1 month follow-up.

Another review into the effectiveness of massage for low back pain conducted in 2002 identified nine studies (eight of which were randomised trials) and showed variable effectiveness of massage in patients with lower back pain. The authors concluded that massage might be of benefit to patients with subacute and chronic non-specific lower back pain, especially if combined with exercise and acupuncture (Furlan *et al.* 2002).

Ernst (2004) reviewed six randomised controlled trials and seven clinical trials of the effectiveness of massage therapy for relieving lower back pain and management of delayed onset muscle soreness (DOMS) within a systematic review of chiropractic and massage manual therapies for pain control. He described 'serious methodological flaws' in many of these studies which described 'often contradictory' findings. Further examination of these studies identified: small sample sizes; no blinding; inadequate outcome measurements; short follow-up periods; and low volumes of data, as reasons for these contradictory findings and weak evidence of the effectiveness of manual therapies for the treatment of pain (Ernst 2004).

Massage and pain will be reviewed further under the musculoskeletal and psychological headings.

Physiological effects on the musculoskeletal system

The focus in this section is on the possible effects massage may have on muscles. Inevitably there will be some reference again to pain, as muscular pain and soreness are not uncommon.

In a 1989 study by Balke *et al.* researchers investigated how massage might affect muscle fatigue. Subjects performed a gradual exercise test on a treadmill and this was then followed by either rest or manual or mechanical massage of the legs for about 15 minutes. Exercise performance was retested and this improved in both the manual and mechanical massage groups. The sample group was very small, but the researchers considered that massage assisted recuperation from fatigue 'more effectively than total rest alone'. This finding is reinforced in a small way by another study investigating a number of modalities with respect to treatment of subacute low back pain. Incorporated in their procedures was the Sorensen fatigue test, which examined trunk extension and how long this might be maintained in seconds to the point of fatigue. Subjects in the massage grouping received 15 minutes' back massage three times a week over a period of 3 weeks. The massage group showed the greatest improvement in best extension effort and fatigue time when compared with the other modalities used such as corset, spinal manipulation (Pope *et al.* 1994).

A 1990 study investigated percussive vibratory massage on short-term recovery from muscle fatigue. The experimental group received 4 minutes' percussive vibratory massage and 1 minutes' rest compared with 5 minutes' rest only for the control group. The procedures for the two groups were interspersed between three periods of exercise and rate of fatigue measurements. It was found that there was no significant benefit from massage in the terms of these study conditions. The length of massage time, the type of massage and the timing of the intervention could all be questioned; however, it does not convincingly negate the use of massage for the effects on muscle under different circumstances (Cafarelli *et al.* 1990).

A 1995 cross-over study (Rinder and Sutherland 1995) was more positive about the effect of massage on muscle fatigue. Subjects were exercised to the point of fatigue and on one occasion allotted to the massage group and on the next occasion to the rest group. Massage in the form of effleurage and petrissage was applied for 3 minutes to this fatigued quadriceps muscle. Other subjects rested for 6 minutes. Following immediately after either massage or rest, subjects were asked to complete as many leg extensions as possible against their individual half load maximum. The results showed that massage had significantly improved quadriceps performance compared to rest. The discussion of this study points out that even where no significant effect of massage was elicited, no study has found detrimental effects of massage on muscle fatigue. It also considered that not all effects might be of a purely physical nature and psychological factors could not be ruled out.

DOMS can occur in any individual who performs some unaccustomed exercise. It is considered to appear 8–24 hours post exercise, building to its height of discomfort at about 48 hours post exercise and resolving over a few days (Smith *et al.* 1994). DOMS may present as slight discomfort localised to myotendinous areas, to stiffness and extreme pain throughout the muscle. It commonly occurs in association with eccentric muscle activity. It is thought that such activity sets up an acute inflammatory reaction in the muscle and massage intervention may be able to moderate the injury response. Two 1994 studies examined this area, producing variable findings. Smith believed that massage applied 2 hours after exercise could hinder the delivery of neutrophils to the 'injury site', i.e. the exercised muscle, and so reduce the inflammatory response and resultant soreness. Fourteen untrained male subjects exercised elbow flexors and extensors isokinetically and eccentrically. The experimental group was given 30 minutes' 'athletic' massage 2 hours post exercise. The control group was rested. DOMS, creatine kinase and neutrophil levels were assessed before exercise and at intervals up to 120 hours post exercise. It appeared that massage reduced DOMS and creatine kinase levels. It produced prolonged elevation of circulating neutrophils, leading to the assumption that these had not accumulated in the muscle so the inflammatory response and subsequent soreness were reduced (Smith *et al.* 1994).

The second study by Weber *et al.* (1994) examined DOMS from a slightly different perspective. Muscle soreness and force deficits following high-intensity eccentric exercise were investigated using 40 untrained female subjects. These were randomly assigned to one of four groups – therapeutic massage, upper body ergonomics, micro current electrical stimulation and control which took the form of 8 minutes' rest. Soreness was measured using a visual analogue scale. Maximum voluntary isometric contraction (at 90° elbow flexion) and peak torque were assessed using a Cybex isokinetic dynometer. Readings were taken before exercise and at 24 and 48 hours post exercise. The elbow flexors were eccentrically exercised to exhaustion. The massage group was given 2 minutes' light effleurage, 5 minutes' petrissage followed by 1 minute's effleurage immediately after exercise and after 24 hours at reassessment. No differences were noted between the massage and other groups. The results from this study do not support the use of massage immediately post exercise or 24 hours after exercise to relieve DOMS or the force deficits associated with it.

Some earlier research studies have also produced contradictory findings but often studies are not comparing like with like. There are great variations in types of massage used and the length of time it is applied. There is much work to be done to refine study design and consistency. Maybe then tangible proof of the effects of massage will be found.

Muscle tension can lead to pain and soreness. Massage has been used to promote relaxation of muscle and is a means of dealing with or offsetting the development of such discomfort. An early study postulated that tension in muscles on the posterior aspect of the trunk and lower limbs would limit trunk forward flexion. The flexion was measured on a 'fingers to floor' basis. Measurements were taken before and after a 30-minute rest period, and before and after a 30-minute massage. The massage was to the whole of the back and lower limbs. All 25 study subjects showed gain in trunk flexibility after undergoing massage compared to the pre- and post-rest readings. It was concluded that massage can create relaxation in voluntary muscles, although mechanisms were not clear. Comment was made that almost all subjects reported a feeling of relaxation and this may implicate higher centre nervous activity relative to spinal circuitry. Local vascular metabolic changes were also proposed as possible contributors (Nordschav and Bierman 1962).

Hopper *et al.* (2005) reported significantly increased hamstring muscle lengths ($p < 0.001$) in 36 female hockey players following classic massage ($n = 19$) and following dynamic soft tissue mobilisation ($n = 16$) techniques. However, 24 hours later the significant lengthening of the hamstrings of these hockey players was no longer demonstrable in either of the treatment groups ($p > 0.160$).

Danneskiold-Samsoe *et al.* (1982) studied 13 women with regional back and shoulder(s) muscle pain and tension. Subjects were given a course of 10 massage treatments each lasting between 30 and 45 minutes. After each massage, plasma myoglobin and the extent of the area of muscle tension were measured. Plasma myoglobin levels rose following the early massage treatments, reaching a peak some 3 hours after the treatment. It was noted that as muscle tension declined with further treatments, so did the plasma myoglobin levels. The researchers concluded that release of plasma myoglobin occurs from muscles that exhibit tension and that massage assists in the normalisation of muscle tension. Plasma myoglobin showed no change from normal levels when muscles without pain or tenderness were massaged. This suggests that regional muscle tension and pain may be due to disorders of muscle fibres rather than involvement of connective tissue. Proposed mechanisms for these findings were not forthcoming.

Van Dolder and Roberts (2003) reported improved range of motion (ROM), pain and function in patients with shoulder pain using soft tissue massage of the shoulder ($n = 15$). Although their various outcome measurements reached statistical significance (all at $p < 0.05$) these authors concluded that 'the mechanisms behind these effects remain unclear' (Van Dolder and Roberts 2003).

Hernandez-Reif *et al.* (2001) reported improved pain outcomes (as measured using the Short-Form Pain Questionnaire (Melzack 1987)) in their massage treatment group and in their relaxation control group ($p < 0.001$). However, pain reduction was reported to be maintained in the treatment group, but not in the relaxation control group, suggesting that massage therapy may be more effective at reducing pain than relaxation over time.

A very recent review of the literature regarding the effectiveness of massage therapy on musculoskeletal pain conducted by Lewis and Johnson (2006) examined the quality and findings of some 20 studies. Their conclusions were equivocal in describing 9 out of the 20 massage therapy studies reviewed as being effective in reducing musculoskeletal pain, whereas 11 of the 20 studies reviewed were reported as being ineffective.

This brief survey of some of the available research on the effects of massage on muscles has identified both positive and negative findings.

Psychological effects

A question that comes to mind under this heading is, does this warrant a separate section or are the effects to be discussed just an extension of physiology? Much debate is possible, but the contents of this chapter are considered to be either psychological or psychophysiological. Research papers to date have not been very successful in clarifying such matters as it is suggested that much evidence is based on 'anecdotal testimony and practical field experiences' as to the 'positive effects of massage on psychological wellbeing' (Cafarelli and Flint 1992).

An interesting study by Weinberg and Kolodny (1988) investigated the relationship between exercise, massage and mood enhancement. The subjects were 183 students of physical education and they were divided into six groups. These groups were swimming, jogging, racquetball, tennis, a control rest condition and a massage (full body) condition group. The psychological measurement tools used were the profile of mood states (POMS) after McNair (1971), the state anxiety inventory (SAI) of Spielberger (1970), and the Thayer adjective checklist (1967), all cited in Weinberg and Kolodny (1988).

The POMS questionnaire is used to measure mood fluctuations. It contains six subscales: tension–anxiety (somatic tension), depression–dejection (feelings of personal inadequacy), anger–hostility (feelings of intense overt anger), vigour–activity (mood of high energy), fatigue–inertia (mood of weariness and low energy) and confusion–bewilderment (cognitive inefficiency). The SAI questionnaire is designed to assess the state of anxiety. Thayer's adjective checklist is used to examine anxiety and activation, these recognised respectively through the subscales of high activation (feelings of tension and anxiety) and general activation (feelings of calm and relaxation).

Each subject completed these questionnaires prior to and immediately after their 30-minute period of either exercise, Swedish massage or rest. The results showed that the massage and the running groups were consistently more related to positive mood states and psychological wellbeing immediately after the 'activity'. However it was noted that the benefits were much more marked in the post-massage group.

Results from the other groupings generally did not produce significant change. All the subscales of the POMS questionnaire, except the vigour subscale, showed a positive relationship to massage. The beneficial relationship was also demonstrated with regard to the high activation and general activation subscales of Thayer's adjective checklist. The researchers concluded that massage was 'consistently related to transitory positive mood enhancement' and psychological wellbeing even if only demonstrated in the setting of the study. It would seem to go part way to justifying subjective comments often made post massage on its use in the sports context as well as in many other areas of life.

The tension–anxiety part of mood states has been investigated in a number of studies. Some studies have also attempted to link changes in psychological state to altered physiology. Many different subject groups have been used and findings have been of infinite variety. It appears almost easier to assess mood psychological state changes by the different, available inventories than to predict physiological responses relative to those changes in psychological dynamics.

Different markers are used to monitor physiological changes. These are commonly blood pressure (systolic and diastolic), heart rate, skin temperature (often of the fingers), galvanic skin response, respiratory rate, saliva composition and somatic electromyography (EMG) on muscles like the masseter and trapezius, which are often identified as having high levels of tension. There is thought to be much interrelationship between the continuum of arousal–relaxation and levels of anxiety. High levels of arousal may occur in emotionally stressful situations, and often, but not always, this manifests as raised levels of blood pressure, heart rate, EMG activity and constriction of blood vessels in peripheral circulation as demonstrated by reduction of temperature in the fingers (Longworth 1982). Some of these physiological changes will undoubtedly involve adjustments via the autonomic nervous system (ANS).

The following is a brief sampling of studies that have dealt with psychophysiological effects and massage.

Longworth (1982) investigated the effects of slow stroke back massage (SSBM) in 'normo-tensive females' who were nursing students and staff with an age range from 19 to 52 years. This quite complex study attempted to monitor many changes. Anxiety was assessed by use of the state (trait) anxiety inventory of Spielberger, as mentioned previously. A number of physiological readings were taken. Six minutes of uninterrupted slow stroke massage were administered during the approximately 27-minute experimental period, which also contained baseline rest and final rest periods. At the end of the experimental period subjects generally stated they felt rested and relaxed. The researcher believed that the SSBM had been successful in lowering the psycho-emotional and somatic arousal level of subjects into the rest period post massage. This finding was reinforced by significant decreases in SAI scores, demonstrating a reduction in anxiety state. It was also noted during the period that EMG levels were reduced, indicating lower levels of muscle tension.

Changes in other physiological markers were more difficult to explain. No significant differences were noted for systolic/diastolic blood pressure or heart rate between the baseline rest and final rest periods of experimental time. It was assumed the massage between the rest periods produced no prolonged effect on the ANS even though changes had occurred during the experimental time, e.g. an initial rise in systolic blood pressure during the first 3 minutes of massage, and increased heart rate in the last 3 minutes of the 6-minute massage.

A study by Barr and Taslitz (1970) examined the effects of back massage on autonomic functions in 19 college students aged 19–21 years. Each student underwent three massage sessions of 20 minutes with pre- and post-massage rest periods and three separate control periods of corresponding duration. Some of the physiological findings correspond to those of the Longworth study and others do not. Heart rate did tend to increase during massage; however, systolic and diastolic blood pressure decreased during the initial period of massage, the latter apparently conflicting with the Longworth findings. Barr considered that back massage did have an influence on autonomic functions, mainly an increase on sympathetic activity and a smaller effect on parasympathetic action. It was speculated further whether the changes were primarily as a result of the massage or the mental state of the subjects. This highlights again the mysterious interrelationships of higher centre activity in the CNS to autonomic adjustments and pain control. What influence do changes of mood or emotions play in physiological adjustments? Does the afferent input of massage change activity in the limbic system, the subcortical and even the cortical areas and do they in turn instigate changes within body systems? Some consistency does appear to be present in the literature regarding the positive effects of massage on mood-anxiety levels in a range of people.

Ferrell-Torry and Glick (1993) investigated whether massage could modify anxiety and the perception of cancer pain as well as monitoring other physiological changes. The study group comprised nine hospitalised males all experiencing cancer pain. Pain was measured by visual analogue scale and anxiety by Spielberger's SAI, these being used before and immediately 'after massage. Thirty minutes' effleurage, petrissage and myofascial trigger point massage therapy was applied to the neck, back and shoulders. Respiratory and heart rates and blood pressure were measured. Massage produced significant reductions in both pain perception (mean 60%) and anxiety (mean 24%) levels. Feelings of relaxation were enhanced. In this study the physiological measures tended to decrease following massage.

Meek (1993) working with 30 hospice clients used SSBM to achieve relaxation. The duration of the massage was only 3 minutes. Modest but not very prolonged decreases took place in blood pressure and heart rate along with a rise in skin temperature. The researcher took these to be indicative of increased relaxation, which usually means a low arousal level and this suggests a low anxiety state (Longworth 1982; Meek 1993).

Groer *et al.* (1994) studied anxiety levels and took post-massage saliva samples in a group of 18 well, older adults. The control group underwent a 10-minute period of relaxed lying and the experimental group had a 10-minute back rub. SAI questionnaires were completed before and after the intervention. Anxiety levels went down for both the experimental and the control group but not to significant levels. The saliva in the post-massage group showed increased levels of immunoglobulin A. This finding is part of a claim that massage can have beneficial effects on the body's immune system. It is not clear why reduction in anxiety did not reach significant levels on this occasion.

Fraser and Ross (1993) also looked at the effect of back massage on elderly residents in institutionalised care. A similar format of monitoring physiological markers, blood pressure, etc. and anxiety levels via Spielberger's self-evaluation questionnaire were used pre and post intervention. Three experimental subject groups were given either back massage with normal conversation, conversation only or no intervention. Post-test scores were all lower in the massage group although not statistically significant; however, there was a statistically significant difference in mean anxiety score between the massage group and the no intervention group. Verbally subjects reported the back massage to be relaxing. It was felt massage as a form of touch was valuable in the care of the elderly person and perhaps assisted communication.

Corley *et al.* (1995) also looked at the effect of back rubs on elderly residents in care. Mood was found to improve in both massage and rest control groups but not to significant levels. Subjectively the residents commented positively on the back rub. Little of significance was found in physiological measures.

Much of the above reinforces the practice of massage, but fully supportive research evidence is as yet elusive.

Snyder *et al.* (1995) looked at the use of hand massage in decreasing agitation behaviours associated with care activities in elderly patients with dementia. Behaviours had been observed for 5 days before massage intervention and 5 days after a 10-day intervention period. There was observed to be some reduction in agitation behaviours such as screaming and punching relative to morning care activities. It was speculated that massage might have achieved the limited effect through bringing a degree of calmness and relaxation to patients' stress levels. This area of study was complicated and much was unexplained.

At the other end of the age spectrum, touch and massage have been examined for effect on children and young people. Some of those effects are taken to be psychological. Ottenbacher *et al.* (1987) reviewed 19 studies on the effects of tactile stimulation on infants and young children. Results were variable and dependent on study design, but it was acknowledged that infants and young children respond to tactile stimulation. Performance in such activities as vocalisation and motor skills was much better than in the control or comparison group.

Field *et al.* (1993) looked at anxiety and mood in 52 hospitalised, depressed and adjustment disordered children and young people. One grouping had 30 minutes' back massage over 5 days and the other group watched relaxing videotapes. The massage group showed immediate decreased anxiety as measured by state anxiety inventory for children (STAIC) questionnaires which were administered before and immediately after treatment. Depressed subjects showed longer-term improvement. Using the POMS scores of both depressed and adjustment disordered subjects a less depressed mood was noted by day 5. Saliva cortisol noticeably decreased during the massage only. This is usually an indication of lowered arousal and anxiety levels.

Two different studies have produced findings regarding changing saliva composition relative to massage when used to create relaxation or reduce anxiety level. Green and Green (1987) comment that stress is known to be immunosuppressive, but how enhancing to the immune system is relaxation? Massage to the back (20 minutes) was one of the study groupings and in the post-test readings immunoglobulin A was increased.

Ironson *et al.* (1996), in their study of 29 homosexual men (20 HIV-positive and 9 HIV-negative), reported that, following a daily massage lasting 45 minutes and given for a month, there were significant decreases in anxiety level and stress hormone levels. Salivary cortisol demonstrated such a decrease. Improvement occurred in immune defence mechanisms, including a significant increase in natural killer cell numbers, but no change was noted in HIV disease progression markers. However, Birk *et al.* (2000) examined the impact of weekly 45-minute whole body massage therapy over a period of 12 weeks and the immune responses of 42 HIV+ participants; these authors found no significant improvements in immune response following treatment (all immunological measures failed to reach significance at $p < 0.05$).

The randomised clinical trial reported by Hasson *et al.* (2004) also examined patients' mental energy and self-rated health outcomes before massage therapy, immediately after intervention and at 3 months follow-up. Similar to the previously described findings by these authors on patient pain outcomes, mental energy and self-rated health improved in the treatment group immediately post intervention (compared with baseline scores; $p < 0.01$ and $p < 0.03$ respectively). However, these improvements were not evident at the 3-month follow-up, with both of these psychological outcomes returning to baseline levels (Hasson *et al.* 2004).

Preyde's (2000) study into the effectiveness of comprehensive massage therapy and soft-tissue manipulation over exercise and sham laser control treatments indicated a significant improvement in state anxiety over the course of treatment and as measured at 1 month follow-up. These findings have been corroborated by Walach *et al.* (2003) who described massage therapy for chronic pain patients as being at least as effective as standard medical care, but with improvements lasting for longer in massage patients, particularly in the psychological domains of pain ratings, depression and anxiety (Walach *et al.* 2003). These findings support those of Smith *et al.* (1999), who reported psychological improvements in the areas of relaxation, wellbeing and positive mood changes in their group of 114 hospitalised patients receiving one to four massages per day whilst in hospital (Smith *et al.* 1999). They also support the work of Hernandez-Reif *et al.* (2001) who described reduced anxiety, depression and improved sleep outcomes in a massage treatment group over relaxation control participants. A large meta-analysis of massage therapy research conducted by Moyer *et al.* (2004) identified 37 studies examining nine dependent variables for the effectiveness of massage therapy. These authors concluded that single applications of massage therapy effectively reduce state anxiety, blood pressure and heart rate, but not negative mood, immediate pain assessment and cortisol levels. Multiple applications of massage therapy were reported to reduce delayed pain assessment. These authors report the largest effects of massage therapy on reducing depression and trait anxiety (Moyer *et al.* 2004).

Some interesting findings regarding patient expectations and the effectiveness of Swedish massage and acupuncture for low back pain were reported by Kalauokalani *et al.* (2000). These authors reported increased improvement in function (as assessed using the Roland Disability Scale) in participants who had higher expectations of the treatment they were about to receive than those with lower expectations (86% versus 68% improvement respectively; $p < 0.01$), and this discrepancy was also shown for those expecting to improve more with massage than with acupuncture (and vice versa). These data suggest that patient expectations have a significant influence on clinical outcomes regardless of treatment with acupuncture or with Swedish massage (Kalauokalani *et al.* 2000).

The research papers that have been reviewed here demonstrate some difficulty in attaining consistency of findings. However, massage does appear to produce positive and beneficial responses, or no significant response, rather than having any detrimental effects.

Summary of the mechanisms of massage therapy

A recent and extensive review of the effects and mechanisms of massage conducted by Weerapong *et al.* (2005) concluded that there is 'limited empirical data on the possible mechanisms of massage'. These authors suggest that several studies reporting increased flexibility and range of motion lacked methodological rigour and that a further range of studies into the physiological effects of massage on blood circulation, hormone levels, blood pressure and heart rate are still inconclusive (Weerapong *et al.* 2005). These findings support those of Ernst (1999) who reviewed massage therapy for lower back pain. This review only identified four randomised controlled trials for massage therapy in lower back pain patients. Each of the studies reviewed was criticised in a number of areas for: not adequately describing participants in sufficient detail; not accounting for drop-outs; not adequately describing randomisation procedures; not conducting power calculations; not describing the massage therapy in detail; using inappropriate outcome measurements to examine efficacy of the treatment (two studies); and not applying enough massage for effects to be observed (one study). The author concludes that the paucity of findings may not be limited by potential ineffectiveness of massage therapy, but more by a lack of rigour being applied to the study of such effects (Ernst 1999).

Cherkin *et al.* (2003) make the point that massage, like acupuncture, chiropractic and osteopathic manipulation, are not well-defined monotherapies; they are in reality collections of numerous interventions tailored to the individual requirements of the patient depending on the experience and training of the practitioner. With this in mind, it is difficult to standardise procedures for rigorous scientific enquiry and to stipulate treatment procedures that will be efficacious for certain types of patient/condition. It is this 'umbrella nature' of massage that has prevented firm conclusions from being drawn from the multitude of studies that have attempted to examine the various impacts of massage therapy. Future work could usefully be directed at very specific and reliably repeatable massage techniques in larger-scale randomised controlled study designs. Alternatively, a more Bayesian approach could be adopted by collecting together data from numerous studies employing the various massage techniques in a range of patients to examine the probability of massage therapy being effective, and effective for which groups of people or conditions. This, though, could well prove problematic owing to the range of conditions, patient groups and massage techniques that have been applied, and to the generally low sample sizes reported in many of the studies examining the various aspects of massage therapy. The current state-of-the-art yields too many variables for useful analyses to be conducted. However, the fact that massage therapy is so popular and that it is conducted so frequently and so widely reinforces the conclusion that massage therapies are beneficial – it may be that the effects of massage are so subtle that we have yet to design outcome measures that are sensitive enough to detect any potential benefits of the therapy.

Massage in vulnerable groups – risk awareness and contraindications

The definition of a vulnerable patient for massage will always present with difficulties as it implies a certain fragility and susceptibility to harm that may be present in many different circumstances. However, there are some individuals who can be grouped together as being potentially vulnerable, either because they are less able to understand the intention of massage and what it entails, and thus cannot give informed consent, or they have suffered some previous trauma that is associated with touch, for example, physical harm or torture. Groups within the former category include young children and babies, individuals with significant learning disabilities, people with dementia or cognitive deficiencies including some mental illnesses, and those unable to communicate, perhaps either because they are in a coma or under deep sedation. People in the latter category who have been subject to some form of physical abuse (including extreme neglect and avoidance of physical contact) could present at any age or in any medical category and the therapist may not be aware of their full history on the first, or subsequent, meetings. It is therefore very important that the therapist is sensitive to subtle verbal or body language messages that the client may convey indicating that massage may not be a welcomed intervention and could cause physical or psychological harm if implemented.

The question then arises as to the appropriateness of performing massage on these patients and the research literature is somewhat sparse in addressing these issues.

The justification for introducing massage should be based on the known benefits as already discussed, such as reducing anxiety and stress, relieving pain and promoting beneficial physiological changes, or additional positive effects such as enhanced self esteem. There is much written about how bonding between parent and baby is enhanced by baby massage, including where the mother is suffering from post-natal depression (Onozawa *et al.* 2001), and several studies report beneficial effects in reducing symptoms in children with a variety of disorders (e.g. asthma (Field *et al.* 1998a), arthritis (Field *et al.* 1997) and atopic dermatitis (Schachner *et al.* 1998)) and young people with eating disorders, behavioural problems and mental illness (Field *et al.* 1992, 1998b). These could all be described as vulnerable groups where insight and informed consent may not be fully available. However, it is beholden upon the therapist to evaluate the clinical risk–benefits of any situation, involve the individual or his/her advocate in shared decision making, record all actions and interventions accurately and fully, and be mindful of the quality of evidence supporting the choice of massage intervention (Cohen and Kemper 2005; Cohen 2006).

Additional contraindications to massage with any vulnerable patient must include refusal, an aversion to the prospect of massage and the presence of distress when massage is instigated. It is likely that when these responses occur the decision to include massage in a treatment regime will be discussed by a larger multidisciplinary team, involving the patient or advocate, with the possible introduction of massage on a more gradual basis such as hand touch only or clothed back massage.

Contraindications for massage therapy

There are several situations where massage is contraindicated, and even specifically ill-advised. Ernst (2003) reported in a review of the safety of massage therapy that adverse events associated with massage are reported very infrequently, and so an adequate risk–benefit evaluation of massage therapy is not possible. However, he does suggest that massage therapy is not devoid of risks and, although the incidence of adverse events is not known, it is probably low.

Duimel-Peeters *et al.* (2005) suggest that massage is contraindicated where tissues are inflamed, or when there is a risk that malignant cells might be spread along the skin, through the lymph or bloodstream as a result of massage therapy. These authors also contraindicate the use of massage in patients who have disorders of the circulatory system, those who are prone to bleeding, and those who have abnormal sensations resulting from stroke, diabetes or side effects of medication. Duimel-Peeters *et al.* (2005) also suggest that patients who are not in good health, those who are elderly, those with thin or fragile skin and those with underlying tissue damage will not benefit from massage therapy, particularly the more invasive techniques such as tapotement. However, the massage practitioner should make an informed risk assessment of where benefits may outweigh the risks within these suggested groups, especially within the broad category of older massage recipients, with the massage approach and techniques adjusted accordingly.

Broadly speaking, massage is contraindicated in patients in the following circumstances or with the following presentations:

- Skin disorders that would be irritated by either an increase in warmth of the part or the lubricants that might be used, e.g. eczema.
- When superficial infections are suppurating.
- In the presence of malignant tumours.
- Early bruising – although at about the fourth day massage will be of use in treating a haematoma.
- In the presence of recent, unhealed scars or open wounds.
- Adjacent to recent fracture sites and especially at the elbow or mid-thigh.
- Over joints or other tissues that are acutely inflamed, especially joints with tubercular infections.
- A history of or suspected deep vein thrombosis.
- Burns.
- Skin infections.
- Advanced osteoporosis.

Below are listed situations and patient groups where the use of massage should be performed with caution:

- Older people.
- Those with fragile skin.
- Those with circulation disorders of the blood or lymph.
- Those with early stage osteoporosis.
- People recovering from skin infections or bone fractures.
- Children.
- Adults with learning disabilities.
- Adults with physical disabilities not previously described but which may impact on the quality experience of receiving massage therapy.

A recent study by Cherkin *et al.* (2001) described 13% of their massage group (n = 74) as experiencing 'significant discomfort or pain' either during or immediately following massage therapy; however, no serious adverse events were recorded in this study. This again highlights the need for thorough assessment of patients/clients and their situation when selecting and evaluating massage therapy.

The words of Pemberton (1950), cited in Rinder and Sutherland (1995), sum up the essence of this chapter justifying the continued use of massage: 'Successful forms of treatment often run ahead of precise knowledge of the premises from which they arise'. However, despite the variation/discrepancies in evidence for and against massage, its continued popularity with practitioners and numerous client groups demands continued research to establish its efficacy as a therapeutic option.

References

Arkko, P.J., Pakarinen, A.J. and Kar-Koskinen, O. (1983) Effects of whole body massage on serum protein, electrolyte and hormone concentrations, enzyme activities and hematological parameters. *International Journal of Sports Medicine*, **4**, 26–57.

Balke, B., Anthony, J. and Wyatt, F. (1989) The effects of massage treatment on exercise fatigue. *Clinical Sports Medicine Journal*, **3**, 89–96.

Barr, J.S. and Taslitz, N. (1970) The influence of back massage on autonomic functions. *Physical Therapy*, **50**(12), 1679–91.

Birk, T.J., McGrady, A., MacArthur, R.D. and Khuder, S. (2000) The effects of massage therapy alone and in combination with other complementary therapies on immune system measures and quality of life in human immunodeficiency virus. *Journal of Alternative and Complementary Medicine*, **6**(5), 405–14.

Cafarelli, E. and Flint, F. (1992) The role of massage in preparation for and recovery from exercise. *Sports Medicine*, **14**(1), 19.

Cafarelli, E., Sim, J., Carolan, B. and Liebesman, J. (1990) Vibratory massage and short-term recovery from muscular fatigue. *International Journal of Sports Medicine*, **2**, 474–8.

Carreck, A. (1994) The effect of massage on pain perception threshold. *Manipulative Therapist*, **26**(2), 10–16.

Cherkin, D.C., Eisenberg, D., Sherman, K.J., *et al.* (2001) Randomised trial comparing traditional Chinese medical acupuncture, therapeutic massage, and self-care education for chronic low back pain. *Archives of Internal Medicine*, **161**, 1081–8.

Cherkin, D.C., Sherman, K.J., Deyo, R.A. and Shekelle, P.G. (2003) A review of the evidence for the effectiveness, safety and cost of acupuncture, massage therapy and spinal manipulation for back pain. *Annals of Internal Medicine*, **138**, 898–906.

Cohen, M.H. (2006) Legal and ethical issues relating to use of complementary therapies in pediatric hematology/oncology. *Journal of Pediatric Hematology and Oncology*, **28**(3),190–193.

Cohen, M.H. and Kemper, K.J. (2005) Complementary therapies in pediatrics: a legal perspective. *Pediatrics*, **115**(3), 774–80.

Corley, M.C., Ferriter, J., Zeh, J. and Gifford, C. (1995) Physiological and psychological effects of back rubs. *Applied Nursing Research*, **8**(1), 39–43.

Danneskiold-Samsoe, B., Christiansen, E., Lund, B. and Andersen, R.B. (1982) Regional muscle tension and pain ('fibrositis'), effect of massage on myoglobin in plasma. *Scandinavian Journal of Rehabilitation Medicine*, **15**, 17–20.

Day, J.A., Mason, R.R. and Chesrown, S.E. (1987) Effect of massage on serum level of B-endorphin and B-lipotropin in healthy adults. *Physical Therapy*, **67**(6), 926–30.

Duimel-Peeters, I.G.P., Halfens, R.J.G., Berger, M.P.F. and Snoeckx, L.H.E.H. (2005) The effects of massage as a method to prevent pressure ulcers. A review of the literature. *Ostomy Wound Management*, **51**(4), 70–80.

Ebel, A. and Wisham, L.H. (1952) Effect of massage on muscle temperature and radiosodium clearance. *Archives of Physical Medicine*, July, 399–405.

Eliska, O. and Eliskova, M. (1995) Are peripheral lymphatics damaged by high pressure manual massage? *Lymphology*, **28**, 21–30.

Ernst, E. (1999) Massage therapy for low back pain: a systematic review. *Journal of Pain and Symptom Management*, **17**(1), 65–9.

Ernst, E. (2003) The safety of massage therapy. *Rheumatology*, **42**, 1101–106.

Ernst, E. (2004) Manual therapies for pain control: chiropractic and massage. *Clinical Journal of Pain*, **20**(1), 8–12.

Ernst, E., Matrai, A., Magyarosy, I., *et al.* (1987) Massage causes changes in blood fluidity. *Physiotherapy*, **73**(1), 43–5.

Ferrell-Torry, A.T. and Glick, O.L. (1993) The use of therapeutic massage as a nursing intervention to modify anxiety and the perception of cancer pain. *Cancer Nursing*, **16**(2), 93–101.

Field, T., Morrow, C., Valdeon, C., Larson, S., Kuhn, C. and Schanberg, S. (1992) Massage reduces anxiety in child and adolescent psychiatric patients. *Journal of the American Academy of Child Adolescent Psychiatry*, **31**(1), 125–31.

Field, T., Morrav, C., Valdeon, C., *et al.* (1993) Massage reduces anxiety in child and adolescent psychiatric patients. *International Journal of Alternative and Complementary Medicine*, July, 23–7.

Field, T., Hernandez-Reif, M., Seligman, S., *et al.* (1997) Juvenile rheumatoid arthritis: benefits from massage therapy. *Journal of Pediatric Psychology*, **22**(5), 607–17.

Field, T., Henteleff, T., Hernandez-Reif, M., *et al.* (1998a) Children with asthma have improved pulmonary functions after massage therapy. *Pediatrics*, **132**(5), 854–8.

Field, T., Schanberg, S., Kuhn, C., *et al.* (1998b) Bulimic adolescents benefit from massage therapy. *Adolescence*, **33**(131), 555–63.

Fraser, J. and Ross, J. (1993) Psychophysiological effects of back massage on elderly institutionalized patients. *Journal of Advanced Nursing*, **18**, 238–45.

Furlan, A.D., Brosseau, L., Imamura, M. and Irvin, E. (2002) Massage for low-back pain: a systematic review with the framework of the Cochrane Collaboration Back Review Group. *Spine*, **27**(17), 1896–1910.

Goldberg, J., Sullivan, S.J. and Seaborne, D.E. (1992) The effect of two intensities of massage on H-reflex amplitude. *Physical Therapy*, **72**(6), 449–57.

Goldberg, J., Seaborne, D.E., Sullivan, S.J. and Leduc, B.E. (1994) The effect of therapeutic massage on H-reflex amplitude in persons with a spinal cord injury. *Physical Therapy*, **74**(8), 728–37.

Green, R.G. and Green, M.L. (1987) Relaxation increases salivary immunoglobulin A. *Psychological Reports*, **61**, 623–9.

Groer, M., Mozingo, J., Droppleman, P., *et al.* (1994) Measures of salivary secretory immunoglobulin A and state anxiety after a nursing back rub. *Applied Nursing Research*, **7**(1), 26.

Guyton, A.C. (1992) *Human Physiology and Mechanisms of Disease*. W.B. Saunders, Philadelphia.

Hansen, T.I. and Kristensen, J.H. (1973) Effect of massage, shortwave diathermy and ultrasound upon the disappearance rate from muscle and subcutaneous tissue in the human calf. *Scandinavian Journal of Rehabilitation Medicine*, **5**, 179–82.

Hasson, D., Arnetz, B., Jeveus, L. and Edelstam, B. (2004) A randomized clinical trial of the treatment effects of massage compared to relaxation tape recordings on diffuse long-term pain. *Psychotherapy and Psychosomatics*, **73**, 17–24.

Hernandez-Reif, M., Field, T., Krasnegor, J. and Theakston, H. (2001) Lower back pain is reduced and range of motion increased after massage therapy. *International Journal of Neuroscience*, **106**, 131–45.

Holey, E. and Cook, E. (1997) *Therapeutic Massage*. W.B. Saunders, London.

Hollis, M. (1998) *Massage for Therapists*. Blackwell Publishing, Oxford.

Hopper, D., Conneely, M., Chromiak, F., Canini, E., Berggren, J. and Briffa, K. (2005) Evaluation of the effect of two massage techniques on hamstring muscle length in competitive female hockey players. *Physical Therapy in Sport*, **6**, 137–45.

Hovind, H. and Nielsen, S.L. (1974) Effect of massage on blood flow in skeletal muscle. *Scandinavian Journal of Rehabilitation Medicine*, **6**(2), 74–7.

Ironson, G., Field, T., Scafidi, F., *et al.* (1996) Massage therapy is associated with enhancement of the immune system's cytotoxic capacity. *International Journal of Neuroscience*, **84**(1), 205–17.

Kalauokalani, D., Cherkin, D.C., Shennan, K.J., Koepsell, T.D. and Deyo, R.A. (2000) Lessons from a trial of acupuncture and massage for low back pain. *Spine*, **26**(13), 1418–24.

Lakhani, S.R., Dilly, S.A. and Finlayson, CJ. (1993) *Basic Pathology – An Introduction to the Mechanisms of Disease*. Edward Arnold, London.

Lewis, M. and Johnson, M.I. (2006) The clinical effectiveness of therapeutic massage for musculoskeletal pain: a systematic review. *Physiotherapy*, **92**, 146–58.

Longworth, J.C.D. (1982) Psychophysiological effects of slow back massage in normotensive females. *Advances in Nursing Science*, **4**, 44–61.

Mancinelli, C.A., Davis, D.S., Aboulhosn, L., Brady, M., Eisenhofer, J. and Foutty, S. (2006) The effects of massage on delayed onset muscle soreness and physical performance in female collegiate athletes. *Physical Therapy in Sport*, **7**, 5–13.

Meek, S.S. (1993) Effects of slow stroke back massage on relaxation in hospice clients. *Image: Journal of Nursing Scholarship*, **25**(1), 17–21.

Melzack, R. (1987) The Short-Form McGill Pain Questionnaire. *Pain*, **30**, 191–7.

Melzack, R. and Wall, P.D. (1965) Pain mechanisms: a new theory. *Science*, **150**, 971–9.

Morelli, M., Seaborne, D.E. and Sullivan, S.J. (1990) Changes in H-reflex amplitude during massage of triceps surae in healthy subjects. *Journal of Orthopaedic and Sports Physical Therapy*, **12**(2), 55–9.

Morelli, M., Seaborne, D.E. and Sullivan, S.J. (1991) H-reflex modulation during manual muscle massage of human triceps surae. *Archives of Physical Medicine and Rehabilitation*, **72** (October), 915–19.

Mortimer, P.S., Simmonds, R., Rezvani, M., *et al.* (1990) The measurement of skin lymph flow by isotope clearance reliability, reproducibility, injection dynamics, and the effect of massage. *Journal of Investigative Dermatology*, **95**(6), 677–82.

Moyer, C.A., Rounds, J. and Hannum, L.W. (2004) A meta-analysis of massage therapy research. *Psychological Bulletin*, **130**(1), 3–18.

Nordschav, M. and Bierman, W. (1962) The influence of manual massage on muscle relaxation: effect on trunk flexion. *Journal of the American Physical Therapy Association*, **42**, 653–7.

Onozawa, K., Glover, V., Adams, D., Modi, N. and Kumar, R.C. (2001) Infant massage improves mother–infant interaction for mothers with postnatal depression. *Journal of Affective Disorders*, **63**(13), 201–207.

Ottenbacher, K.L., Muller, L., Brandt, D., *et al.* (1987) The effectiveness of tactile stimulation as a form of early intervention: a quantitive evaluation. *Development and Behavioural Paediatrics*, **8**(2), 68–76.

Pope, M.H., Reed, B., Phillips, D.C., *et al.* (1994) A prospective randomized three week trial of spinal manipulation, transcutaneous muscle stimulation, massage and corset in the treatment of subacute low back pain. *Spine*, **19**(22), 2571–7.

Preyde, M. (2000) Effectiveness of massage therapy for subacute low-back pain: a randomized controlled trial. *Journal of the Canadian Medical Association*, **162**(13), 1815–20.

Puustjarvi, K., Airaksinen, O. and Pontinen, P.L. (1990) The effect of massage in patients with chronic tension headache. *International Journal of Acupuncture and Electrotherapeutics*, **13**, 159–62.

Rinder, A.N. and Sutherland, C.L. (1995) An investigation of the effects of massage on quadriceps performance after exercise fatigue. *Complementary Therapies in Nursing and Midwifery*, **1**, 99–102.

Schachner, L., Field, T., Hernandez-Reif, M., Duarte, A.M. and Krasnegor, J. (1998) Atopic dermatitis symptoms decreased in children following massage therapy. *Pediatric Dermatology*, **15**(5), 390–5.

Scull, C.W. (1945) Massage physiologic basis. *Archives of Physical Medicine*, March, 159–67.

Severini, V. and Venerando, A. (1967) Effect of massage on peripheral circulation and physiological effects of massage. *Europa Medicophysica*, **3**, 165–83.

Shoemaker, L.K., Tiidus, P.M. and Mader, R. (1997) Failure of manual massage to alter limb blood flow: measures by Doppler ultrasound. *Medicine and Science in Sports and Exercise*, **29**(5), 610–614.

Smith, L.L., Keating, M.N., Holbert, D., *et al.* (1994) The effects of athletic massage on delayed onset muscle soreness, creatine kinase, and neutrophil count: a preliminary report. *Journal of Orthopaedic and Sports Physical Therapy*, **19**(2), 93–9.

Smith, M.C., Stallings, M.A., Mariner, S. and Burrall, M. (1999) Benefits of massage therapy for hospitalised patients: a descriptive and qualitative evaluation. *Alternative Therapies in Health and Medicine*, **5**(4), 64–71.

Snyder, M., Egan, E.C. and Burns, K.R. (1995) Efficacy of hand massage in decreasing agitation behaviours associated with care activities in persons with dementia. *Geriatric Nursing*, **16**(2), 60–63.

Sullivan, S.L., Williams, L.R.T., Seaborne, D.E. and Morelli, M. (1991) Effects of massage on alpha motoneuron excitability. *Physical Therapy*, **71**(8), 55–9.

Sullivan, S.L., Seguin, S., Seaborne, D.E. and Goldberg, L. (1993) Reduction of H-reflex amplitude during the application of effleurage to the triceps surae in neurologically healthy subjects. *Physiotherapy Theory and Practice*, **9**, 25–31.

Tiidus, P.M. and Shoemaker, L.K. (1995) Effleurage massage, muscle blood flow and long-term post-exercise strength recovery. *International Journal of Sports Medicine*, **16**, 478–83.

Van Dolder, P.A. and Roberts, D.L. (2003) A trial into the effectiveness of soft tissue massage in the treatment of shoulder pain. *Australian Journal of Physiotherapy*, **49**, 183–8.

Wakim, K.G., Martin, G.M., Terrier, L.C., *et al.* (1949) The effects of massage on the circulation in normal and paralysed extremities. *Archives of Physical Medicine*, March, 135–44.

Walach, H., Guthlin, C. and Konig, M. (2003) Efficacy of massage therapy in chronic pain: a pragmatic randomised trial. *Journal of Alternative and Complementary Medicine*, **9**(6), 837–46.

Weber, M.D., Servedio, F.L. and Woodall, W.R. (1994) The effects of three modalities on delayed onset muscle soreness. *Journal of Orthopaedic and Sports Physical Therapy*, **20**(5), 236–42.

Weerapong, P., Hume, P.A. and Kolt, G.S. (2005) The mechanisms of massage and effects on performance, muscle recovery and injury prevention. *Sports Medicine*, **35**(3), 235–56.

Weinberg, R.L.A. and Kolodny, L. (1988) The relationship of massage and exercise to mood enhancement. *The Sport Psychologist*, **2**, 20–22.

Weinrich, S.P. and Weinrich, M.C. (1990) The effect of massage on pain in cancer patients. *Applied Nursing Research*, **3**(4), 140–45.

II

The application of massage

4 Examination and assessment

Ann Thomson

Treatment planning

The topics covered in this chapter are:

- Examination of patients
- Assessing findings
- Clinical reasoning
- Determining the indications for massage
- Measuring change and outcome measures
- Palpation and skill

Examination of patients

This comprises a subjective component and an objective component. The subjective part identifies the history, onset, behaviour, nature, intensity, aggravating factors and easing factors of the patient's symptoms and clinical features. This involves asking questions that enable the patient to describe the problem(s). The symptoms are feelings described by the patient such as pain, pins and needles, feelings of weakness, numbness or heaviness.

Problems are the restrictions in activities of the patient's lifestyle that the patient attributes to the clinical features, e.g. stiffness, actual weakness, and loss of balance and co-ordination. The subjective component informs the therapist's planning of the objective component, enabling the therapist to observe and measure the patient's function and to determine the impact or relationship of any restrictions on the patient's symptoms and problems. Objective examination involves observation of posture and functional activities, testing range of joint movement, muscle power, balance and co-ordination, observation of gait and activities of daily living, and palpation of skin, fascia, muscles, nerves and joint accessory movements for musculoskeletal problems.

For patients with neurological dysfunction the emphasis is on proprioception, balance, sensory deficit, co-ordination, state of muscle tone and functional analysis. For patients with respiratory problems the emphasis is on lung function tests, thoracic cage mobility, breathing patterns, nature of secretions, and ability to cough or huff, for which specialised massage techniques are indicated.

For the purpose of this text emphasis will be on neuro-musculoskeletal problems. The therapist must examine every patient thoroughly because each patient is different. This may seem obvious, but it is important to recognise that patients with the same diagnosis or similar clinical features will react to pathology in different ways.

These differences will result from a number of factors, for example:

- A stoical/non-stoical nature.
- Attitudes to touch – some patients do not like being touched, possibly associated with history of abuse or torture. Other patients respond to the caring, educated, thinking hands of the therapist.
- Locus of control – some patients want to be independent and be advised on what they can do for themselves (internal locus); others wish to have therapy administered to them by someone else (external locus).
- Impact of occupation – e.g. physical demands, attitudes of fellow workers, employer attitudes. Tension and anxiety at work can inhibit progress and diminish treatment effects.
- Sometimes the major part of the treatment programme is to enable the patient to rearrange the work set-up, order of activities or work/rest ratio.
- Family and social background – patients in secure relationships with happy supportive relatives and friends will on the whole respond better to treatment more quickly than those who are less fortunate. There is also some evidence with back pain sufferers that the over-sympathetic spouse/partner can contribute to prolongation of pain whereas the spouse/partner who encourages activity contributes to a speedier recovery.
- Life experiences and culture – the past experiences of the patient have a bearing on the outcome of treatment, as does culture.
- Previous treatment – it is important to understand the patient's perceptions of previous treatment as this can have a large impact on the outcome, particularly where the patient has great belief in a particular treatment.
- Health beliefs and psychosocial influences have a large bearing on the patient's response to treatment, in particular to massage, because stressors or unhappiness is reflected in the state of relaxation or tension in the soft tissues.

Comprehensive examination identifies:

- The patient's problems, clinical features and symptoms.
- Any limitation of function.
- The relationship of symptoms, e.g. pain to activities.
- The impact of pathology on these activities.
- The patient's expectations and goals of treatment.

Assessing findings

On completion of the examination the therapist assesses the findings and plans treatment according to indications and contraindications for the possible therapy skills that might be appropriate for the patient. Objective tests are identified for measuring change, together with overall outcome measures and the patient's expectations. The therapist will also establish a prognosis. Skills are then selected and applied according to the best evidence that informs the clinical reasoning of the therapist.

Clinical reasoning

Types of clinical reasoning are hypothetico-deductive, pattern recognition, narrative and predictive. As a general rule, novice therapists use a 'template' for examining patients which is developed with clinical experience to form hypotheses that are then tested and retested. As expertise and experiential learning (enhanced by reflective learning) develop, pattern recognition becomes an integral part of the clinical reasoning process. Narrative reasoning relates to enabling the patient to express the problem in his or her own way so that the therapist understands the patient as a person. The 'genics' (see below) are designed to facilitate advancement of clinical reasoning. Predictive reasoning relates to estimating outcomes and prognosis (Jones and Rivett 2004).

Factors that assist in prediction (prognosis) are:

- Patient's perspectives and expectations.
- Patient's motivation and adherence.
- Locus of control.
- Social, occupational and economic status.
- Patient's past experiences.
- General health and comorbidity.
- Irritability – how easily stirred and time to settle.
- Severity – impact on patient's lifestyle.
- Nature – inflammatory, mechanical 'dysfunction', trauma.
- Mechanisms and patterns of clinical features ('genics').

Clinical features that may guide the therapist towards the possible sources/causes of patients' problems (the 'genics')

Arthrogenic joint related

Includes all structures that constitute a joint – bony surfaces, cartilage (hyaline and fibro cartilage), intervertebral discs (discogenic), synovium and ligaments.

- Degenerative changes, mal tracking.
- End feel – bony block, crepitus, hard rubbery resistance.
- Movement faulty.
- Deformity.
- X-ray – diminished joint space, shape of joint surfaces, density of bone.
- Palpation – stiff, tender, effusion, passive physiological intervertebral movements (PPIVM), passive accessory intervertebral movements (PAIVMs). Combined movements are diminished and may reproduce some of the patient's clinical features; similarly passive physiological and accessory movements of peripheral joints are abnormal. Heat, oedema, effusion and instability may be detected.
- Active and functional movements – locking, catching, block.
- Painful arc.
- Trauma; feeling of giving way; morning stiffness.
- Family history of rheumatoid arthritis (RA), osteoarthritis (OA), ankylosing spondylitis (AS).
- Blood tests.
- Pain related to movement; joint compression – distraction; nature of pain: local, referred, distal, proximal, deep burning aching pain.
- Discogenic relating to intervertebral discs – aggravated by repeated movements of the spine. Centralisation/peripheralisation, i.e. with patient in prone position over pillows: if pain in leg diminishes and is perceived more in the spine, then prognosis is good; if pain in leg increases, the recovery may be slow; aggravated by flexion and prolonged sitting; eased by rest, straight leg raising (SLR) positive; history – onset gradual after trauma; lateral shift of pelvis.

Myogenic fasciogenic

Related to muscles, sheaths, aponeurotic attachments, and deep and superficial fascia.

- Delayed onset muscle soreness (DOMS).
- Myofascial shortening.
- Palpation – fascial torsion; cramp; trigger points.
- Weakness; imbalance within group action; lengthened/shortened.
- Torn/ruptured/bruised – haematoma.
- Spasm – limiting movement, hard feel or 'string type thickenings' indicating chronic spasm.
- Denervated – no voluntary contraction; diminished spinal reflex.
- 'Compartment syndrome'; fascial compartments and attachments tight stretched and tender; overdeveloped muscle is restricted when fascia does not expand to accommodate the extra bulk of the muscle tissue.
- Fascial tightness – motion barriers on palpation (Fig. 4.1)
- Adherent; tender (myositis).
- Contracture – includes contractile and non-contractile elements.
- Myotendinous junctions and tenoperiosteal junctions tender.
- Thickenings.
- Tendonitis, tendonosis.
- Altered architecture, clicking/clunking of joints – poor motor control.

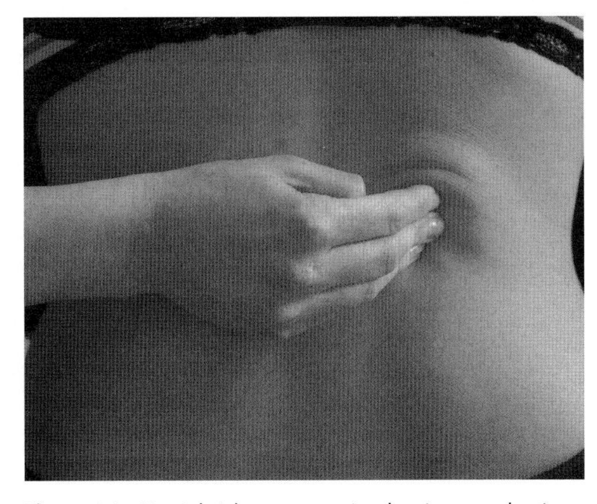

Figure 4.1 Fascial tightness – motion barrier on palpation.

- Crepitus between joint surfaces or between fascial planes – felt under the palpating hand during contraction or passive joint movement.

Neurogenic

All aspects of neural tissue including the peripheral nervous system (PNS) (lower motor neuron lesion, LMNL), central nervous system (CNS) (upper motor neuron lesion, UMNL) and autonomic nervous system (ANS).

- Neuropathic pain (diffuse limb pain aggravated by work, especially repetitive tasks) – nerve sheath inflammation without axonal damage.
- Diminished neural mobility and altered dynamics; nerve/tissue interface compromise.
- Hypoanaesthesiae, hyperalgia, allodynia, hyperpathial.
- ANS – skin temperature/colour/sweat/ texture/ health (trophic skin changes). Sympathetically maintained pain.
- Somatic pain – arising from structures that receive a nerve supply including joints, synovial membrane, ligaments, muscles, dura mater, intervertebral discs, altered dynamics, fascial torsion and restrictions. Somatic referred pain is pain perceived in a region separate from the primary source.
- Radicular pain – generation of ectopic impulses in nociceptive afferents in the affected nerve root.
- Central – brain, spinal cord, peripheral sensory/motor/reflexes.
- Anterior primary rami, posterior primary rami, 'double crush'.
- Unsteadiness, weakness, intracranial pressure, spinal stiffness (possibility of meningitis).

Osteogenic

Relating to disease, pathology or injury of bone.

- Includes poor union/torsion and remodeling following fracture.
- Night pain; deep; sclerotomal; unremitting.
- Aggravated by exercise and weight bearing; difficult to ease.
- Deformity; bone density altered.
- Systemic/vascular insufficiency.
- X-ray; magnetic resonance imaging (MRI) changes.
- History of recent sudden trauma – fracture.
- Prolonged unaccustomed exercise – stress fracture; local heat; blood tests.

Cardiovasculogenic

Relating to the heart and all blood and lymph vessels plus fascial torsion and restrictions.

- Exercise-related pain; throbbing in nature; ischaemic pain.
- Pain with rest.
- Family history; heavy smoker.
- Restless legs; night and daytime cramp.
- Previous history – on anticoagulants/blood pressure tablets.
- Pins and needles – 'unpleasant numbness' (as opposed to warm and pleasant).
- Trophic changes.
- Pain not provoked or relieved by specific movements.
- Pulsating mass (aneurysm – especially abdomen).
- Buttock puckering (connective tissue massage, CTM).
- Diet.
- Light headedness (blood pressure, diabetic, hypoglycaemic); fatigue.

Viscerogenic, genitourinary, gastrointestinal, endocrine, pulmonary

Relating to any organ/system other than those above.

- Single/recurrent operations.
- Affected by food intake.
- Cyclical pain with unusual patterns – not associated with movement.
- Heartburn.
- Bladder/bowel abnormalities – frequency, pain, blood, excess. Diminished urinary flow.
- Stress, depression.
- Prolonged non-steroidal anti-inflammatory drugs (NSAIDs).
- Poor diet.
- Visceral tenderness (liver, kidney, spleen).
- Muscle guarding, e.g. abdominal muscles.
- Breathing pattern apical – diminished air entry (e.g. Pancoast's tumour).

- Altered hormonal activity, e.g. thyroid under- or overactive.
- 'Indigestion' – related or unrelated to eating.
- Stomach cramps.
- Not ill/not well.
- Muscle aching (food allergy?).
- Fatigue; listlessness.

Psychogenic

Relating to the state of the patient's mind, which may also be linked to other sources of the problem.

- Stress; anxiety; depression; aggression; anger.
- Non-verbal communication, 'body language'.
- Reaction to people; reaction to physiotherapist.
- Description of pain – focus, catastrophising.
- Locus of control: external – wants others to help/treat; internal – wants to take charge of own management.
- History, e.g. eating disorders.
- Non-compliance.
- Previous psychiatric history; previous illnesses; operations.
- Regular or frequent last-minute cancellation of appointments (unable to attend, UTA); does not attend (DNA); late for appointment.
- Addictions – alcohol, drugs; coping strategies; legal case in progress.
- Concentration/memory problems; irritability.
- History of torture or abuse.

Ergogenic

Relating to work and leisure conditions, which may be contributing to or maintaining the problem.

- Posture in work position; work related – better on holiday.
- Daily pattern; repetition/sustained movement.
- Diffuse; non-specific; may ease with movement or activity.
- Environment/equipment – awkward.
- Stress/unhappy/worried/bullied.
- Several minor injuries – repeated.

Sociogenic–socioeconomic

Relating to the patient's social or economic conditions.

- Financial situation; employment; relationships.
- Socioeconomic class; culture/ethnic origin/religion.
- Accommodation.
- Role in family.
- Hobbies/sport; legal case; grievances.
- Life changes; diet; age; gender; alcohol intake; drug abuse.

As therapists advance in professional autonomy and self-referral for patients becomes the norm, it is essential that therapists can identify clinical features that arise from sources other than the neuromusculoskeletal systems. The guide above is not comprehensive but is designed to facilitate the recognition of the effect other systems and factors may have on the presenting clinical picture. It is also important to note that aspects of the psychosocial background to the patient's problems may be gathered over two to three visits and not on the first day of treatment.

Determining the indications for massage

Aspects of examination and assessment that relate to massage

The decision to apply massage and to select particular techniques is based on an understanding of how the assessment of examination findings relates to the therapeutic effects of massage. These have been described in Chapter 3 and will be considered under the same headings.

Observation and palpation using massage strokes to identify indications

It is important that therapists practise palpating and describing tissue response and end feel in asymptomatic normals so that a database is built up in the brain that acts as a standard by which to judge tissue responses.

Determining the nature of the tissues guides the therapist's choice of intervention. For example, tissues that have lost elasticity may respond to kneading, picking up and wringing, whereas stiff

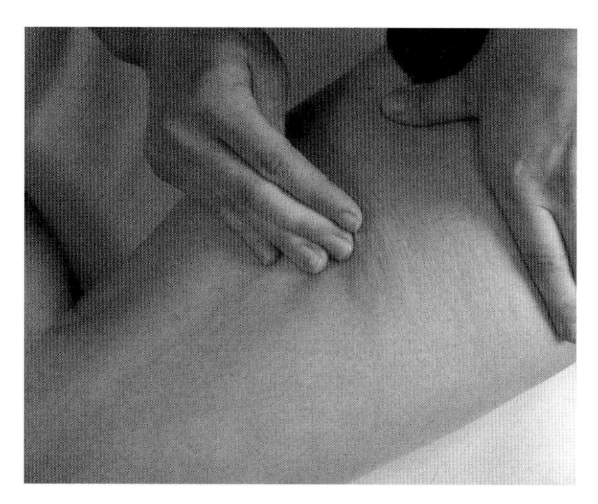

Figure 4.2 Modified stroking to produce a localised stretch.

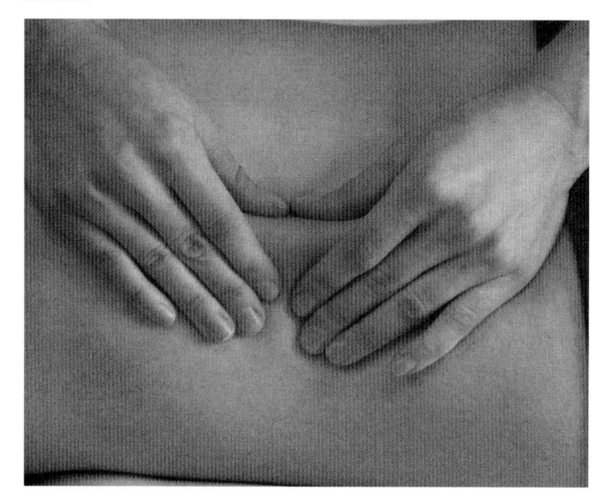

Figure 4.3 Skin rolling on lower back.

tissues may respond to stretch (modified stroking; Fig. 4.2) and possibly skin rolling (Fig. 4.3).

Maher *et al.* (1998) studied the descriptors used to describe palpation of spinal stiffness. Tables 4.1–4.3 summarise the descriptors used that may be helpful in describing abnormal and normal tissue response to palpation.

Other abnormal descriptors include crunchy, crackly, reactive, guarding, spasm (US physiotherapists); cement-like, grotty, hard, immobile, jumpy, spasmy, stuck, woody (Australian physiotherapists).

Table 4.1 Palpation descriptors through range feel.

Abnormal responses	Normal responses
Stiff	Smooth
Tight	Free running
Restricted	Resistance free
Firm	Soft
Inelastic	Spasm free
Non-compliant	Springy
Thick, non-springy	Well oiled
Blocked	Yielding
Limited	Elastic
Hypo mobile	Friction free
Active recoil	
Undue give	
Spongy	
Squashy	
Boggy	

Table 4.2 Palpation descriptors through end feel.

Abnormal responses	Normal responses
Abrupt	Yielding
Bony	Gradual
Capsular	Elastic
Elastic	Patient and therapist agree comfortable limit
Firm	
Hard	
Muscle spasm	
Non-reactive	
Non-springy	
Resilient	
Rubbery	
Soft	
Springy	
Sudden	
Unyielding	

Skin

On observation skin may appear ischaemic, whitish-blue in colour, shiny, stretched, puckered, pitted, dry or flaking (e.g. after removal of fixation). All of these signs indicate underlying pathology. On palpation resting the hands on the skin, the temperature may be cold and the skin may appear dry or oily. On stroking the back of the hand over the skin the therapist feels stickiness due to perspiration indicative of increased metabolic activity or inflam-

Table 4.3 Palpation descriptors through overall impression.

Abnormal responses	Normal responses
Abnormal	Pain free
Symptomatic	Perfect
Bad	Good
Comparable	Ideal
Disadvantaged	Smooth purposeful
Imperfect	co-ordinated movements
Non-pathological	
Old	
Average	
Painful	
Pathological	
Uncharacteristic	
Unphysiological	

mation. Palpation of the skin using varieties of kneading including using the finger and thumb reveals loss of mobility of the skin on underlying fascia, sometimes described as non-compliance of the skin.

The skin may feel 'thickened', immobile or dry, indicating dehydration of the tissues. Where there is excess fluid in the tissue layers the descriptions spongy or boggy may be appropriate. Provided that there is no acute inflammation, massage would be the technique of choice – with or without base oil or a non-allergic cream – to mobilise the tissues, redistribute arterial circulation, facilitate venous and lymphatic drainage and restore tissue fluid to the tissue spaces.

Scar tissue

On observation, healed scars may be puckered or adherent reddish-blue or white. Picking up and wringing are used to examine a scar for mobility (Fig. 4.4). Adherent scar tissues limit joint movement, and the traction on C fibre nerve endings causes pain (Fig. 4.5a,b).

There is increasing clinical evidence of the effects of deep scarring in the fascia and for the relief of this by myofascial release techniques, of which massage techniques are a component.

In a study by Lewitt and Olsanka (2004) problem scars are described as 'active scars' detected by skin drag (sweating) and thicker skin fold. They indicate

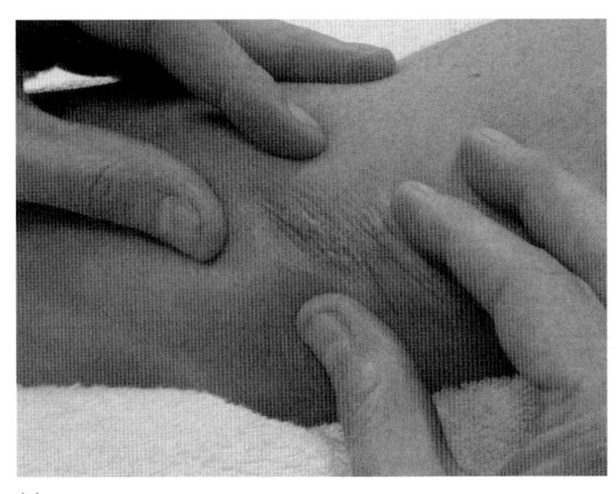

(a)

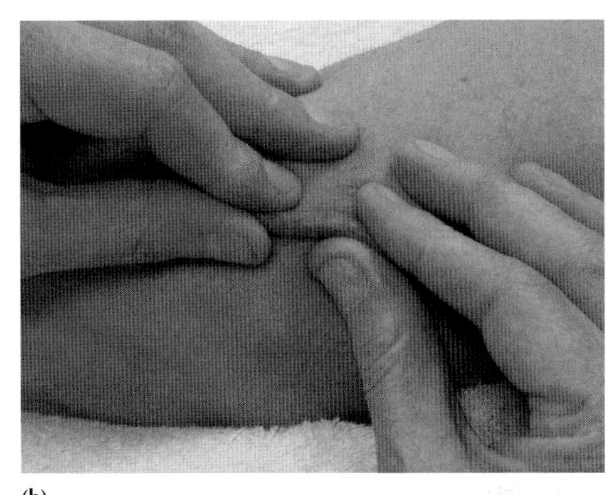

(b)

Figure 4.4 (a) Examining a scar for mobility. (b) Wringing to demonstrate mobility.

the nature of clinical features attributable to various areas of scar tissue:

Scars	Clinical features
Appendicectomy	Low back pain
Breast surgery	Neck pain
Gynaecological surgery	Headache
Thoracic surgery	Vertigo
Extremity injury	Root pain
Rectal surgery	Abdominal pain
Cholecystectomy	
Inguinal hernia	
Laminectomy	
Thyroidectomy	
Orchidectomy	
Hip replacement	
Umbilical hernia	

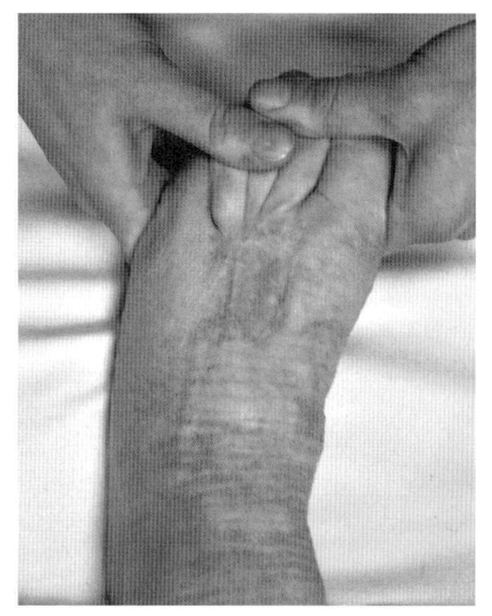

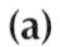
(a)

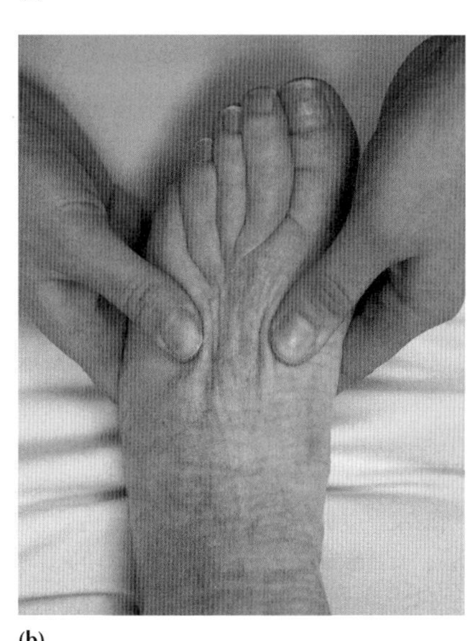

(b)

Figure 4.5 (a) Adherent scar demonstrating stretch on tissues and limitation of plantar flexion of the metatarsophalangeal joints. (b) Combination of thumb kneading and modified picking up to mobilise the scar.

According to this study it is important for the therapist to explore the possible influences of scarring at a site quite a distance from the clinical feature, e.g. headache arising from a tethered appendicectomy scar.

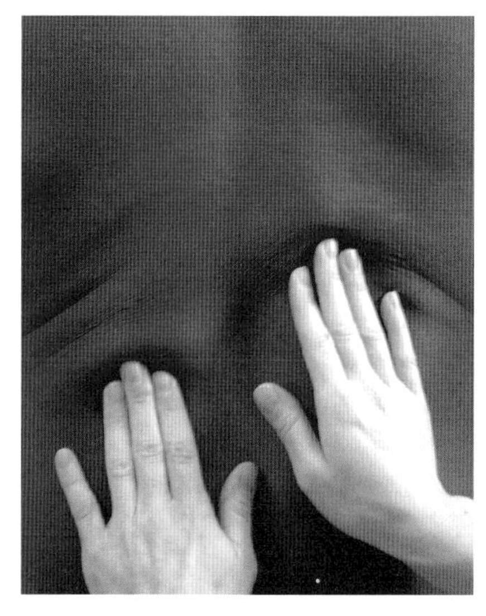

Figure 4.6 The tissues on the right are 'running free'. On the left there is a motion barrier.

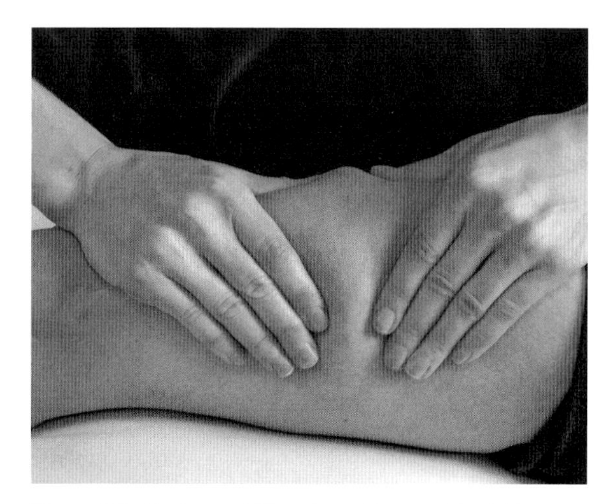

Figure 4.7 Testing mobility of quadriceps with picking up.

Muscles and fascia

These tissues can become adherent, resulting in loss of tissue fluid flow, drainage of lymph is impaired, and nutrition and vital membrane transport are inhibited. Mobility is tested with deep stroking to identify 'tissue barriers'. In Fig. 4.6 the tissues on the right of the patient's back are running free (normal mobility). On the left there is restriction and the therapist has detected a motion barrier.

In Fig. 4.7 the mobility of the quadriceps is being examined with picking up and with wringing in

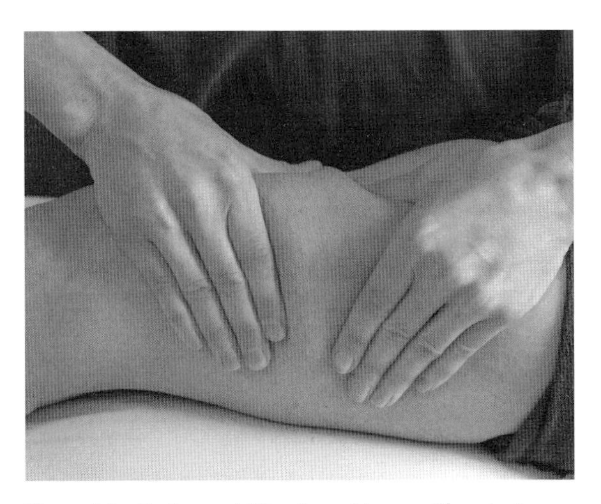

Figure 4.8 Testing mobility of quadriceps with wringing.

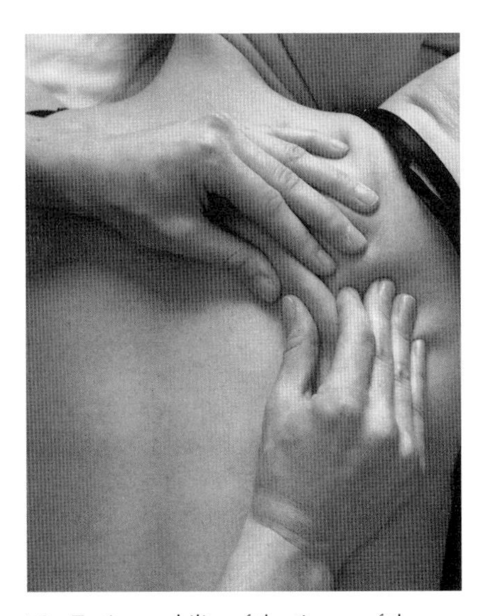

Figure 4.9 Testing mobility of the tissues of the upper back with skin rolling.

Fig. 4.8. In Fig. 4.9 the tissue mobility of the upper back is being tested with skin rolling. Trigger points are detected within muscle tissue as nodules that on palpation reproduce some of the pain pattern with which the patient is familiar or on quick stretch may produce the classical jump sign (Travell and Simons 1992; Mense *et al.* 2001). Figure 4.10 shows the position of the hands on gastrocnemius muscle ready to sink in slowly and detect trigger points. This approach also enables the therapist to detect deep local thickenings – to be differentiated

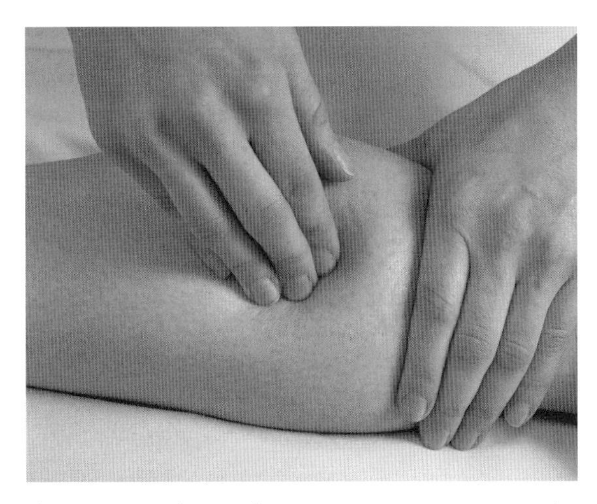

Figure 4.10 Palpating for trigger points in gastrocnemius muscle.

from trigger points -that lie within the muscle belly and that result from minor tears/strains in the tissue. Deep transverse frictions, finger kneading or specific soft tissue mobilisations (Hunter 1998) will mobilise these thickenings, enabling the muscle fibres to glide smoothly again.

Tendons

It is important to note the role of tendons in contributing to force output, as they store and release energy to enhance the force of muscle contraction. The Achilles' tendon may become shortened in people who wear high-heeled shoes and is curved convex medially in patients with hind foot valgus. Techniques that apply stretching are appropriate for tight tendons, e.g. wringing, deep stroking and kneading to surrounding tissues.

Nerve tissue

There is substantial evidence that nerves glide within their fascial bed and that they can become adherent to adjacent tissues especially at interfaces where they pass through muscles and across joints, e.g. in the carpal tunnel across the joints of the wrist and carpus. (Greening *et al.* 1999).

Palpation of the nerves in position of tension can reveal adherent tissues and mobility can be restored with deep stroking along the line of the nerve or at particular interfaces with deep stroking and kneading/wringing, and connective tissue massage technique. In this case the massage techniques are used to both test and treat, i.e. the technique is applied and then the response is tested.

Muscles that are in spasm feel hard and non-compliant. Massage –slow deep stroking or effleurage and slow rhythmical kneading – may be used to modify the H-reflex (see Chapter 3), reducing the efferent neural impulses and therefore reducing tension/spasm. This prepares the patient and the tissues for improved active exercise.

Pain and soreness

Pain and soreness associated with the patient's description of prolonged or awkward activity may be indicative of muscle fatigue or possible overuse. Kneading and slow effleurage are indicated. There is increasing evidence that massage relieves this problem and that if the patient is sensible in returning to graded activity the improvement is maintained.

Oedema

Following removal of fixation, oedema may have formed in the tissue spaces and this responds readily to effleurage kneading, picking up and wringing, in conjunction with active exercise in elevation. This combination is essential to prevent the fluid from fibrosing and becoming chronic thickening – resulting in permanent impairment.

Pitting oedema, where palpation leaves an indentation for 50–60 seconds, may be associated with renal or cardiac failure. Massage can be effective in reducing this oedema, but the benefit will be maintained only if the underlying condition is treated. Manual lymphatic drainage is highly effective in reducing lymphoedema. Once the therapist has established the depth, techniques and time required for effect, the patient or a relative must be taught the techniques as this type of massage needs to continue often on a daily basis. For example, the patient can have a normal functioning arm following mastectomy instead of a heavy swollen arm that is too heavy for the muscles to move.

Observation and palpation using massage strokes to identify contraindications

See Chapter 3.

Skin disorders

Open wounds are not contraindications for specialised massage directed at promoting healing. However, open areas must be avoided because of the risk of infection. Suppurating or hot inflamed areas must be avoided.

Eczema is contraindicated because of the possibility of increasing the irritation and spreading the problem.

Malignant tumours

Diagnosed malignancy may not be contraindicated where oncology and palliative care is being given. Massage by therapists with specialist knowledge may bring great relief and increased quality of life. Undiagnosed malignancy is a problem and the therapist must be aware of 'alarm bells' that present during the examination, for example:

- Sudden unexplained weight loss.
- Pale pallor.
- Night pain.
- Unremitting pain – not eased or aggravated by any activity or rest.
- Examination findings that do not point to any clear source of pain.
- Vague unexplained pain.
- Patient may respond to treatment at first but improvement is not retained.

Bruising

Early bruising is identified by the colours of red/purple/blue. It is also important to note that if there is a history of a blow or twist there may be exquisite tenderness before the bruising appears, and this is a contraindication to massage. Later when the blood is being dispersed by macrophages the colour changes to yellow and massage facilitates the removal of the exudate and blood cell remnants.

Recent fractures

These are usually diagnosed before the patient presents to the therapist. However, stress fractures (e.g. metatarsal or tibia) must be kept in mind where there is a history of prolonged exercise and exquisite tenderness on palpation possibly with the presence of a hard immobile lump; then massage is contraindicated.

Acute inflammation of joints

Joints that are hot and swollen (e.g. due to acute rheumatoid arthritis) must not be massaged.

Swellings

Palpation may reveal soft unexplainable swellings not related to bursitis or tendonitis within soft tissues or over joints; these may be tubercular or developing infection sites and the patient must be referred to a doctor.

Measuring change and outcome measures

Measurements used to monitor change in patients' tissues after massage and therefore claimed to be as a result of the intervention include the following:

- Heart rate.
- Blood pressure.
- Respiratory rate.
- Sweating.
- Salivary composition.
- H-reflex activity.
- Electromyography.
- Mood measures.
- Anxiety indices.
- Measures of pain threshold.
- Vital capacity, energy levels, posture – measured with photography, sit to stand (Davis *et al.* 2002).
- Pain: Visual Analogue Scale (VAS) 0–10 rating scale – no pain, discomfort, mild, moderate, severe.
- Goniometer to measure joint range where tight tissue or muscle spasm/tension are determined as the limiting factors.
- Spasm/tension is determined as the limiting factor.
- Tape measure for swelling/oedema.
- Patient and therapist judgement of range of movement – increased range, easier to move, smoother movement, can be held at end range for longer.
- Proprioception – can patient return to an exact position after movement?
- Functional activities, e.g.
  - hand behind back (HBB), hand behind neck (HBN)
  - speed and ease of sit to stand
  - timed walking over measured distance.
- Validated outcome measure.

The Patient-Specific Functional Scale (PSFS) (Stratford *et al.* 1995). This useful questionnaire can be used to quantify activity limitation and measure functional outcome for patients with any orthopaedic condition.

Examination and assessment recording

Recording of examination results varies according to the individual therapist's recording methods. Examples are given in Petty and Moore (2001) as well as Holey and Cook (2003).

The important results to record in relation to massage are given below.

Body chart

This is commonly used in physiotherapy clinics (Fig. 4.11). It is helpful to have more than one body chart, e.g.

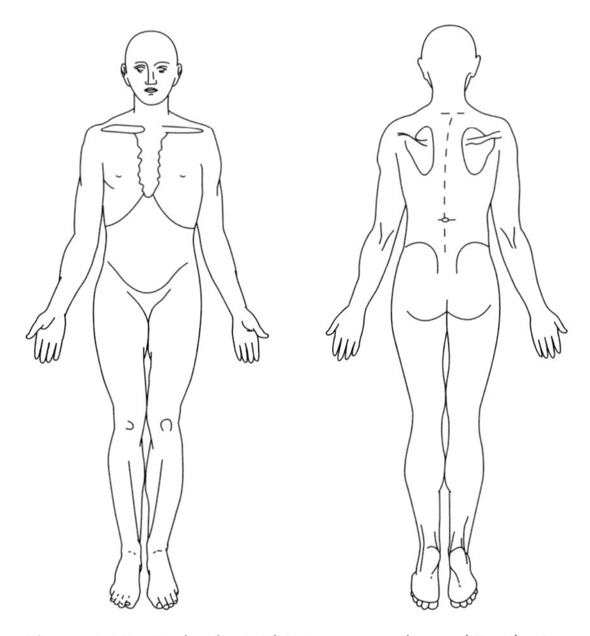

Figure 4.11 Body chart. This is commonly used in physiotherapy clinics. (Courtesy of Elizabeth Sharp, Director, ES Physio, London.)

- one for recording the patient's main problems, i.e. pain site and distribution, pins and needles, areas of numbness, abnormal muscle bulk, abnormal curves (scoliosis in the spine), bruising, swelling.
- a second for recording palpation findings, i.e.
  - sites of scars
  - areas of puckering
  - tenderness
  - trigger points
  - tethering
  - area of injury where tissues feel 'knotted'.

Samples of symbols that might be used to denote abnormalities detected:

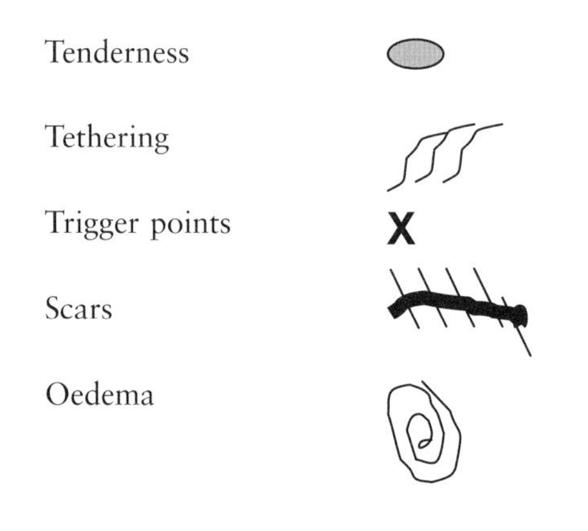

Body image drawings

Good use of body image representation is illustrated by Lederman (2005) (Fig. 4.12). These are powerful demonstrations of the change in body image that follows a manual experience.

SOAP notes

SOAP notes are a common way to write records:

- S Subjective
- O Objective
- A Assessment
- P Plan

This can be illustrated with short case studies where only the essential details are given.

Case study 1

A 70-year-old lady presenting with painful arc.

Subjective

Painful arc on abduction through to elevation of the right shoulder 80–110° aggravated by active abduction and eccentrically controlled adduction.

Objective

Painful arc aggravated by resistance to abduction and slowly returning the arm to the side. Eased by passive or assisted elevation through abduction and by resisted adduction to return the arm to the side.

Palpation – supraspinatus tendon (SST) thickened and immobile. Humeral head sits anteriorly in the glenoid.

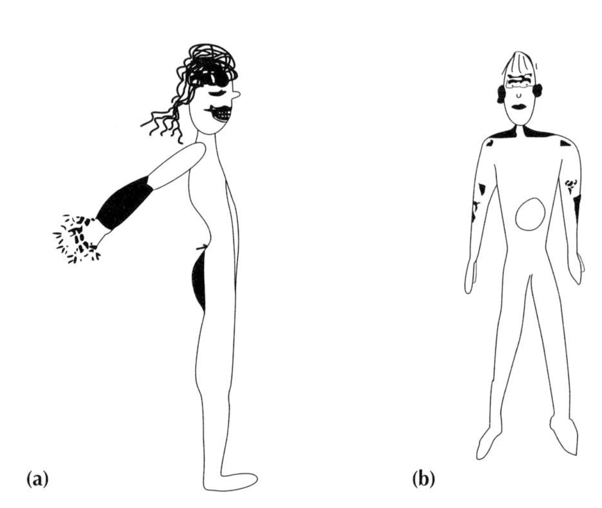

Figure 4.12 A more balanced representation of the body (a) before and (b) after a manual experience. Drawings were made during a workshop run by Tsafi Lederman (wife of Eyal Lederman) during a CPDO (Centre for Professional Development in Osteopathy) weekend course on 'Touch as a Therapeutic Tool'. (Reprinted from Lederman (2005) *The Science and Practice of Manual Therapy*, Elsevier Churchill Livingstone, with permission from Elsevier and the author.)

Assessment

Is massage indicated?

Yes, possibly SSTM or slow deep transverse frictions to mobilise the tendon, improve the subacromial microcirculation, and create space and tendon glide to prevent the impingement during elevation. However, the thoracic spine is very kyphotic with the chin poking posture of the cervical spine that compensates. Therefore the scapula is downwardly rotated with the glenoid facing down and the inferior angle prominent. This poor biomechanics has led to reactive fibrosis in the SST tendon as the humeral head tends to 'fall out of the glenoid'.

Plan

Teach repositioning of the spine – sternum up and forward, stretch head up out of shoulders, stretch and release pectorals and clavi pectoral fascia.

Reposition and hold scapula – teach elevation through abduction with lateral rotation. Assess effect on painful arc.

Treatment

Patient was taught to hold position of realigned thoracic spine sternum and cervical spine. Kneading, hold and release plus stretching was applied to pectorals and fascia. Scapula was held in neutral rotation and acromion in elevation/retraction. Patient reported 70% reduction in pain; after six repetitions patient repeated the movement positioning the scapula with its own muscles – pain continued to be 70% reduced. Anterior to posterior mobilisations were applied to the heads of the humerus. On testing, the movement was 90% pain reduced.

Three exercises were taught to retain the positional alignment and mobility of the spine, to stretch pectorals and fascia, to relocate the head of the humerus more centrally in the glenoid and retrain lateral rotation of the humeral head during elevation.

Reflection

Massage alone to SST may have had temporary relief. However, the whole spinal, shoulder girdle, shoulder complex needed to be addressed to realign the humeral head and for glenoid mechanics to have any long-term benefit.

This illustrates how local massage to the tendon was not the optimum treatment and any randomised controlled trials that purported to test massage, e.g. frictions versus ultrasound versus steroid injection for SST impingement, would be doomed to produce 'inconclusive results' with this patient's clinical features as entry criteria.

Case study 2

A 34-year-old lady presented with a fracture of the fibula. Six weeks after the injury when bony fusion had been established she was in great pain when walking and moving the foot past 90 degrees dorsiflexion. A lot of boggy swelling was palpated around the ankle, tendo Achilles and hind foot. Having had a variety of exercise and manual therapy she was still in pain aggravated by walking. She needed two elbow crutches to get about. Twenty minutes of massage to mobilise the lower leg muscles and stimulate lymphatic/venous drainage (kneading, picking up, wringing) plus squeezing, squeeze kneading and effleurage to clear the oedema from the ankle and foot resulted in immediate pain reduction, normal gait pattern and no need for crutches. Three more sessions of this massage cleared the oedema. At review 12 weeks post injury she was pain free and independent with a good gait pattern.

Reflection

Massage was the optimum treatment in this case. Oedema of the lower leg, ankle and foot does not clear with movement – active or passive – alone. The oedema inhibits tissue mobility, impairs neural transmission and creates a microenvironment that activates the C fibres. It accumulates in the superficial fascia from where the muscle pump action has little influence. Without massage therefore the only other possibility for oedema control is to put on two layers of 'Tubigrip'. However, it is important to avoid dependency on this. After the first massage treatment she was able to tolerate heel raising exercises which were progressed as the pain diminished.

Case study 3

A 28-year-old man suffered from repeated sprained ankle (inversion plantar flexion). He complained of feeling insecure in that the joint felt like it would give way, although it had not in fact done so. He also felt the ankle was weak and there was no spring in his step. Although the ankle had almost full range of movement he felt it to be stiff.

His lower end of fibula was forward on the talar facet. He was given anterior postero mobilisation on the lateral malleolus and strapping to emphasise the relocation of the fibula facet squarely on the talar articular surface. Immediately his gait was more even with effective push off. The strapping was continued for 14 days after which he progressed to advanced rehabilitation and complete recovery.

Reflection

It would be reasonable to give slow transverse frictions to restore elasticity to the anterior band of the lateral ligament of the ankle as it feels thickened and adherent. However, this alone would not achieve long-term gain as the joint surfaces need to be realigned; no doubt this is easier if the ligament is mobile and elastic. Massage is therefore not the optimum treatment but an adjunct to the overall management.

Summary

Assessment of examination findings provides powerful evidence for reasoning. This is in turn informed by many sources, e.g. 'academic' and scientific databases, textbooks, journals, friends, colleagues, patients and media. It is important for massage therapists to develop a broad spectrum of experience as this will enable them to relate well to all patients.

Permission to touch with an explanation as to how it is going to benefit is also an important part of preparing the patient.

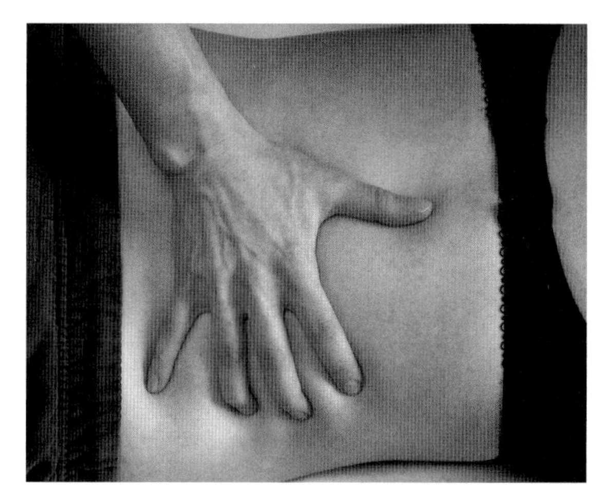

Figure 4.13 Hard tight hand – associated with poor technique and lack of sensitivity.

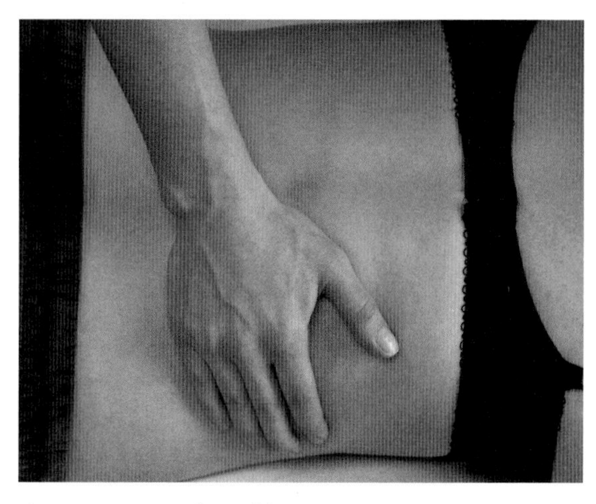

Figure 4.14 Hand moulding to part – sensitive to patient tissue response.

Palpation and skill

The most vital part of examination to determine indications for massage is palpation and it is essential that the tissues are palpated in a way that is repeatable, reliable and valid. This means paying particular attention to the patient's and therapist's position and ensuring that the hands are accurate, sensitive and testing what the therapist claims they are testing. As the three patients above illustrate, the therapist must be able to decide accurately when to apply massage and when to definitely not apply massage.

The method of palpating is going to have a large bearing on tissue response. Figure 4.13 illustrates the therapist with hard tight hands, while Fig. 4.14 illustrates the difference when the hands mould to the part. This will give the patient a feeling of care and therapy. In turn, the mind-set of the therapist will have a huge effect on the tissues' response. If the therapist is angry or upset then this tension is transmitted to the hands which are then less sensitive and possibly provide wrong information regarding the tension, tightness or mobility of the patient's tissues.

Specific soft tissue mobilisations (SSTMs)

SSTMs (Hunter 1998) are oscillatory manual techniques applied to soft tissues. The techniques are graded in a manner similar to that described in Maitland (1986). Pressure is applied to the structure at right angles to the longitudinal axis of the structure to be treated in such a way as to create a bowing and therefore lengthening effect. These techniques are very effective for lengthening and releasing scar-type collagen in healed, tight or adherent structures such as muscles, tendons and ligaments.

Effectiveness is dependent on thorough examination in order to identify the problem structure, requiring the therapist to have a sound in-depth knowledge of applied anatomy and sensitivity in palpation.

Acknowledgements

The author thanks the following people for advice, information on patients, photographs and proof reading: University College London (UCL) MSc in Advanced Physiotherapy students Stephen Bramson, Irit Endelman, Jonathan Kenyan, Justine Pettifer and David Stanley; UCL Physiotherapy Skills Course Leader Alison Skinner; Kings College London (KCL) MSc in Advanced Physiotherapy students Andrea Havill, Leanne Priestley and Andrew van Blommenstein; and KCL Lecturer in Physiotherapy Isaac Sorinola.

References

Davis, C.M., Doerger, C., Rowland, J., Sauber, C. and Eaton, T. (2002) Myofascial release as complementary in physical therapy for two elderly patients with osteoporosis and kyphoscoliosis; two case studies. *Journal of Geriatric Physical Therapy*, **51**(Suppl), 4.

Greening, J., Smart, S., Leary, R., O'Higgins, P., Hall-Craggs, M. and Lynn, B. (1999) Reduced movement of the median nerve at the carpal tunnel during wrist flexion in patients with non specific forearm pain: a magnetic resonance imaging study. *Lancet*, **354**, 217–18.

Holey, E.A. and Cook, E.M. (2003) *Evidence-Based Therapeutic Massage*, 2nd edn. Churchill Livingstone, Edinburgh.

Hunter, G. (1998) Specific soft tissue mobilization in the management of soft tissue dysfunction. *Manual Therapy*, **3**(1), 2–11.

Jones, M.A. and Rivett, D.A. (2004) *Clinical Reasoning for Manual Therapists*. Butterworth Heinemann, London.

Lederman, E. (2005) *The Science and Practice of Manual Therapy*. Elsevier Churchill Livingstone, Edinburgh, p. 244.

Lewitt, K. and Olsanka, S. (2004) Clinical importance of active scars: abnormal scars as a cause of myofascial pain. *Journal of Manipulative and Physiological Therapies*, **27**, 399–402.

Maher, C.G., Simmonds, M. and Adams, R. (1998) Therapists' conceptualisation and characterisation of the clinical concept of spinal stiffness. *Physical Therapy*, **78**(3), 289–300.

Maitland, G.D. (1986) *Vertebral Manipulation*, 5th edn. Butterworth, London.

Mense, S., Simons, D.G. and Russell, I.J. (2001) *Muscle Pain: Understanding its Nature, Diagnosis and Treatment*. Lippincott/Williams and Wilkins, Philadelphia.

Petty, N. and Moore, A. (2001) *Neuromusculoskeletal Examination and Assessment*, 2nd edn. Churchill Livingstone, Edinburgh.

Stratford, P., Gill, C., Westaway, M. and Binkley, J. (1995) Assessing disability and change on individual patients: a report of a patient specific measure. *Physiotherapy Canada*, **47**, 258–63.

Travell, J.G. and Simons, D.G. (1992) *Myofascial Pain and Dysfunction: The Trigger Point Manual*, Vol 2. Williams and Wilkins, Baltimore.

Further reading

Bullock-Saxton, J., Chaitow, L., Gibbons, P., *et al.* (2002) The palpation debate: the experts respond. *Journal of Bodywork and Movement Therapies*, **6**(1), 18–36.

Comeux, Z., Eland, D., Chila, A., Phebey, A. and Tate, M. (2001) Measurement challenges in physical diagnosis: refining inter-rater palpation, perception and communication. *Journal of Bodywork and Movement Therapies*, **5**, 245–53.

Robertson, S. (2001) Integrating the fascial system into contemporary concepts on movement dysfunction. *Journal of Bodyworks and Manipulative Therapy*, **9**(1), 40–47.

Schleip, R. (2003) Fascial plasticity – a new neurobiological explanation. Part 1 and Part 2. *Journal of Bodywork and Movement Therapies*, **7**(1), 11–19 (part one); 7(2), 104–116 (part two).

Wikipedia (2006) http://en.wikipedia.org/wiki/myofascial release.

5 Preparation for massage

Margaret Hollis and Elisabeth Jones

Massage has been referred to as an art, because its practice involves co-ordination of a high order and the use of great skill to achieve the integrated body movements that allow the application of the appropriate manipulations at the correct depth and speed to achieve maximum effect. To this end potential practitioners must practise each manipulation with great awareness of their own contact with the subject, whether model or patient, so that any discomfort is immediately noticed and the cause detected. Uncomfortable massage is usually born of failure of co-ordinated performance by the practitioner. Minor adjustment of foot position and trunk posture will change the relationship of the practitioner to the support and the subject; and the totality of hand contact and the angle of contact will be altered by the posture of the trunk and arms. Finally, weight transference from the practitioner's feet to the subject will control depth. Rhythm must then be considered, as uneven movement of any one of the practitioner's body components will cause uneven contact, jerky movements of the whole line of work and angular patterns that will cause uneven compression or dragging by some part of the working hand.

Thus when starting to perform and practise massage check that you can:

- Reach all parts.
- Stand in walk or lunge standing to do so.
- Change position from that shown in Fig. 5.1 to that shown in Fig. 5.2a without impedance or hesitation.

Adaptations of these main positions may be made to ensure correct massage application (see Fig. 5.2b, c).

Self preparation

The practitioner should start preparation of himself or herself long before contact with the patient/client. Attention to personal appearance, hygiene and manicure are all important. As close contact will inevitably occur, the practitioner should wear protective clothing which is easily laundered and which allows freedom of movement while maintaining decency. Long hair must be restrained so that it cannot come into contact with the subject and, equally, necklaces or other jewellery which can dangle should be discarded, as should a wristwatch.

Rings should be removed as they can cause discomfort to the practitioner when performing some manipulations and to the patient during most manipulations. Thin wedding rings may be the exception to this rule, provided they do not cause

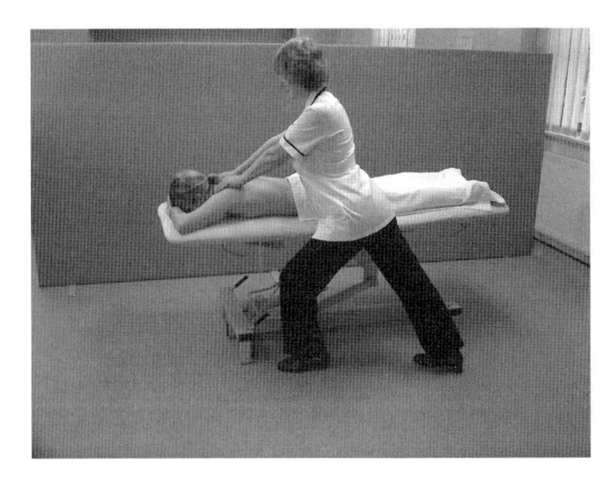

Figure 5.1 Lunge standing reaching along the length of the body.

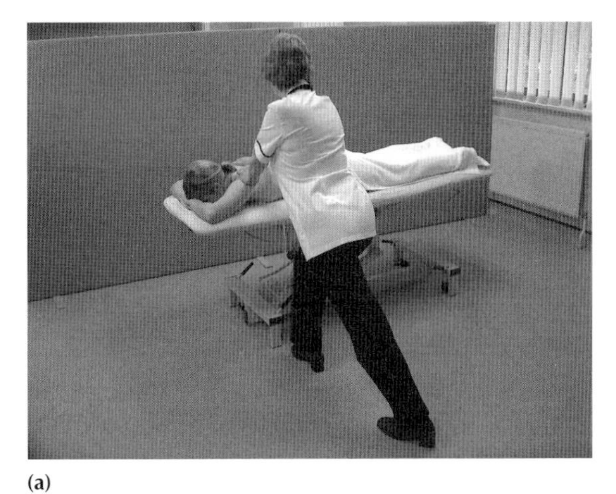

(a)

Figure 5.2 (a) Walk standing reaching across the body.

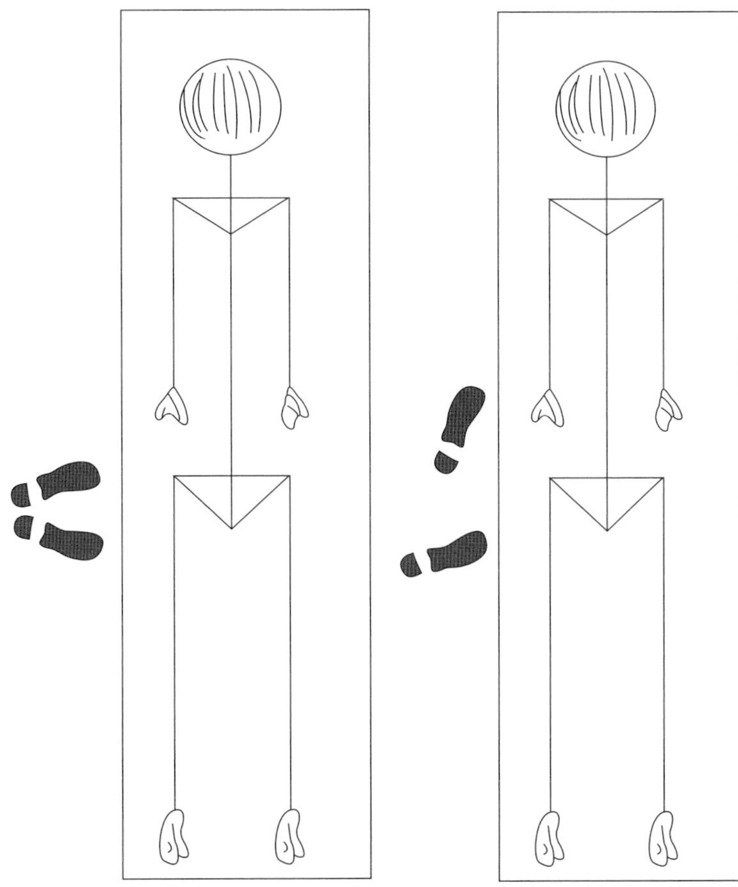

(b)

(c)

Figure 5.2 (b) and (c) Adaption of position from lunge or walk standing for transverse manipulations across the body, anterior or posterior.

discomfort to anyone. Well-cared-for hands which are smooth with short, clean nails are essential.

Cleanliness is important to avoid cross infection so wash your hands before and after each treatment. Cultivate warm hands by always using warm water for washing and by keeping your hands covered when outside in the cold.

The range of movements of all the joints of your forearm and hands should be full. If you have stiff hands, do a series of stretching exercises aimed at increasing your range of movement. The most important large range movements are:

- Full abduction/extension of the thumb to give a wide grasp – an octave.
- Full flexion and extension of the wrists or at least 80° of each movement.
- Full pronation and supination of the radio-ulnar joints.

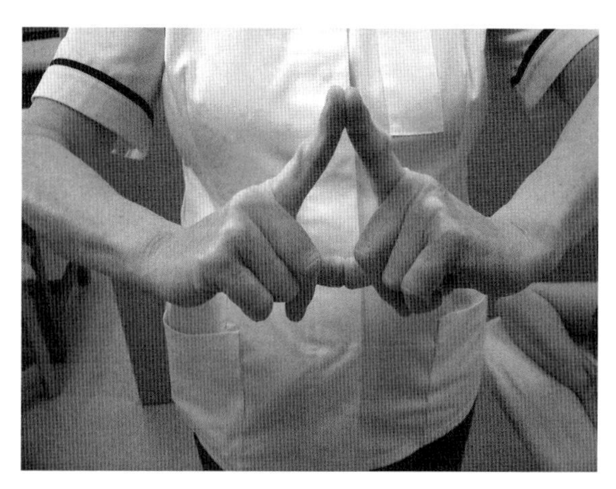

Figure 5.3 Exercise to increase hand span.

Hand exercises

To obtain these ranges of movement the following exercises should be practised. Before each exercise check your shoulder relaxation:

(1) Touch the index finger tip of one hand with the index finger tip of the other and at the same time put your thumbs together. Press fingers and thumbs so they extend backwards. Do this with middle, ring and little fingers, together with the thumbs as before (Fig. 5.3).
(2) Push the fist of one hand between two adjacent fingers of the other hand so that they are separated into wider abduction. Keep your fingers in the same plane. Repeat for each space.
(3) Place your hands together as in prayer and with your thumbs resting on your chest push your wrists downwards to extend them without separating the heels of your hands.
(4) Reverse your hands, placing the backs together and push your elbows downwards thus flexing your wrists.
(5) Place your hands in the prayer position and, keeping them together, turn them down and up. Try to touch your abdomen and chest alternately at each rotation. When you can hold with your hands just very slightly separated practise the rotation of your two hands, not touching, but simultaneously. Next move your two hands alternately so that they pass one another at mid-point (Fig. 5.4). Observe that the finger tips of each hand will now strike your abdomen at precisely the same point.

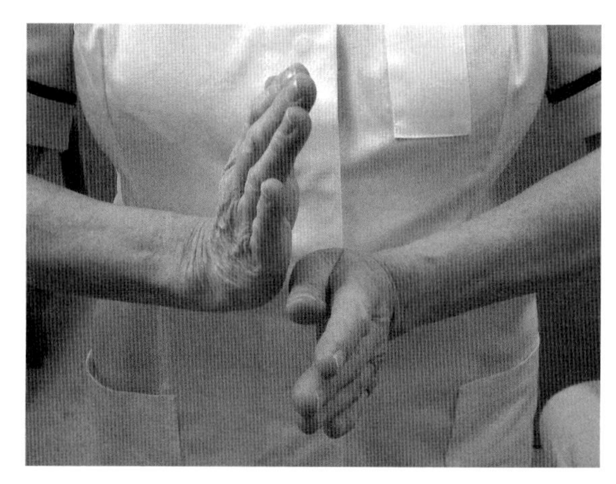

Figure 5.4 The ultimate ability is to maintain wrist extension with a relaxed hand and perform full range pronation and supination with alternate hands.

Relaxation

Relaxation of your hands is very important so that you always use your hands in full contact with your patient, and moulded to the shape of the body you are touching, with awareness of the tissues and of their state.

Relaxed hand contact is one in which the hand conforms to the contour of the part. The natural rest position of the human hand is with the fingers and thumb a little apart and very slightly flexed at each joint and it can easily be adjusted to allow contact with any size of body part. This is the contact that is used in many massage manipulations.

In addition you will need to be able to relax your whole arm to perform some manipulations. You should practise a method of relaxation yourself prior to learning massage. A good method is reciprocal relaxation as you will then become more aware of the position of all your joints and be capable of local relaxation of any body part as needed. Briefly, reciprocal relaxation involves working the opposite muscles to those you wish to relax, then stopping the action and appreciating the new, relaxed position of that body part (Hollis 1993).

Co-ordinated and integrated movement of your body is essential for the comfortable and prolonged performance of massage manipulations without fatigue and physical stress on the practitioner (particularly avoiding back strain).

You should stand and practise transferring your weight forwards and backwards while maintaining your arms stretched away from you:

- Along the couch as in Fig. 5.1.
- Across the couch as in Fig. 5.2a.

These movements, along the length of the patient and across the patient, are key movements in massage. The former allows you to practise long, reaching actions with variable weight from your hands on to the length of the body structures; the latter allows you to practise short, reaching actions with variable weight from your hands across the length of the body structures.

The environment

The treatment area should be quiet, with discreet colours, well heated and well ventilated but not draughty. The padded, adjustable treatment couch or chair should have a washable undercover and towels to cover the areas not being treated. At least two pillows should be available and a disposable paper sheet should cover both pillows and bedding.

Contact mediums

These provide 'glide'. They may be kept in a bottle or small bowl on the table by the couch. Be careful of spillage. Some people prefer not to use a contact medium as they feel they can not only achieve greater palpatory awareness, but also avoid allergy reactions.

Powder

- Talcum powder. It should be non-perfumed if possible, or baby powder may be selected.
- Corn starch BP, which is sterilisable, is a heavy powder which absorbs sweat very readily and should be used in the presence of profound sweating by either the patient or the practitioner. Ensure it is not inhaled by the therapist or patient and that the patient is agreeable to its use. (It is no longer used in the NHS.)

Oils

- Pure lanolin. This has a 'drag' effect on skin due to its thick and heavy texture and is used to obtain a slight pull on the skin. Lanolin cream which is a water-based cream is used when less 'drag' is required.

Liquid oils

- The most commonly used liquid oil is probably vegetable oil (see Chapter 15).
- Liquid paraffin is sometimes used.
- Baby oil may also be used to provide a 'gliding' effect and to lubricate the skin.

Creams

These are commercial preparations using a variety of ingredients.

Water-based lubricants

The water-based lubricant most commonly used is ung. eucerin. This light cream is used to give moderate lubrication and, as it absorbs rapidly, is mainly of value as an introduction to deeper work. The thinner oils used in massage tend to reduce the depth at which the practitioner can work as the hands glide on the lubricated skin and slide away from the part being treated, instead of working with depth. Thicker oils do not cause this problem. Note also that the smaller the manipulations you perform when using oils, the more likely you are to obtain greater depth.

Ensure the medium is at skin temperature before use and is put into the therapist's palm before transfer to the patient with gentle strokes.

Soap and water

Soap and hot water, with or without the addition of oil, is used for scaly skins which may be caused by prolonged immobilisation in a cast or by use of some medications which promote and increase skin healing but which may cause the skin to become dry and scaly.

Allergic reactions

Some contact mediums can cause mild to severe allergies. Nut and wheat content in a contact medium is contraindicated totally for patients who have allergies to these substances. Always check allergic responses of a medium before use.

Preparation of the patient

Ask the patient to undress so that the part to be treated is free of jewellery and adequately uncovered. Remember that some manipulations, to be effective, must extend to the lymph glands lying in proximal spaces. Thus:

- **For treatment of the upper limb,** unclothe from the neck to finger tips and especially remove all straps.
- **For treatment of the lower limb,** unclothe from the groin to the toe – remove trousers, do not pull them up.
- **For treatment of the back,** unclothe from the head to the buttocks. Pants/briefs can remain on, but must be pulled down to leave the area above the gluteal cleft exposed.
- **For treatment of the neck,** unclothe from the head to the level of the lowest point of origin of trapezius, i.e. 12th thoracic vertebra.
- **For treatment of the face,** unclothe from the hairline to just below the clavicle.

Ensure the patient is kept warm by the use of towels, e.g. if he or she is sitting, wrap him or her in a blanket, keeping only the part to be treated free of coverings (Fig. 6.3). If the patient is to lie down supine, cover him or her immediately, having first placed pillows in position as needed. The patient in lying may need:

- One or two head pillows.
- A pillow under the knees.

If the couch has not got a suitable opening, or small towel (rolled up), and the patient is lying in the prone position, he/she may need:

- Two head pillows crossing one another to create an inverted and open triangle so that the patient's nose rests below the crossing.
- A pillow under the abdomen to raise and thus flatten the lumbar spine or avoid pressure on a large bosom.
- A pillow under the ankles to flex the knees slightly.

The patient in side lying may need:

- One or two pillows under the head, and the upper arm and leg also supported by a pillow.
- A pillow supporting the abdomen in pregnancy.

More pillows will be needed for special positions and these are dealt with in the treatments section.

If you use one large cover initially ensure that smaller covers are on hand so that you can split them to keep the patient covered and warm.

Small towels are very useful for placing in direct contact with the patient and to protect the patient's clothes and coverings, as towels are more easily washed and less likely to retain any contact medium you may use.

Palpation and developing sensory awareness

Palpation is a skill that is acquired by practice (Hollis and Yung 1985). It requires that your hands should be clean, warm and relaxed, in firm comfortable contact, and aware of what is under them. The term 'thinking hands' implies that your mind is envisaging the structures that your hands are feeling and is alert both to identify the structure and become aware of variations from normal in the state of the structure.

To learn how to palpate, practise the following procedures. Place your whole hand on a series of varying size, rounded structures in turn, starting with large ones that require an almost flat hand, for example:

- A cushion or part-filled hot water bottle.
- A smaller bottle or rolling pin.
- A broomstick handle.

Increase your pressure on the object to grasp firmly with your whole hand, modifying your hand posture so that every part of the palmar surface is in contact simultaneously. Then release your pressure very slowly until you are only just grasping – think hard about the quality of this pressure. Next, release your pressure so that the object could start to slip. Think about and appreciate this pressure, as such pressure is likely to tickle the patient.

Following this, enlist the help of a colleague and repeat the procedure, applying in turn very firm, firm and very light contact on the back, the thigh, the calf, the arm, the forearm and the foot. Appreciate what pressure/contact you need to be able to touch and not hurt, and to touch and not tickle.

Again use a colleague and decide to palpate for specific anatomical features. Place more of your hand than you need in contact with the area to be examined, lift your palm a little to reduce the contact, so that only the finger pads are touching firmly enough. Your fingers should be straight so that your nails are unlikely to be in contact. Do not lose contact, but, if you do, refrain from re-establishing it by putting only your finger tips on again. To do so will cause you either to poke and hurt or to tickle by touching again too lightly. Remember that too hard a pressure will feel like a drill digging in (Fig. 5.5) and too light a pressure will feel like a

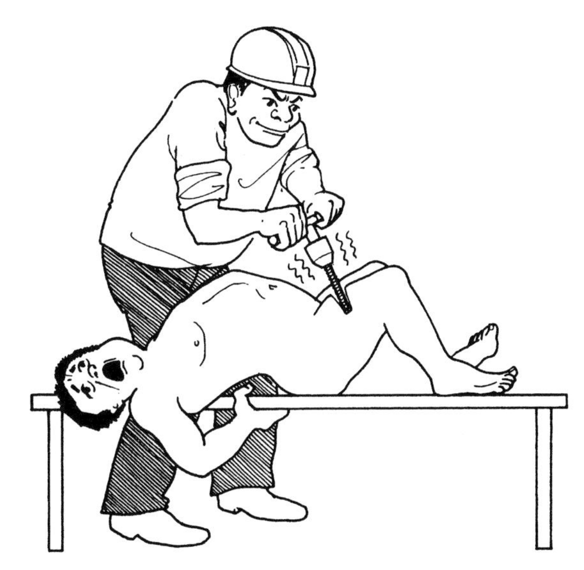

Figure 5.5 Do not palpate at the depth of a drill.

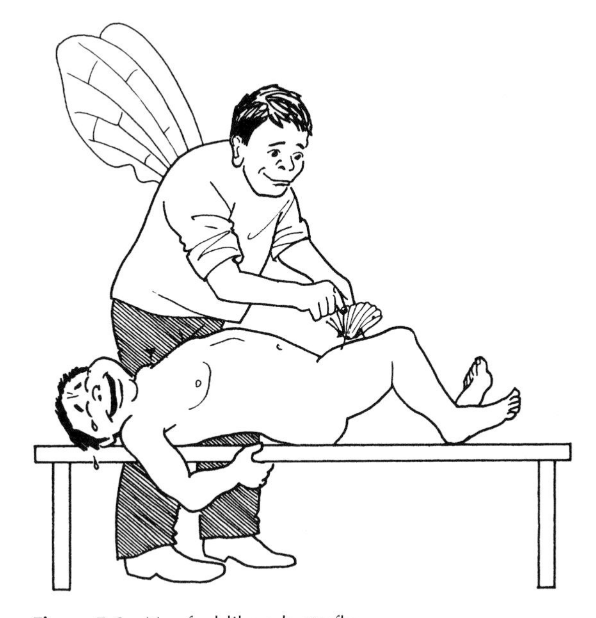

Figure 5.6 Nor feel like a butterfly.

butterfly coming to rest (Fig. 5.6). In neither case will you feel or find anything.

Now slide your fingers towards the structure to be palpated and in doing so ensure that your pressure is such that you neither drag the skin nor skid over it. Mentally count off the anatomical landmarks and apply the check tests that you have learned for identifying that structure, for example:

- Arteries, which can be felt to pulsate.
- Pressure on veins occludes them so that they will appear at their fullest, distally.
- Tendons have muscle tissue attached and may be felt as firm cord-like structures.
- Ligaments, which may be felt as firm bands at joints holding bone ends together.
- Bony prominences.

Examination of the part

See Chapter 4.

Before performing massage on either a model on whom you will practise or a patient whom you will treat you should examine the part on which you are going to work. In the case of a patient you will, of course, have carried out a complete examination and assessment so that you are aware of the problems that the patient presents.

Whether working on a model or a patient, having arranged him or her as described above, you should now examine the part you intend to massage.

Look at the skin state for dryness, oiliness, wetness, hairiness and completeness – thus you may observe bruises, abrasions and lacerations. Look also at the state of subcutaneous tissues – is the skin emaciated or well padded and, if the former, is it taut? Is there any oedema or excess reddening?

Feel – run your hand down the length of the part on every aspect. Think as you do so and be aware not only of the temperature of each area, the degree of muscle tension and joint posture but also of any flinching as painful or ticklish areas are touched. Make mental notes so that problem areas can be approached with caution.

Ticklish subjects

People who are ticklish can be massaged without discomfort to them provided you observe the rules of always putting your hands in very firm contact as you start work and never lifting your hands off by 'trickling', i.e. by lifting your palms off first, then each phalanx, until only your finger tips are in contact.

You should also never move one hand component, especially fingers, in relation to one another once you have placed your hands in contact.

Light work tickles, so always perform the manipulations at the maximum depth tolerable by the model/patient and to produce the required result.

References

Hollis, M. (1993) *Practical Exercise Therapy*, 3rd edn, pp. 33–4. Blackwell Science, Oxford.

Hollis, M. & Yung, P. (1985) *Patient Examination and Assessment for Therapists*, pp. 12–15. Blackwell Science, Oxford.

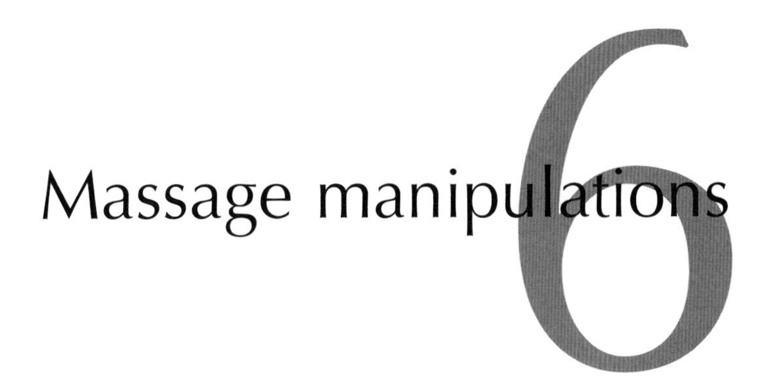

6 Massage manipulations

Margaret Hollis and Elisabeth Jones

The manipulations described in this chapter and Chapters 7–11 are relevant for what may be called 'classical massage'. They are as follows:

- Effleurage/stroking manipulations.
- Petrissage manipulations.
- Friction manipulations.
- Percussive (tapôtement) manipulations.

The word 'effleurage' means to stroke, and the manipulations in this group may be divided into:

- Those in which the intention is primarily to assist venous and lymphatic drainage and in which the direction of the work is from distal to proximal – usually called effleurage.
- Those in which the intention is primarily to obtain a sensory reaction either sedative or stimulative and in which direction is not important but is often from proximal to distal – usually called stroking.

In this book the words effleurage and stroking will apply to the above respective descriptions.

Effleurage

Aims:

- Assist venous and lymphatic drainage.
- Assist fluid interchange.
- Assist in relaxation of the client through sedative effect.
- Help decrease muscle tone (light) or increases muscle tone (deep).
- Help with passive stretch of muscle fibres.

Effleurage is a unidirectional manipulation in which the practitioner's hand passes from distal to proximal with a depth compatible with the state of the tissues and the desired effect. Thus, the manipulation may start at one end and proceed to the proximal space, draining the part to be treated, e.g. finger tips to axilla, toes to groin, buttocks to axilla, neck to supraclavicular glands. The depth should be such as to push fluid onwards in the superficial vessels. This may be observed especially in the veins of the forearm. The manipulation is performed with the whole hand softly curved and relaxed to fit the part, or with any part of the hand which fits the part. Both hands may be used together (Fig. 6.1) on opposite aspects of a part, or may follow one another (Fig. 6.2). Each hand may be used singly while the opposite hand supports the part in an appropriate position (Fig. 6.3). As the manipulation proceeds over the part, the hand(s) must change shape to maintain perfect contact.

The stance of the practitioner is very important as these manipulations often proceed over a considerable length of the body, and it must be possible for the practitioner to transfer body weight to and fro. Lunge standing (Fig. 5.1) adapted to the part is the usual stance adopted, with the weight being

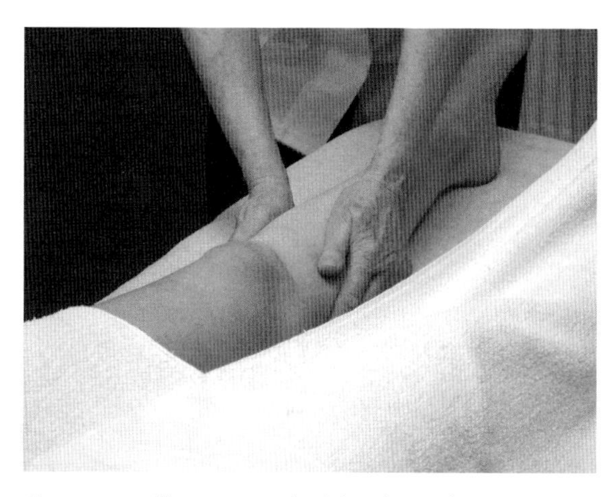

Figure 6.1 Effleurage using both hands together on opposite sides (stroking if proximal to distal).

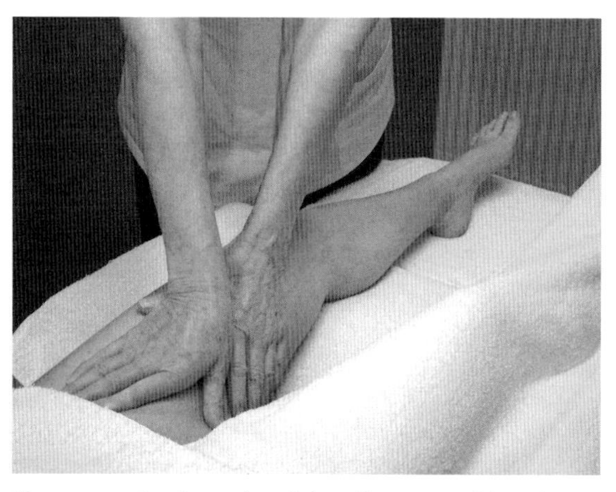

Figure 6.2 The lines of work for effleurage and kneading.

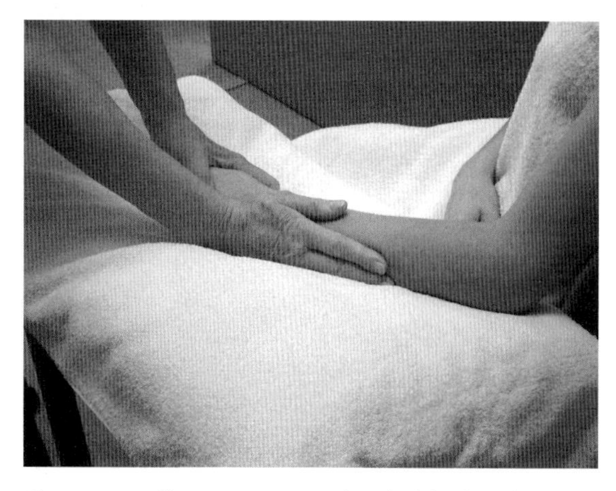

Figure 6.3 Effleurage using one hand while the other hand supports.

transferred from the rear to the forward foot, accompanied, if need be, by either or both lifting of the heel of the rear foot and flexion and extension of the knees and hips. The arms will initially be flexed and become more extended, especially at the elbows as the reach is made. Integration of the arm and body movements must be maintained to ensure a smooth movement of the hand along the part; this is achieved if the arms stretch first, followed by body weight transfer. At the end of every line of effleurage there should be a small increase in depth (often called overpressure) and a slight pause (in the space) before the hand is lifted off with minimum flourish and returned to the distal part to start the next line of work. Some people advocate stroking the hand back to the start.

When the whole hand is used for effleurage, it does not maintain equal contact over its whole surface and should be placed obliquely on the skin so that the leading edge is the 'C' formed by the thumb to forefinger cleft. This edge is formed by the border of the forefinger and the border of the thumb linked by the adjacent web; however, the main pressure is exerted by the 'C' formed by the border of the thumb, the thenar eminence, the hypothenar eminence and the little finger. The pressure is graded from the index to little fingers and adjacent parts of the palm so that the hand operates in the manner of a ski.

If the pressure is exerted by the leading edge, it can be uncomfortable or jerky, or can cause sticking. Lack of control of the modulation of the pressure as the hand proceeds up the part is more usually caused by:

- *Either* standing too near the finish of the stroke (step back to cure this)
- *Or* failing to synchronise the arm movements with the weight transfer.

Stroking

Aims:

- Assists in creating a sedative effect (slow).
- Assists in creating a stimulating effect (fast).
- Assists in application of contact medium.

Stroking is a unidirectional manipulation in which the practitioner's hand passes, usually, from proximal to distal down the length of the tissues at a depth and speed compatible with the required effect, but direction of the stroke may be varied to give greater comfort.

The stroke should start with firm contact (try not to trickle your fingers on) and finish with a smooth lift off of your hands. The hands may be positioned obliquely or so that the heel travels first, but can adjust its position down the length of the part so that comfortable contact is maintained.

The slower strokes are more sedative. Try a speed of one stroke per 5 seconds. The faster strokes are more stimulating. Try a speed of four strokes every 5 seconds, i.e. four times faster.

Obviously greater depth can be achieved at the slower rate, but the need for sedative effects may limit your depth when pain and muscle spasm prevent firmer contact. If this is so, the depth is increased as relaxation occurs and pain diminishes, but the tempo should still be maintained. The faster stroking is often used to complete a more stimulating massage.

The whole area under treatment should be covered by a sequence of strokes. Stroking may be performed using:

(1) One hand – usually on a narrow area.
(2) Two hands simultaneously – one each side on a broad area. Be careful not to pull on the part (Fig. 6.1).
(3) Right and left hands following one another on a narrow area.
(4) Thumb(s) or fingers(s) on confined areas one-handed, two-handed or alternately.
(5) A technique called 'thousand hands' in which one hand performs a short stroke, the second hand does the same overlapping the first, and the hands pass over one another to gain contact as the manipulation proceeds down the length of the part under treatment.

Petrissage

Aims:

- Assists venous and lymphatic return.
- Assists fluid interchange.
- Increases mobility of underlying tissue.
- Has an effect on somatovisceral reflexes.

Petrissage manipulations are those in which the soft tissues (mainly muscles) are compressed either against underlying bone or against themselves. They are divided into:

- Kneading manipulations – when the tissues are compressed against the underlying structures.
- Picking up manipulations – when the tissues are compressed then lifted and squeezed.
- Wringing manipulations – when the tissues are lifted and squeezed by alternating hand pressure.
- Rolling manipulations – when the tissues are lifted and rolled between the fingers and thumbs as in skin rolling or muscle rolling.
- Shaking manipulations – when the tissues are lifted and shaken from side to side.

Kneading

Kneading is a circular manipulation performed so that the skin and subcutaneous tissues are moved in a circular manner on the underlying structures. The manipulation may be performed with the palmar aspect of the whole hand, with the palm only, with all the fingers, or with the pads or tips of the thumb or of the fingers. Whatever the area used, a circle is described by the part of your hand in contact, with pressure on the upward part of the circle but only for a small segment. The actual range or number of degrees for which pressure is exerted varies with the part treated.

On flat areas, e.g. the back, the pressure with the right hand is from 8 o'clock to 11 o'clock with that hand circling clockwise. The left hand circles counter-clockwise and exerts pressure from the 4 o'clock to the 1 o'clock line (Fig. 6.4a).

On the limbs, the pressure is exerted from 6 o'clock to 9 o'clock with the right hand and from 6 o'clock to 3 o'clock with the left hand. On the non-pressure phase of the circle the hand maintains contact but glides on to the next area of skin a small enough distance to allow the next circle to cover at least half the previous area. The right hand moving clockwise will slide downwards from 4 o'clock, while the left hand will glide downwards from 8 o'clock (Fig. 6.4b). Great care must be taken to transmit the required pressure to get the necessary depth through the whole hand and not just the heel of the hand. This is effected by correct foot position

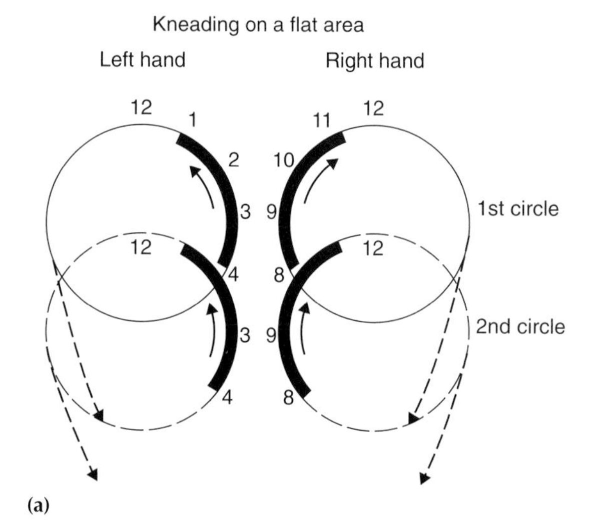

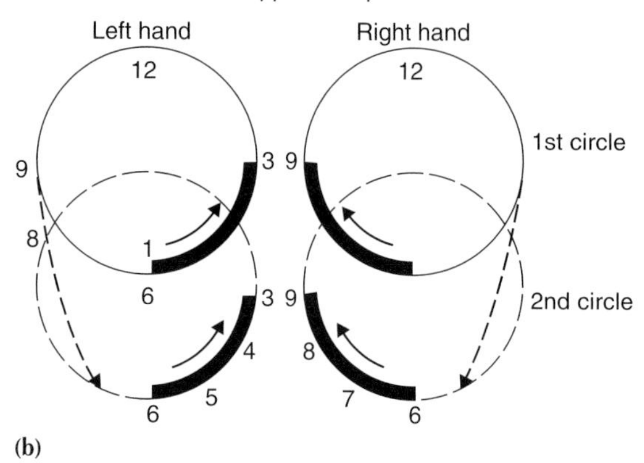

Figure 6.4 Kneading: the right hand works clockwise and the left hand counterclockwise. Pressure is exerted for the shaded part of the circle only: (a) on a flat area (the back); (b) on a round area (the limbs). The hands move on at the down-pointing arrows.

and body position giving a correct relationship to the part under treatment, plus integrated flexion of the hips, shoulders and elbows to transfer and use body weight. In performing all kneading manipulations, stand so that your body weight can move easily from one foot to the other.

Kneading may be performed with:

- The whole hand – whole hand kneading (Fig. 6.5).
- The palm only – palmar kneading (Fig. 6.6).
- The fingers only:
  - flat finger kneading (Fig. 6.7)
  - finger pad kneading (Fig. 6.8)
  - finger tip kneading (Fig. 6.9).
- The thumb:
  - thumb pad kneading (Fig. 6.10)
  - thumb tip kneading (Fig. 6.11).
- Both hands when one is superimposed on the other – superimposed (reinforced) kneading (Fig. 6.12).
- Heel of hand kneading (Fig. 6.13).

In the case of the first four options, the manipulation may be performed:

- Single-handed.
- Double-handed – alternately or simultaneously.

The choice is dictated to some extent by the size of the part under treatment and by the state of the tissues. For example, superimposed kneading has considerable depth and is used on the back and gluteal regions, while thumb and finger tip kneading is used on narrow muscle groups such as the interossei or peronei. However, subjects with very mobile skins may not be suitable for simultaneous double-handed kneading as it is too easy to perform a large range manipulation and cause the subject to slide up and down on the bed. This is especially so when working on the back with the subject in prone lying.

Whole hand kneading

Place your hand obliquely to the long axis of the part and maintain full contact using all of the palmar surface to perform the manipulation (Fig. 6.5).

Palmar kneading

Use only the palm of your hand and allow your fingers and thumb to relax off-contact with the subject. Great depth can be gained using the palm, so take care not to dig in with the bony prominences of the carpus (Fig. 6.6).

Flat finger kneading

This is performed with the palmar surfaces of the second to fifth digits while the palm and thumb

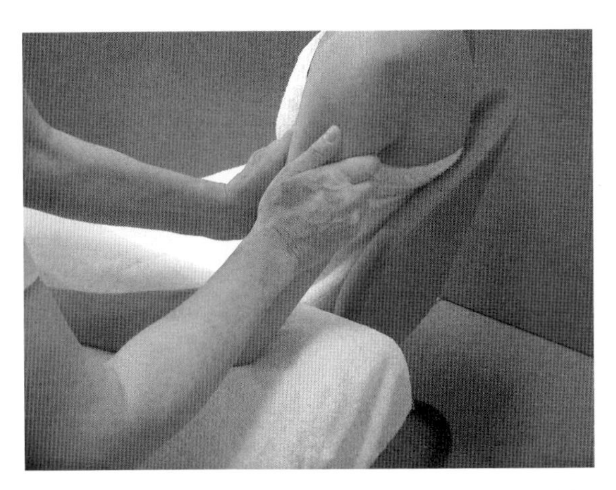

Figure 6.5 Kneading using the whole palmar aspect of the hand.

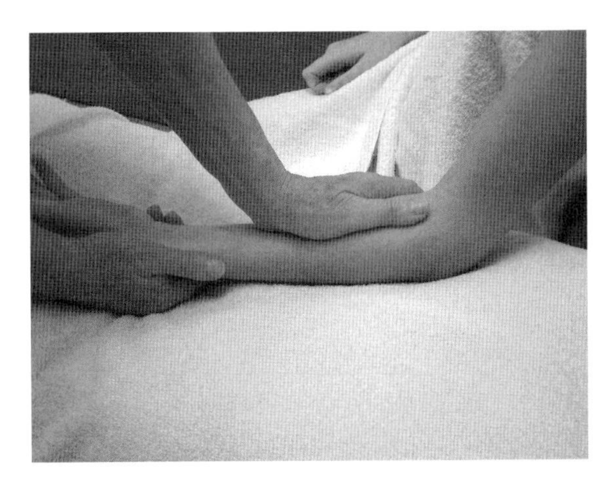

Figure 6.6 Kneading with the palm only – palmar kneading.

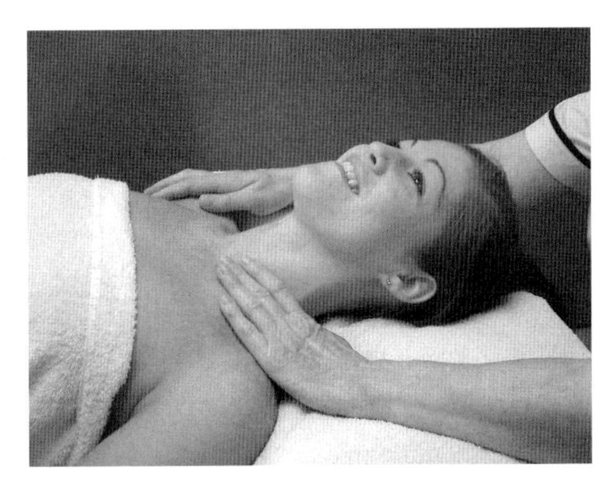

Figure 6.7 Flat finger kneading.

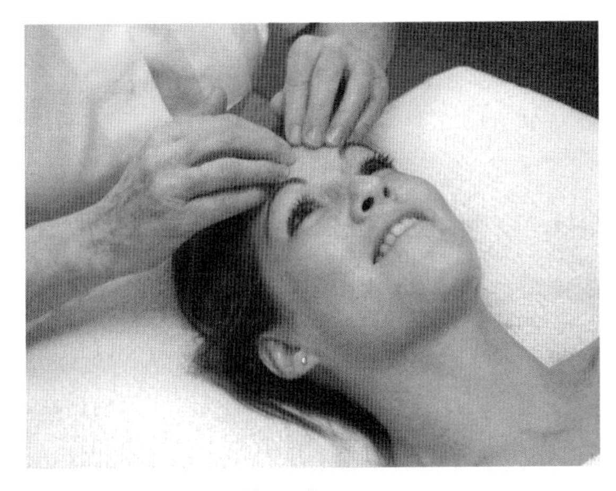

Figure 6.8 Finger pad kneading.

remain off-contact. It is often used to work on less muscular or poorly padded areas (Fig. 6.7).

Finger pad kneading

This is performed with the finger pads either individually, when index or middle fingers are more commonly used, or with several finger pads together to provide a linear contact (Fig. 6.8). The little finger may be too short on most people so the index, middle and ring fingers are bent sufficiently to allow the pads to create a contact line. These manipulations are often used round joints, along the line of ligaments and in treating scars.

Finger tip kneading

This is performed in the same way as finger pad kneading but using only the tip of the pad, taking care to keep your nails off-contact (Fig. 6.9). Narrow, linear areas are dealt with using several finger tips, and one finger tip should be used on small structures or to work on painful areas when the patient will tolerate only very small contact and no movement of the part.

Thumb pad kneading

This is performed with the thumb pads. The size of the area to be treated dictates the amount of the

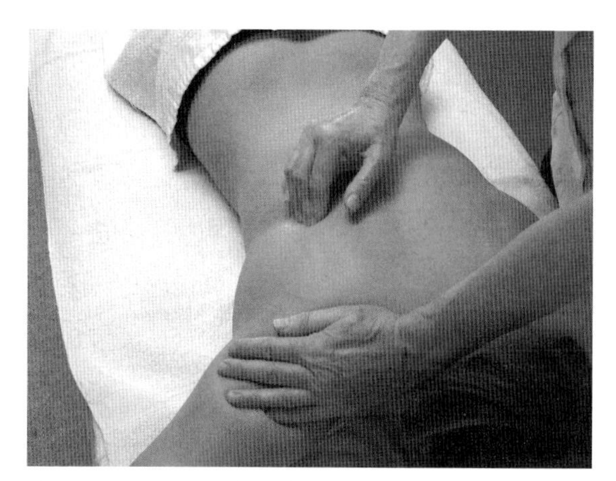

Figure 6.9 Finger tip kneading.

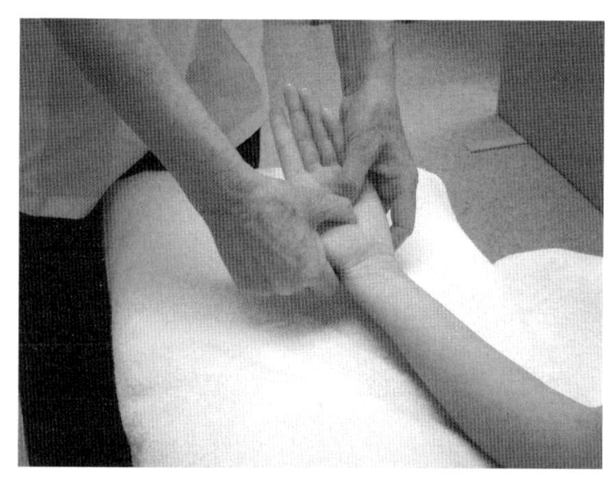

Figure 6.11 Thumb tip kneading.

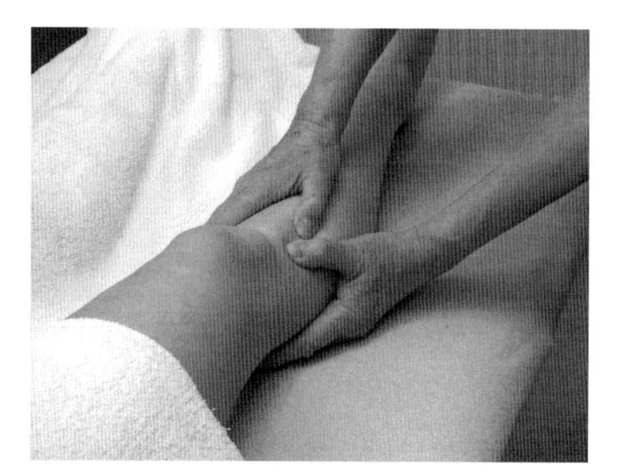

Figure 6.10 Thumb pad kneading.

pad that is in contact with the subject's skin. On larger areas, such as the forearm, back and leg, the whole pad is used (Fig. 6.10). The manipulation is usually performed by resting your fingers on the opposite side of the limbs or more laterally on the back, but when working on the face, or in the presence of any contraindications, the fingers should not rest on the subject. The skin and subcutaneous tissues should be moved on the underlying tissues so as to produce a wrinkle on the outer sides of the working thumb. Mobile, well-padded skin allows a greater range circle to be performed.

Note also the position of the working and resting thumbs. Both lie at an angle to the long axis of the limb, the resting thumb in position ready to start the next circle, while the working thumb maintains the same angle but describes a circle. In other words, the thumb angles to the limb or part only to accommodate the size of the part and the thumb should never slide into adduction.

The working thumb will almost invariably have to pass the resting thumb and should do so by slipping past its tip in contact. If the thumb is lifted to move on, then a 'cat walking' effect is produced, the length of the thumb contact is lost and the pressure of the manipulation will more likely be too deep, uneven and less effective.

Thumb tip kneading

Thumb tip kneading (Fig. 6.11) is performed more frequently with the side of the thumb tip and is useful when the part to be treated has a long, narrow shape, such as the interosseous spaces. Your fingers act as counter supports on the opposite aspect of the part and your thumb should lie in adduction so that your lateral thumb tip is in contact without involving your nail.

Superimposed (reinforced) kneading

This type of kneading can be very deep and is usually performed when greater depth is required. The contact hand is rested fully on the part; the superimposed hand rests on top of it either obliquely across when working on the opposite side of the body (Fig. 6.12) or palm over fingers when working on the adjacent side of the body. The upper hand must not exert such constant pressure that the

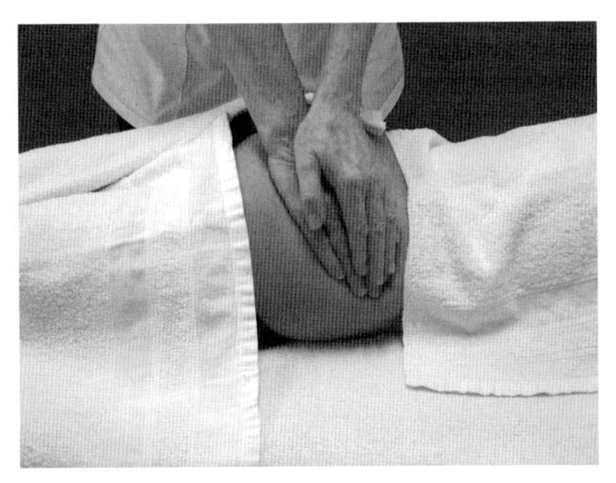

Figure 6.12 Superimposed (reinforced) kneading.

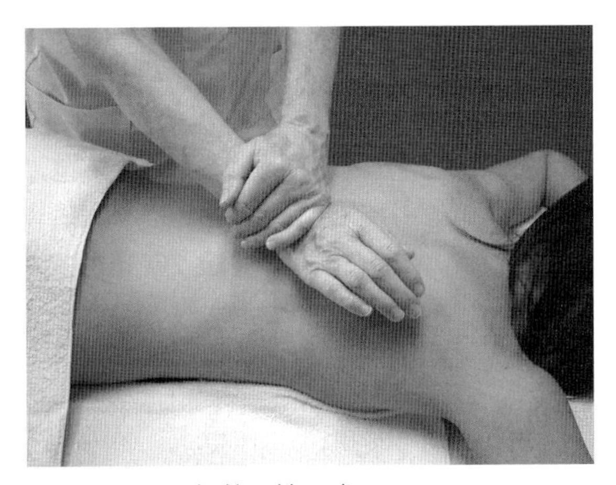

Figure 6.13 Heel of hand kneading.

kneading by the under hand is distorted. Both hands work together. The body movements of the operator are a forward and backward sway from the feet, to enhance depth, but control must be exerted to prevent the circle of the kneading developing a sharp point at the moment of maximum pressure combined with the movement of the hands as they perform the most distant part of the circle.

Heel of hand kneading (for greater depth)

The whole heel of the hand is used in heel of hand kneading, being careful not to dig in. This means thin hands may perform painfully. The remainder of the palm and fingers are held off-contact and a small circular manipulation is performed. Greater depth can be achieved by reinforcing with the palm of the other hand on top of the working palm or by holding the wrist with the other hand, as in Fig. 6.13. This manipulation can be used as an alternative to deep finger and thumb kneading on any well-padded area. It is thus useful on muscle bellies but not on tendinous areas where the heel of the hand will 'bounce' across the tendons.

Picking up

Picking up is a manipulation in which the tissues are compressed against underlying bone, then lifted, squeezed and released. The manipulation is often performed single handed with the thumb and thenar

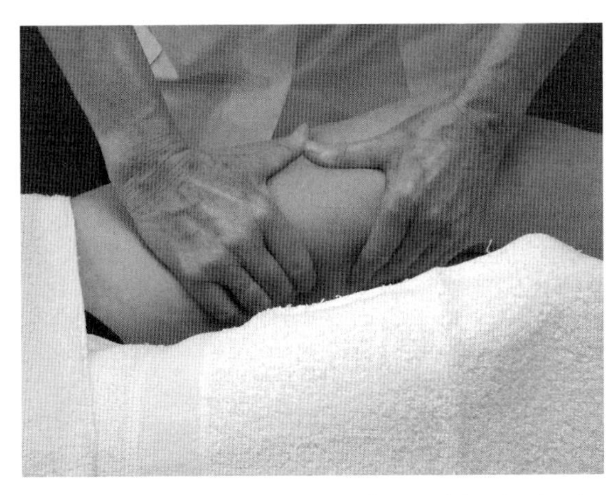

Figure 6.14 Picking up: the 'C' shape of the hand. Also shows double-handed, alternate work.

eminence as one component and the medial two or three fingers and hypothenar eminence as the other component of the grasp. The thumb must be opposed and abducted and the degree of these two movements will produce:

- *Either* a 'C'-shaped grasp (Fig. 6.14) which is wider on larger areas
- *Or* a 'V'-shaped grasp (Fig. 6.15) which is narrower on areas of lesser bulk.

The cleft between the thumb and index finger should always be in contact with the subject's skin, otherwise a pinching effect is produced and depth is lost. As body weight transfer is important, walk standing is the stance required.

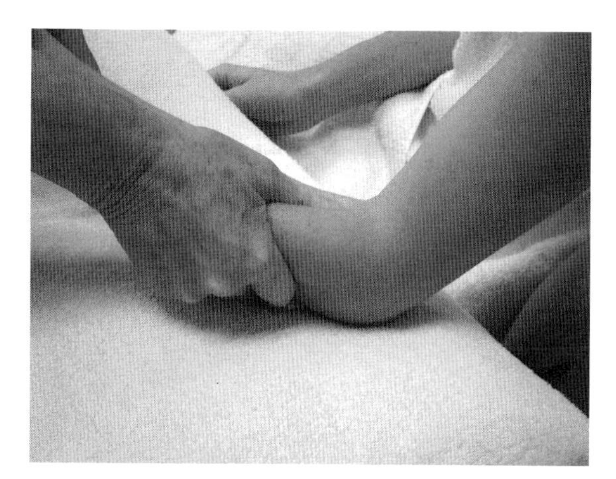

Figure 6.15 Picking up: the 'V' shape of the hand (practise on your own forearm).

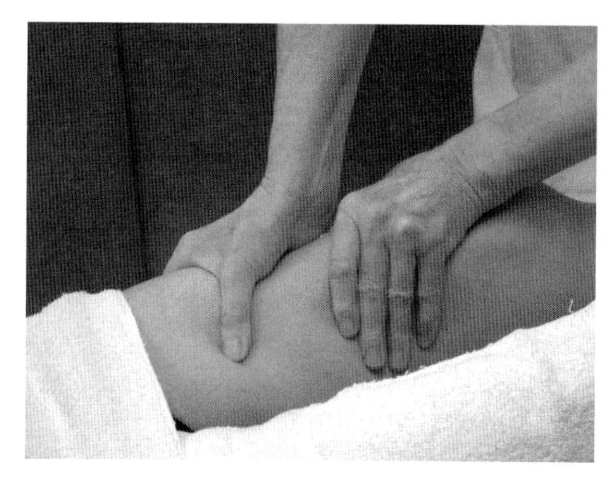

Figure 6.16 Picking up: double-handed simultaneous work.

Picking up should be performed with your arms held in slight abduction and with semiflexed elbows. The wrists are always used initially extended and are more extended as the grasp is effected. Your wrists should never be flexed as this will cause you to pivot on your thumb and finger tips with a screwing action.

Place your hand on the part so that the thumb cleft lies across the centre line of the muscle bulk, with your thumb and thenar eminence disposed on one side and your medial two or three fingers and hypothenar eminence on the other side. Exert compression by transferring your body weight from your feet through your forearm to the whole hand.

Count this as *one*. Then immediately grasp, using the two grasp components equally so that your wrist extends more, but do not further flex any part of your thumb and fingers. This exerts a squeeze, and a simultaneous lift of the tissues will occur. Count this as *two*. Release your grasp – count this as *three*. Your body weight should still be forward, but as you move your relaxed hand on to the next part, maintaining the current conformation, take your body weight back again to your starting position. Count this as *four*. Thus the body weight movement is:

- Forward on count *one*
- Backward on count *four*

while the hand:

- Compresses on *one*
- Grasps on *two* (lift occurs)
- Releases on *three*
- Moves on *four*.

Learning this combination of movements is one of the more difficult tasks in massage training. Practise first with each hand working backward, down the length of a muscle (Fig. 6.15) or up the length of a muscle. Then try travelling in the reverse direction on the longer muscle masses, as in the lower limb, leading up to working one hand travelling backwards as the other hand travels forwards at such a distance that your fingers and thumbs never touch but the muscle is constantly lifted (Fig. 6.14).

Alternatively, on larger muscle masses, such as the anterior aspect of the thigh, your two hands may work as one unit spanning the muscle. Your hands lie so that the thumb of the first hand lies parallel to the index finger of the second hand. The thumb of this second hand lies under the heel and alongside the hypothenar eminence of the first hand (Fig. 6.16). The compression is performed by both hands. The grasp is performed by radial extension of both wrists so that the tissues are lifted and squeezed between the medial part of the palms and medial three fingers of both hands. The tissues are released, and your hands move backwards as one unit for one-third of their length on to a new area.

Wringing

Wringing is a manipulation in which the tissues are compressed against the underlying structures prior

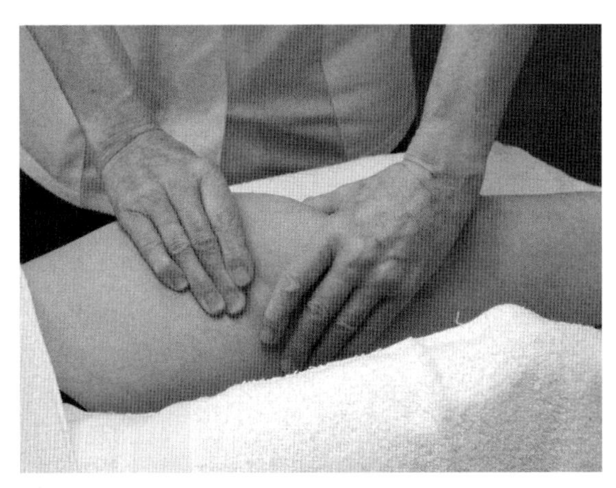

(a)

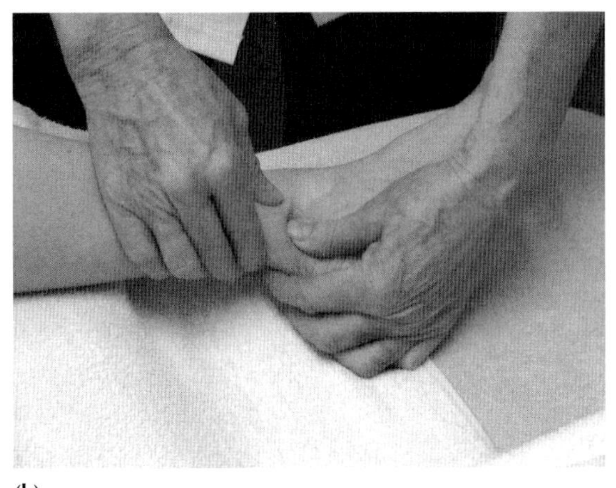

(b)

Figure 6.17 Wringing: (a) on a muscle belly; (b) on the tendocalcaneus.

to lifting them, as in picking up. Then, instead of squeezing the tissues, you pull gently towards yourself with the fingers of one hand while the thumb of your other hand pushes gently in the opposite direction. The tissues are kept elevated and passed from hand to hand by moving the non-pressing component of each hand in turn along the tissues (Fig. 6.17a).

The smaller the tissue, the more the tips of your thumbs and fingers are used, and your arms are more adducted and wrists lifted to be more alongside one another. If your arms are abducted and your wrists and forearms lie more parallel with the long axis of the tissues, then the bigger manipulation can be performed.

When the tissue is very small, as in the case of the tendocalcaneus, the manipulation is performed between your thumbs and finger tips as in Fig. 6.17b.

Rolling

The most common rolling manipulation is skin rolling, but muscles may also be rolled.

Skin rolling

Skin rolling is a manipulation in which the skin is lifted and rolled between the thumbs and fingers of the two hands. The manipulation is most often performed on the back, abdomen and thighs, but it is also used round superficial joints such as the knee, and in modified form on scar tissue which is shortening and thickening.

Stand in adapted walk standing at the side of the area to be treated and facing across it. Place both hands on the surface of the area more distal from you so that your palms are fully in contact, with your thumb tips touching and parallel to the long axis of the part. Your thumbs should be abducted to such an extent that your index fingers do not touch and indeed should have a space between them (Fig. 6.18). Maintain full palmar contact and pull your hands backwards towards yourself, without changing their shape and with sufficient pressure to pull the underlying skin. Next, apply pressure with your thumbs as you adduct and oppose them with some depth so that they remain in line with each other but the skin is pushed in a roll towards the fingers (Fig. 6.19). Almost simultaneously, your palms should gradually lift off the skin but your finger tips should remain in contact. Now roll your thumbs forwards still maintaining the roll of skin in your grasp and the skin will roll against your fingers. As this occurs, the skin is folded over on top of your fingers (Fig. 6.20).

Try not to 'creep' your fingers as you roll as this can tickle. On adherent skins the skin will only lift slightly and the length of the rolling action must be shortened. The model shown in Figs 6.18–6.20 had very mobile skin and half the width of the back could be treated at once. For adherent skin two or three lines of work should be done instead of the one line shown in Figs 6.18–6.20.

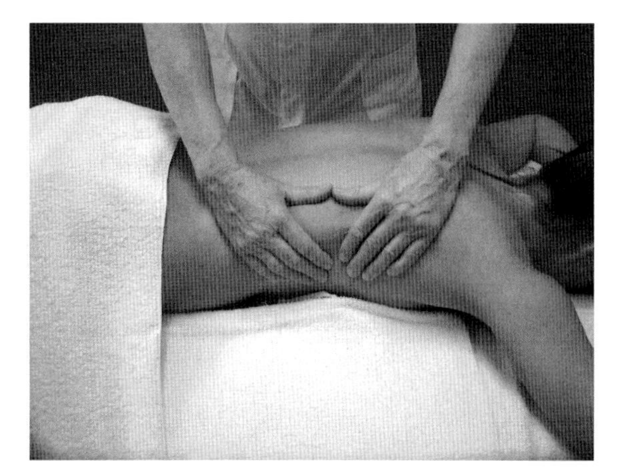

Figure 6.18 Skin rolling – start.

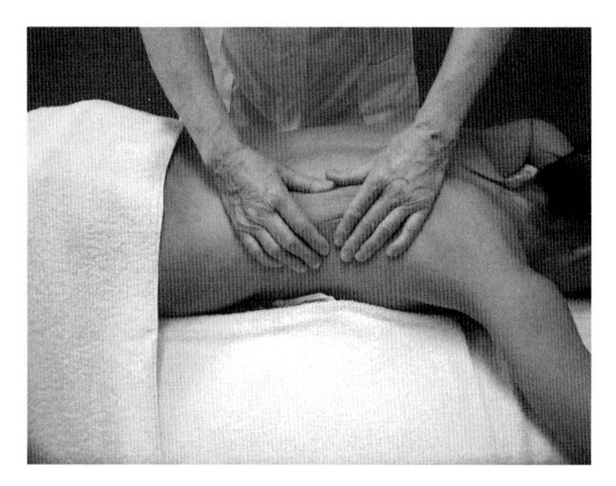

Figure 6.19 Skin rolling – squeeze and lift.

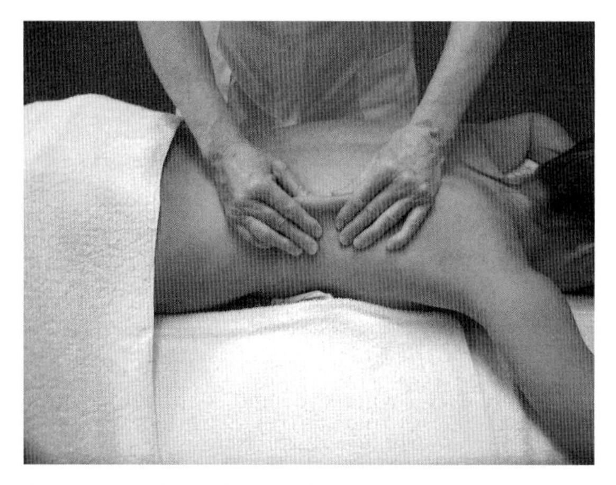

Figure 6.20 Skin rolling – roll.

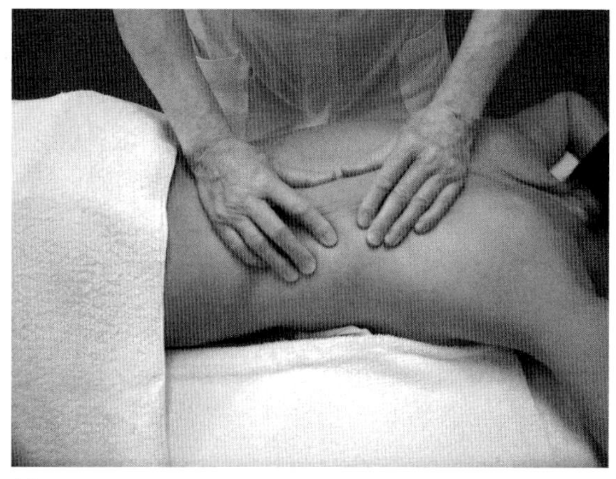

(a)

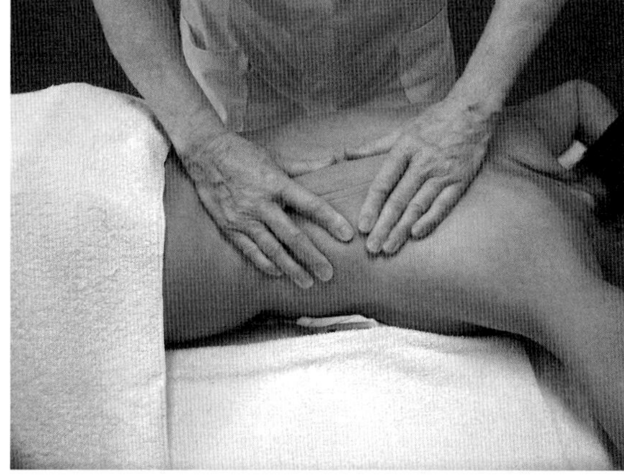

(b)

Figure 6.21 Muscle rolling: (a) push with the flat thumbs; (b) pull back with the finger tips.

Muscle rolling

Muscle rolling is performed by working across the muscle fibres and along the long axis of muscles. You should be in adapted walk standing to allow weight transference. The lateral boundaries of the muscle should be palpated, then your thumbs placed tip to tip along one border with your fingers along the opposite border. Apply a little pressure with both components so that the muscle bulges slightly between your thumbs and fingers. Then push first with your thumbs and release the pressure simultaneously with the fingers which move to an adjacent area (Fig. 6.21a). Rapidly reverse, pressing with the fingers and releasing the pressure of your thumbs which also move to an adjacent area (Fig.

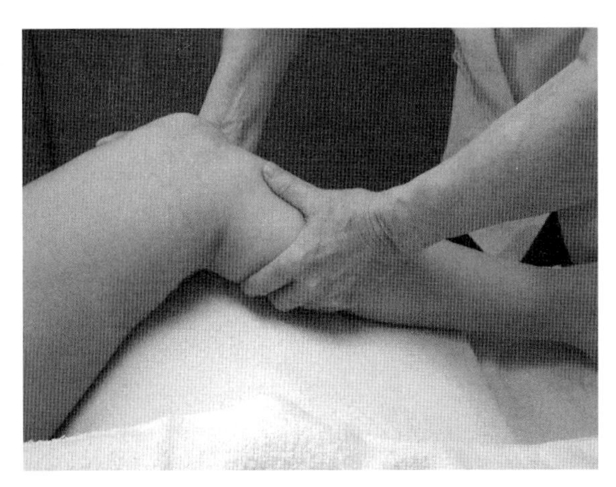

Figure 6.22 Muscle shaking on the calf muscles.

6.21b). It is often a more effective and comfortable manipulation if the pressure is slightly down into the muscle mass rather than back and forth across it. This manipulation can be performed slowly and deliberately to exert a slight stretch, or faster so that there is stimulation to the circulation.

Muscle shaking

All long muscle bellies may be shaken and the manipulation may be performed on the larger muscles such as biceps, triceps, quadriceps and gastrocnemius and also on the small muscles of the thenar and hypothenar eminences.

The manipulation is one in which:

- **For longer muscles** the length of your thumb should be placed on one side of the muscle belly and all your fingers placed on the other side of the muscle belly. Your palm should be slightly off contact (Fig. 6.22). Your hand is then rapidly shaken from side to side as you traverse the length of the muscle belly avoiding contact with the underlying bone. Stand in lunge standing so that your weight is transferred as you work from proximal to distal on the muscle belly. The muscle will be 'thrown' rapidly from side to side and feels very invigorated.
- **For very small muscles** the tip of your thumb should be placed on one side and an appropriate number of finger tips placed on the other side of the muscle belly, and the shaking movement described above is performed.

Frictions

Aims:

- Stimulate local circulation (erythema).
- Mobilise underlying tissues.

Frictions are small range, deep manipulations performed on specific anatomical structures with the tips of the fingers or thumbs. No other part of the practitioner's hand must rest on the part. There are two types of frictions:

- Circular
- Transverse

Circular frictions

Circular frictions are performed with the finger tips. The structure to be treated should be identified by careful palpation and the finger tip(s) placed so that they cover the area. The rest of the hand is kept off-contact. Pressure is applied and a small, stationary manipulation is performed, in a circular manner and at gradually increasing depth for three or four circles. The pressure is released and the manipulation is repeated. One hand may reinforce the other on deeper structures. The manipulation can be over ligaments and myofascial junctions (Fig. 6.23).

Transverse frictions

Transverse frictions were advocated by Dr J. Cyriax in 1941 for treatment of tendons, ligaments, myofascial junctions and muscles. The manipulation is performed with:

- *Either* the thumb tip
- *Or* the finger tip of the index finger
- *Or* the middle finger reinforced by placing the index finger on top of the middle finger nail (more useful when the hand is curved round a limb) (Fig. 6.24)
- *Or* by two finger tips when a long structure is affected (such as a tendon)

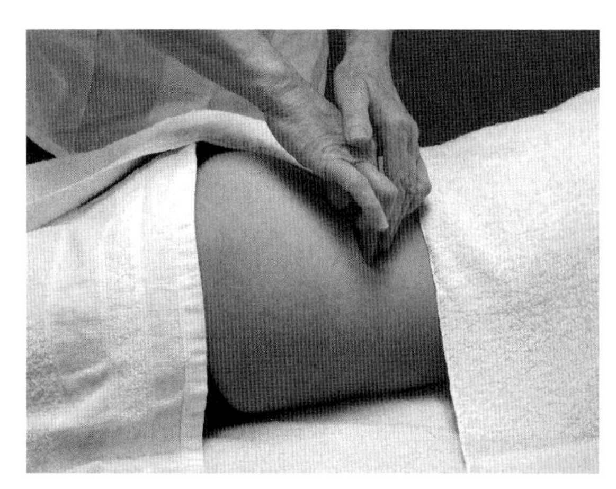

Figure 6.23 Circular frictions to the attachments on the iliac crest.

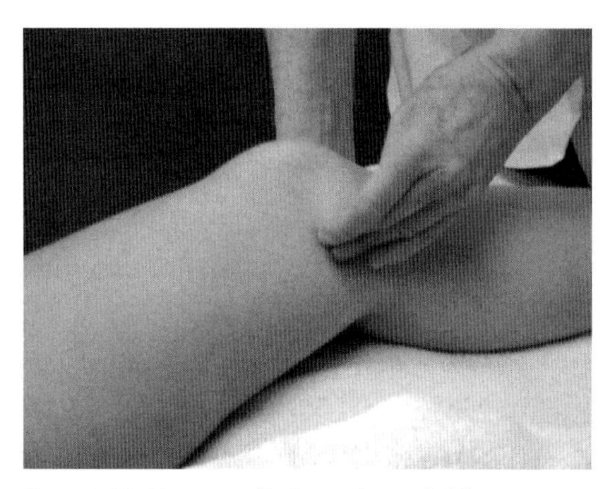

Figure 6.24 Transverse friction to the medial ligament.

- *Or* by the opposed fingers and thumb on structures that can be grasped, e.g. tendocalcaneus.

Identify the structure to be treated and place your fingers across the longitudinal axis of the structure, i.e. across the length of the collagen fibres (Figs 6.24 and 6.25).

Now perform the friction by moving your digit and the client's skin as one, keeping your digit, hand and forearm in a line parallel to the movement to be performed. Do not flex and extend only your digit or wrist. Learn to use both hands so that you lessen your own fatigue. Try to use a movement from your upper arm, trunk or feet so that you

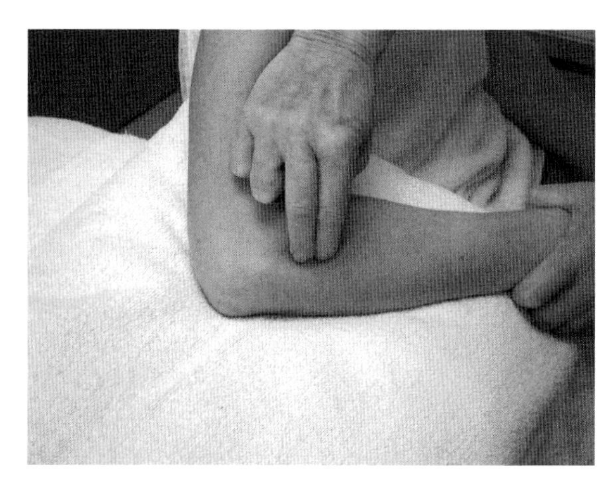

Figure 6.25 Transverse friction to the common extensor tendon.

achieve greater power with less fatigue. Either sit down or stand in walk standing.

Start to move your fingers forwards and backwards across the structure under treatment with sufficient sweep to produce separation of the fibres at a depth to engage the affected tissue rather than at the patient's tolerance. He or she should be warned that the treatment may be painful, but that numbness may supervene as it progresses. The movement must not take place between your fingers and the patient's skin, but between the affected structure and the overlying tissues.

The patient's skin must be dry with no lubricants to ensure your fingers do not slip. If necessary, apply either spirit or a wisp of cotton wool to the part. The wool is kept in position during the treatment.

Keep tendons taut by putting them on the stretch, but keep muscles relaxed by positioning the model so that the part and the attachments of the muscle are approximated during treatment.

Tapôtement (percussion)

Aims:

- Stimulate local circulation.
- Stimulate muscle tone and tendon reflexes.
- Stimulate nerve endings.
- Assist in peristalsis via vibrations.
- Help evacuation of hollow organs.

Stand in adapted walk standing for transverse manipulations. The percussive manipulations are those in 'which the treated part is struck soft blows with the hands'. They are performed either to assist evacuation from hollow organs or to stimulate either skin or muscle reflexes. The manipulations are:

- Hacking
- Clapping
- Vibrations
- Beating
- Pounding
- Tapping

Hacking

Hacking (Fig. 6.26) is a manipulation in which the skin is struck using the back of the tips of the three medial fingers. A correct performance is dependent on:

- The initial posture of the whole of the practitioner's arms and hands with good wrist extension.
- A good range of pronation and supination of the radio-ulnar joints.

The only movement required is that of pronation and supination. The elbows *must not* flex and extend. The hands are held at a small distance apart so that as they rotate alternately, they just clear one another. The arms are in slight abduction, and the elbows are flexed to a right angle with the forearms held far enough above the patient's skin to allow only the backs of the little, ring and middle fingers to touch when the forearm is in supination. The wrists are well extended to about 50° (Fig. 6.26). Note: this manipulation cannot be performed properly with less than 50° extension of the wrists. The fingers are in relaxed flexion, i.e. the posture the relaxed hand adopts spontaneously, and are separated.

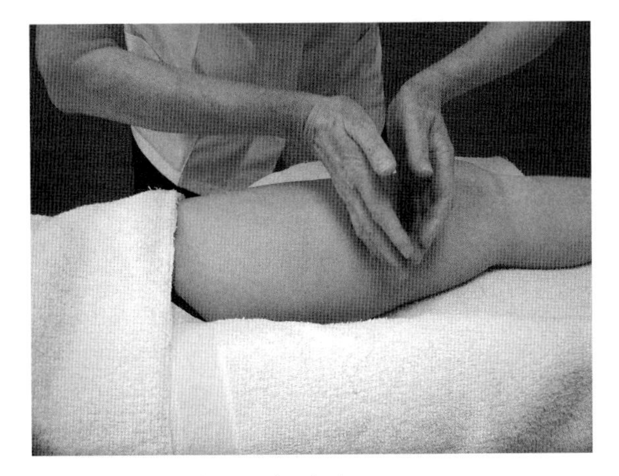

Figure 6.26 Hacking to the thigh.

Experiment by resting the finger tips of your hands on each other with your little finger resting on the patient's skin. Then slightly separate the finger tips – less than 1.5 cm – and check to see if pronation and supination are alternately possible without your finger tips touching those of the other hand.

The 'strike' is modified by the vigour applied to the rotatory movement. A very light hacking produces a susurration, whereas vigorous hacking should sound like a sharp striking noise. Initially, try a slow rate of 10 strikes per 5 seconds with each hand, then work up to a fast rate of 20–30 strikes per 5 seconds with each hand. Single strikes can achieve great depth and can be used to obtain reflex contractions of muscle. Slow, deep hacking may produce mechanical effects on hollow organs. All hacking, but especially fast work, produces effects on the skin circulation, and appropriate subjects demonstrate this by producing distinct erythema (reddening) of the skin at the points of strike.

Clapping

Clapping (Fig. 6.27) is a manipulation in which the whole palmar aspect of the hand is used to strike the body part. The hand is, however, cupped in such a manner that the centre of the hand does not touch the part, but is hollowed. The fingers are slightly flexed, more so at the metacarpophalangeal joints of the index, middle and ring fingers. The thumb is adducted so that it lies just under the index finger and adjacent palm. The hand must be kept in this posture but as relaxed as possible. The wrists should be used to create the difference between striking a hollow sounding blow and a slightly sharper blow. (Slapping sounds very sharp.) The former will have the depth to cause 'jarring' and is used to evacuate hollow organs. The latter is for skin stimulation.

The difference is brought about by the arm movements performed and the effects they have on the hands. The percussive effect is achieved when the

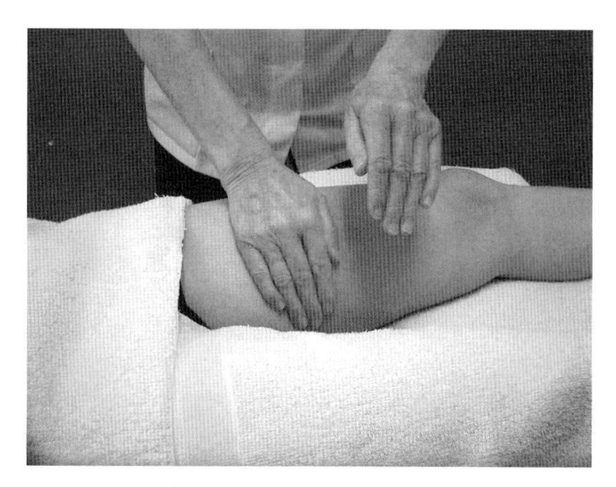

Figure 6.27 Clapping to the thigh.

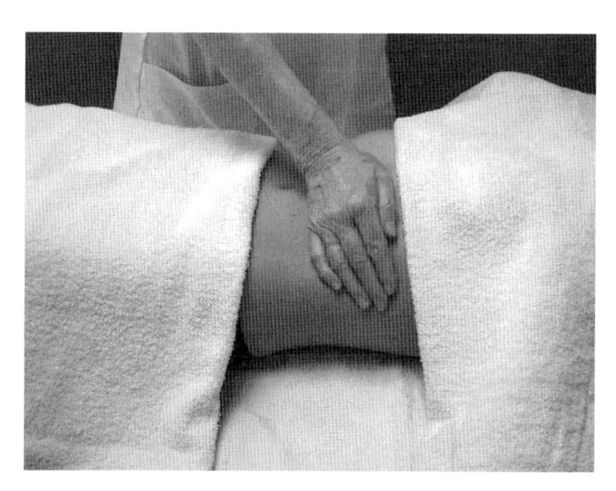

Figure 6.28 Practising vibrations on the abdomen.

heel of the hand is lifted from the part more than the finger tips. The wrist is extended, then flexed (Fig. 6.27). This movement is brought about by lifting the arm into abduction and allowing it to drop. The velocity of the drop (not the height) creates the depth of the work. This deeper manipulation can be performed with the skin lightly covered by a sheet, thin blanket or a single layer of the patient's clothing.

The more stimulating manipulation is also brought about by arm abduction, but with the finger tips raised from the body part without increasing the wrist flexion. In other words, the whole hand is raised. The 'strike' is brought about by actively lowering the arm. The tempo of the action should be slower to obtain greater depth, and faster for skin stimulation.

Vibrations

Vibrations are often wrongly called shakings. The difference is that a vibration involves a movement in which the tissues are pressed and released using an up and down motion (Fig. 6.28). In shaking, the movement on the model is sideways and involves rapid radial and ulnar deviation of your wrists.

Vibrations may be fine or very coarse. Vibrations may be performed with the whole hand or the finger tips. Practise with your hand stationary or slide it backwards and forwards on the area. Vibrations are best practised by placing the whole hand with the arm outstretched and oscillating the whole hand into rapid and minute wrist flexion and extension. The movement is sustained from the shoulder and can be observed to occur spontaneously in some people if the arms are outstretched.

Beating

Beating is a much less used manipulation in which the loosely clenched fist is used for the 'strike'. Its value lies in that the hand is made smaller, but is used as in clapping.

The fingers are flexed at the metacarpophalangeal and proximal interphalangeal joints, but extended at the distal interphalangeal joints so that there is a flat surface composed of the backs of the two distal phalanges and the margin of the palmar surface of the palm. The thumb is kept flat against the lateral part of the flexed hand. The most important part of the practitioner's action is to raise the whole arm into abduction and allow the wrist to droop (Fig. 6.29) in relaxation. The arm is allowed to drop and strike the part. The speed to attain is six strikes per 10 seconds.

Pounding

Pounding is a less used manipulation but also has value in that it is a form of hacking done with a loosely clenched fist.

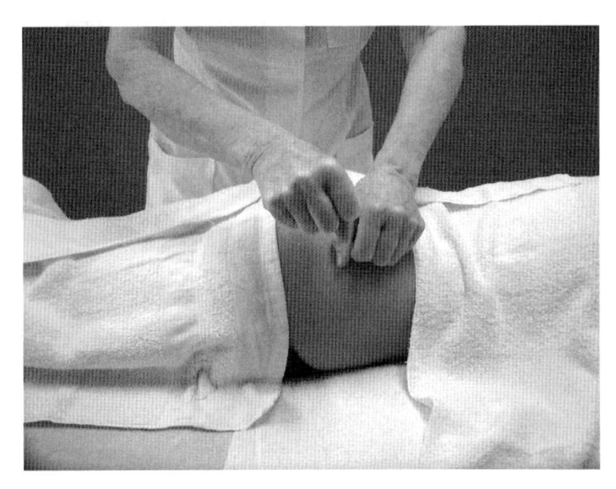

Figure 6.29 Beating.

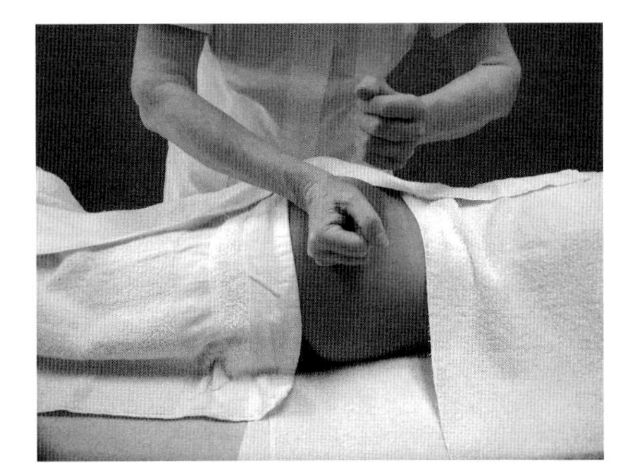

Figure 6.30 Pounding.

The fingers are loosely flexed at all the joints and the thumb lies flat on the lateral side of the hand halfway between adduction and flexion. The action is exactly that of hacking, i.e. pronation and supination of the semi-flexed forearms so that the 'strike' is with the knuckles of the little finger (Fig. 6.30). The rate of 'strike' is slightly slower than in hacking.

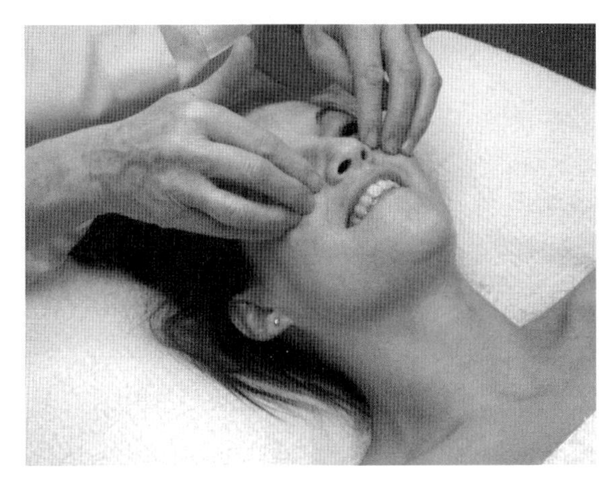

Figure 6.31 Tapping on the face.

Tapping

Tapping is performed with the tips of the finger pads and is used on very small areas such as the face (Fig. 6.31). The hand is held relaxed over the area to be treated and the fingers tap at a depth to produce a slightly hollow sound. The index, middle and ring fingers may be used together or in any smaller number, or these three fingers may be used singly in sequence. Both forms of tapping are seen in restless or irritated people who tap chair arms.

7 Massage to the upper limb

Margaret Hollis and Elisabeth Jones

The whole upper limb is usually treated as one unit. It is so much smaller than the lower limb that it is possible to work all the way down the limb performing the same manipulation in sequence.

Preparation of the patient

Ask the patient to remove all clothing from the appropriate arm and shoulder. Shoulder straps should also be slipped off for women.

For a treatment in sitting position

Offer the patient a towel to put over the other shoulder and wrap it obliquely across both aspects of the trunk to cross under the axilla of the arm to be massaged. The two ends can often be tucked in to secure the towel. Check that the towel does not hang on the floor as the patient sits down. Provide a 76-cm (30-in) or higher table with a top about the size of a standard pillow. Place a pillow on the table and cover with a towel. Place the patient's arm on the pillow so that it rests in a comfortable degree of shoulder abduction and elbow flexion (Fig. 7.1a).

For a treatment in lying position

Prepare a couch as for treatment of the lower limb, and ask the patient to lie supine using only two head pillows. Place a pillow alongside the trunk so that the arm can rest on it in a degree of slight abduction and flexion of the shoulder. Ensure the pronated hand is fully supported on the pillow; if not, pull the pillow down slightly, leaving the shoulder area unsupported.

You should stand in adapted lunge standing just beyond the patient's finger tips with your outer leg forward.

To elevate the arm

Position the patient in supine lying as for an arm treatment, but use additional pillows to ensure that each more distal joint is higher than its proximal neighbour, i.e. the elbow is higher than the shoulder, the wrist is higher than the elbow.

It may be necessary either to lower an adjustable couch or for you to stand on a platform in order to reach. In the absence of either facility it is possible to work backwards, but do remember to keep looking round at the patient's face.

Before starting work, uncover the whole limb in order to examine it. Follow the procedure described

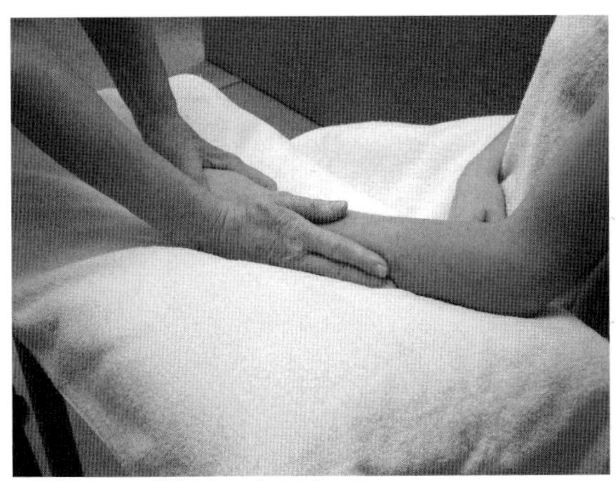

(a)

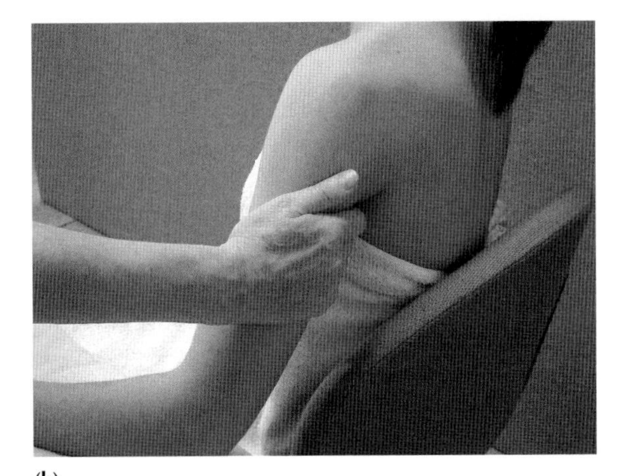

(b)

Figure 7.1 Effleurage – first stroke with the outer hand: (a) on the ulnar aspect of the forearm; (b) at the axilla.

earlier, and especially check by observation the state of the skin for abrasions and dryness, and the posture of the joints, which may need extra support. Then palpate by running your hand down the length of each aspect of the limb and note temperature, tenderness and muscle tone. Ensure only light pressure over bony prominences.

Effleurage

To the whole limb

Effleurage to the upper limb is usually performed with one hand at a time while the other hand controls both the stability of the limb and the position of the hand. The grasp on the hand should be with your own palm cupped so you obtain a contact with only your own palmar margins, so that a 'sticky' grasp does not arise.

Extensor aspect

Grasp the pronated hand as in Fig. 7.1(a) with your hand nearest to the patient. The working hand – the furthest from the patient – is inserted under the little finger and proceeds up the extensor aspect of the forearm to the axilla (Fig. 7.1b). The second stroke starts on the back of the fingers, and goes up the back of the forearm and the posterior surface of the arm to the axilla. Turn the forearm to mid-pronation and start the third stroke on the thumb; continue up the radial border of the forearm and the lateral surface of the arm to the axilla.

Flexor aspect

As your working hand returns, grasp the patient's hand and maintain the mid-pronation. Your former grasping hand works from the thumb (Fig. 7.2a), over the flexor surface of the forearm and the flexor surface of the arm to the axilla (Fig. 7.2b). Turn the palm into more supination and take the fifth stroke from the palmar aspect of the fingers over the front of the forearm and the anterior surface of the arm to the axilla. The sixth stroke goes from under the little finger, up the ulnar border of the forearm and the medial surface of the arm to the axilla.

Every stroke starts with your fingers in most contact and leading the way until you reach the wrist, when your working hand, now in full contact, should lie obliquely on the limb.

At the axilla your hand should proceed with increased depth into the area of the space by at least the length of your working fingers and pause momentarily there.

In effect these strokes have great overlap on one another, but do create a feeling of thorough cover of the part.

Part strokes

The **shoulder** is effleuraged by crossing your hands to rest one each side of the shoulder. As the strokes

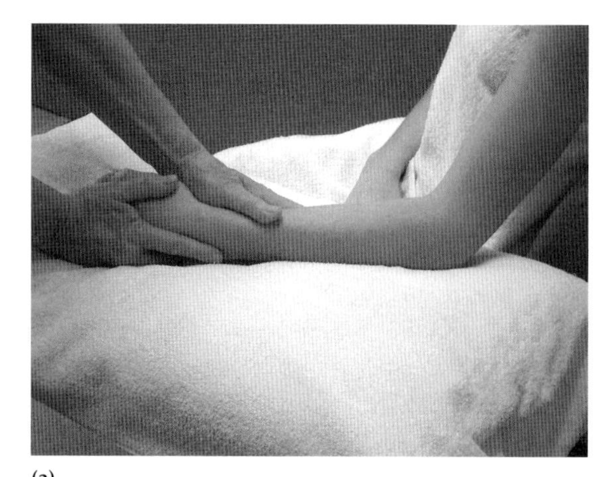

(a)

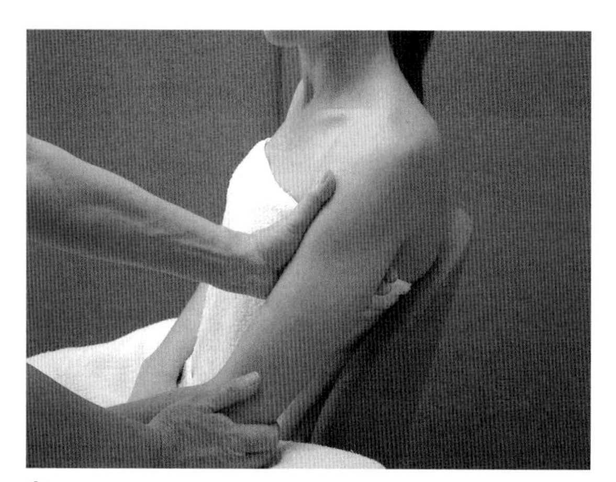

(b)

Figure 7.2 Effleurage with the inner hands: (a) on the wrist; (b) at the axilla.

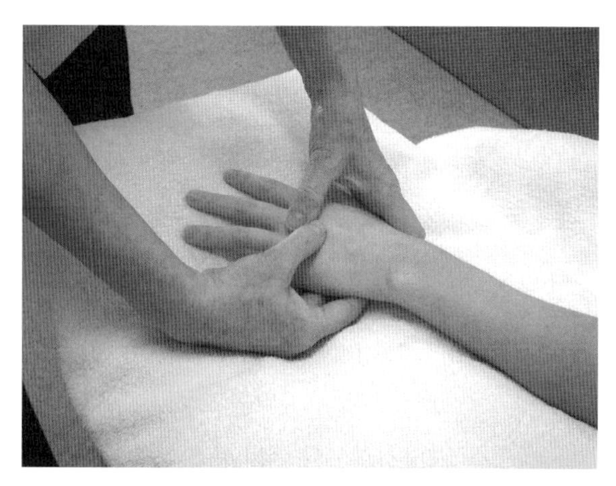

Figure 7.3 Stroking the interosseous spaces. The same hand position is used for kneading the spaces.

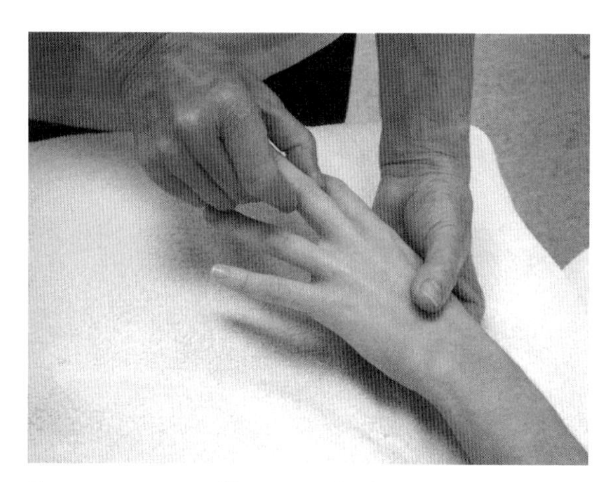

Figure 7.4 Finger effleurage to the digits.

are made, the hands are uncrossed and turned to allow the deltoid to be effleuraged as the fingers enter the axilla.

The **arm** may be effleuraged on its own, starting at the elbow and finishing at the axilla using the pattern of full length strokes described earlier.

The **forearm** may be effleuraged either from the wrist or using the finger tips, to the anterior aspect of the elbow where some glands lie. Use the appropriate parts of the full length strokes described earlier.

The **hand** may be effleuraged using the whole of your hand or individual structures may be treated by using your thumb or finger tips.

The **interosseous spaces** of the dorsum may be effleuraged using your thumbs in alternate spaces and working simultaneously (Fig. 7.3). The palm may be effleuraged using your thumbs or one or more fingers. By selecting anatomical features, such as abductor pollicis brevis and abductor digiti minimi to be treated simultaneously, your two thumbs can work together. The two flexors and then the two opponens muscles can also be treated by your two thumbs, whereas three fingers will cover a less defined field.

The **digits** can be effleuraged in pairs – two with four, and three with five. The thumb can be effleuraged on its own. Balance the tip of each finger on your own middle phalanx and perform a stroke up one side with your index finger (Fig. 7.4) and up the other side with your thumb. This trick keeps the finger under treatment straight. If the fingers are a problem for this method, then grasp the tip gently with one of your index fingers and thumb and stroke up each side with the index finger and/or thumb of your other hand. It is more usual to stroke the sides of digits as the greatest drainage occurs there.

Kneading

All the kneading manipulations described are performed using the circling technique shown in Fig. 6.4b. Always be aware that the size of the circle must be related to the size of the area under treatment. Ensure you are working on muscle or soft tissue and avoid deep, moving pressure over bony ridges and prominences. The pressure on all the manipulations should be inwards towards the centre of the arm and with upward pressure so that you can envisage assisting venous blood and lymph flow from distal to proximal.

Double-handed alternate kneading

Double-handed alternate kneading of the upper limb is usually performed straight down the length of the limb, from the shoulder to the finger tips, rather than sectionally as for the longer and more muscular lower limb. In consequence, the sequence of work involves careful manoeuvring of your hands so as to turn the 'corners' and to maintain full hand contact. Thus the hands start cupped over the shoulder and deltoid, encircle the upper arm to work on triceps and biceps, and turn at the elbow to lie obliquely on the flexor and extensor aspects of the forearm and hand.

Start by reaching high with your arms and your shoulder girdle so that your hands can rest over the shoulder joint, with your finger tips touching on top (Fig. 7.5). Your elbows should be bent. Knead with alternate hand circles and inward pressure, slowly pivoting on your finger tips so that the heels of your hands move to rest over the mid-line of the deltoid – about six to eight circles with each hand.

Next, work down on the deltoid in very small stages, keeping your hands parallel and your thumbs touching, until your fingers can slip into the axilla. Your hands should now rest with the mid-line of each hand on the vertical mid-line of the bellies of the triceps and biceps. Your fingers may overlap over the medial border of the humerus (Fig. 7.6).

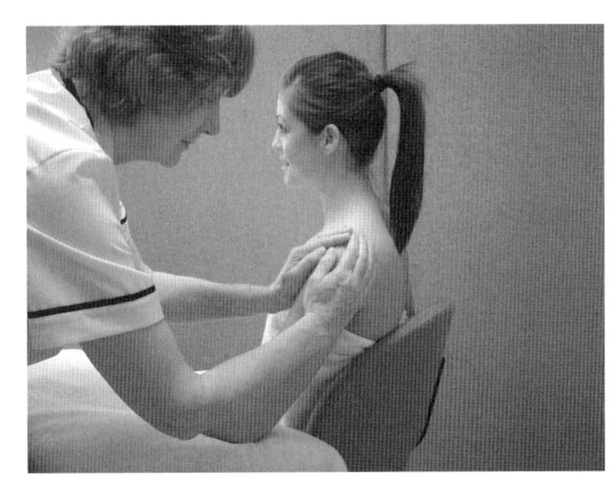

Figure 7.5 Kneading the deltoid.

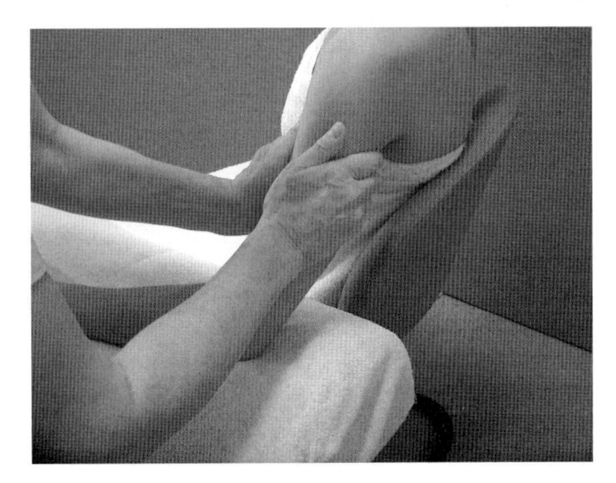

Figure 7.6 Kneading the biceps and triceps.

The kneading should now be less of a compressive manipulation, and have an element of squeeze with each hand, but, as you must keep your thumbs lying vertically and close together on each side of the lateral border of the humerus, the squeeze is effected by the thumb and thenar eminence on one side and the palm and fingers on the other side of each muscle.

Proceed down the upper arm, manoeuvring your hands gradually in the lower third so that the hand on the triceps comes more to the front of the elbow,

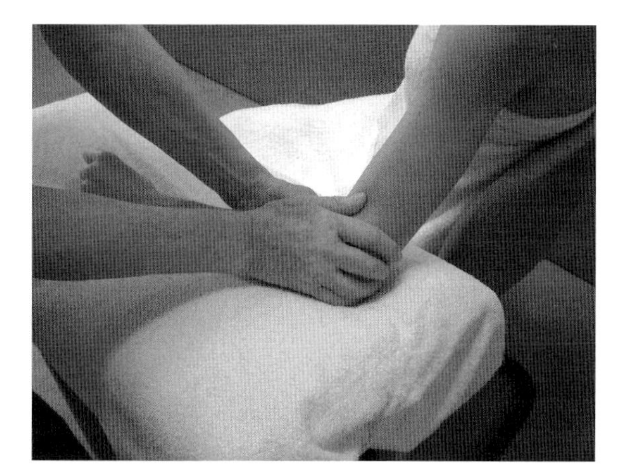

Figure 7.7 Kneading – turning the elbow.

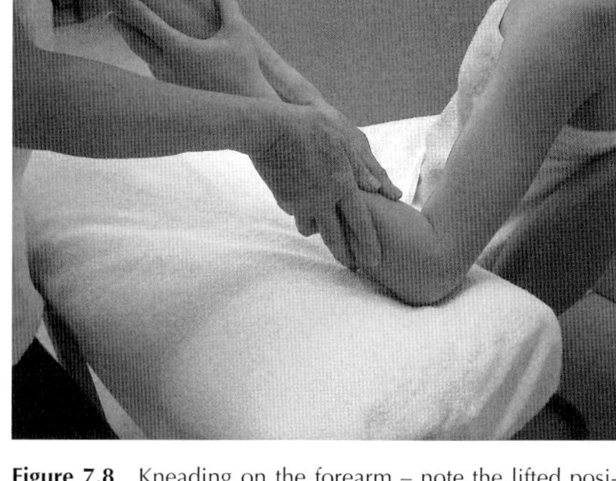

Figure 7.8 Kneading on the forearm – note the lifted position to facilitate the manipulation and the practitioner's hands both in contact yet in different dispositions.

and that on the biceps lies more to the back of the elbow (Fig. 7.7). Let your front hand perform stationary work, while your rear hand works and slides gradually under the medial side of the elbow and on to the flexor aspect of the forearm, followed by the other hand on to the extensor aspect of the forearm.

The kneading on the forearm is done by letting your inner hand on the flexors lie across the limb and the outer hand on the extensors. The latter should lie obliquely but with a more vertical alignment (Fig. 7.8). In this way both your hands can maintain full contact, and the hand on the flexors can slightly lift the forearm to allow your hands to move down more easily. Your hands will catch up with each other to work at the same level on the palm (Fig. 7.9), continuing until the fingers lie in the middle of your palm. Any part of this sequence may be used to treat any specific muscle(s).

Single-handed kneading

The deltoid

The whole of one of your hands may be used to knead the deltoid muscle. The outer hand is the easier to use, and your inner hand should support the arm just below the axilla and on the medial side, in order to give counterpressure and stabilise the area.

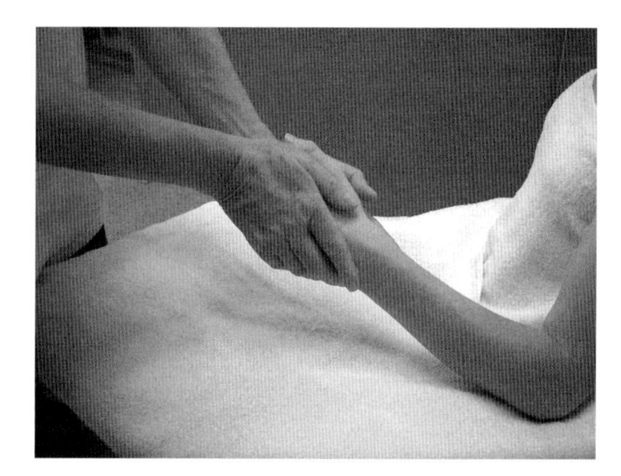

Figure 7.9 Kneading on the hand.

The triceps

The triceps is kneaded with your outer hand, and counterpressure with your other hand is given initially halfway down and then at the distal part of the biceps.

The biceps

The biceps is kneaded with your inner hand, with counterpressure with your other hand over the midpoint and then the distal part of the triceps.

Extensors of the forearm

The forearm extensors are kneaded with your outer hand starting above the elbow flexure (remember some of the muscles take origin above the flexure), and working down to the wrist, eventually using your palm only. Support is given with your inner hand over the wrist to prevent it moving and also to raise the forearm if necessary.

Flexors of the forearm

The forearm flexors are treated in a similar way, using your inner hand starting in the elbow flexure with the whole hand, and gradually using only your palm as you work down to the wrist. The wrist is supported with your outer hand.

The hand

The dorsum of the hand is kneaded using the palm of your outer hand, while supporting the patient's palm with the palm of your inner hand. Try to cup this palm so that sticky contact of the middles of the two palms is avoided. The supporting hand should be placed across the supported palm so that your fingers lie on one side and your thumb on the other side.

Some people find it easier to learn single-handed kneading before learning to use both hands.

Finger kneading

The palm of the hand is more usually kneaded with either all or most of the fingers, using flat fingers to fit over the muscle areas. Your outer hand supports the supinated hand on the dorsum to allow the middle of the palm and then the hypothenar area to be treated. Your hands change roles and the hypothenar eminence is grasped to allow your outer hand to work on the thenar area. Finger pad kneading can be performed on each small area and eventually on individual intrinsic muscles working from proximal to distal.

Thumb kneading

Thumb kneading is more usually performed on the flatter or smaller muscle groups of the upper limb.

Flexors and extensors of the forearm

The flexors and extensors of the forearm are treated similarly. Hold the forearm a little elevated from the pillow so that your fingers can lie on the opposite aspect. Obtain maximum contact with the length of your thumbs by keeping your forearms low and parallel with the patient's forearm. Then perform maximum size circles without skin drag, and be aware that the appearance of a wrinkle above the working thumb means that your range is enough, and skin drag will follow if you continue with pressure. Ensure your thumbs pass one another 'off-contact' just sufficiently to allow the relaxed thumb to pass adjacent to the lateral border of the working thumb. **Do not press most with the metacarpophalangeal joint** of your thumb – avoid this by maintaining **very slight** flexion at this joint, thus avoiding hyperextension of your thumb. The manipulation is deeper on the muscle bellies, and much lighter on the distal half to third of the forearm. The extensors are treated from above the elbow flexure anterior to the lateral epicondyle, and the flexors from below the elbow flexure and distal to the medial epicondyle.

Interosseous spaces

The interosseous spaces are kneaded on the dorsal aspect using the sides of your thumbs. The manipulation has a long, narrow, oval shape and is usually performed in alternate spaces, i.e. 1 and 3, 2 and 4. Support the palm with your fingers and work from proximal to distal, having determined the length of the space by stroking up it (Fig. 7.3).

The thenar and hypothenar eminences are thumb kneaded by supinating the hand and:

- *Either* using both your thumbs alternately on each eminence in turn
- *Or* using one thumb on each eminence and selecting the appropriate pairs of small muscles (Fig. 7.10).

Then the centre of the palm is kneaded with both thumbs alternately (Fig. 7.11). This sequence prevents the wrist from being rocked sideways as the manipulations are performed. Use your thumb pads or tips for these manipulations.

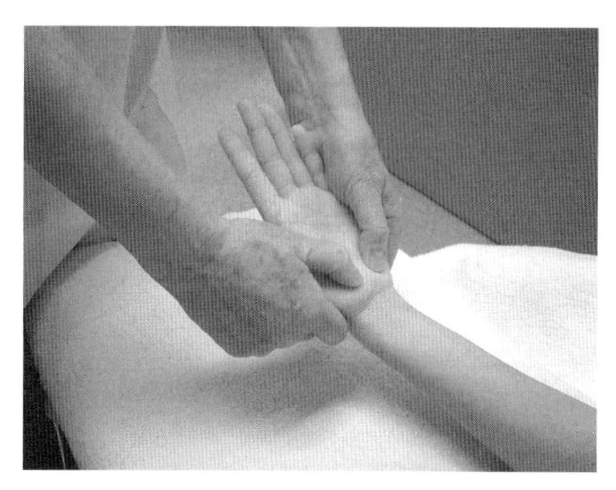

Figure 7.10 Simultaneous thumb kneading to the abductor pollicis brevis and abductor digiti minimi.

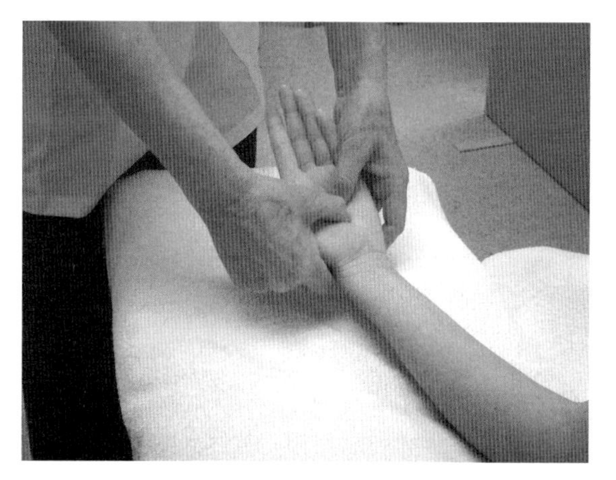

Figure 7.11 Alternate thumb kneading to the centre of the palm.

Fingers

The fingers can be kneaded in two ways. Turn the hand into pronation and:

- *Either* hold the patient's hand in one of your hands, and use the thumb pad and pad of the index finger of the other hand, one on the front and one on the back of the finger near the cleft, to knead both aspects at once.
- *Or* knead first one aspect, then the other (Fig. 7.12).
- *Or* hold the proximal phalanx of two alternate fingers cupped on the middle phalanx of your index finger.

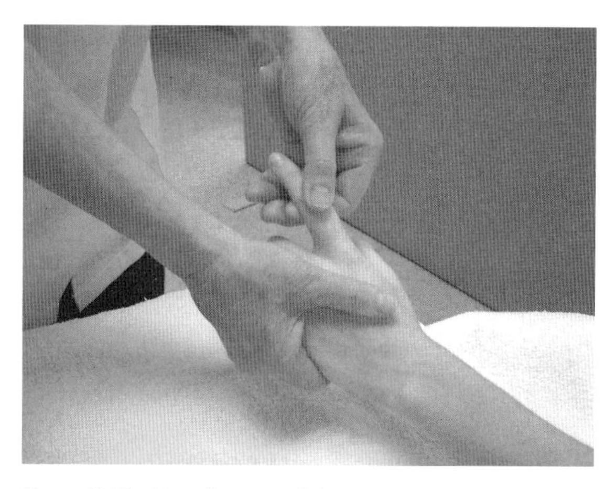

Figure 7.12 Kneading one digit at once.

Picking up

Picking up on the upper limb muscles is usually performed with one hand at once, and from proximal to distal. The practitioner's outer hand works on the deltoid, triceps and brachioradialis, and the inner hand on the biceps brachii and the forearm flexors. The free hand stabilises the limb adjacent to the working hand. Progress should be in small stages of about 1–2 cm (0.5–0.75 in) at a time.

The deltoid

The deltoid is picked up using your outer hand with your inner hand stabilising on the medial side of the arm near the elbow. Find the bony margins of the spine of the scapula, the acromion process and anterior border of the clavicle. Now slip down on to the deltoid and totally off the bone. Keep your palm in contact with the deltoid all the time so that you compress the whole muscle but pick up rather less of it. Your forearm should be parallel with the patient's forearm and remain so as you work. The 'pick up' is performed by extending your wrist after you have grasped the muscle, and you should neither pivot on your thumb and finger tips nor lever on the heel of your hand (Fig. 7.13). A vulnerable bony area is the lateral border of the bicipital groove and your thumb should always lie lateral to it and not on it.

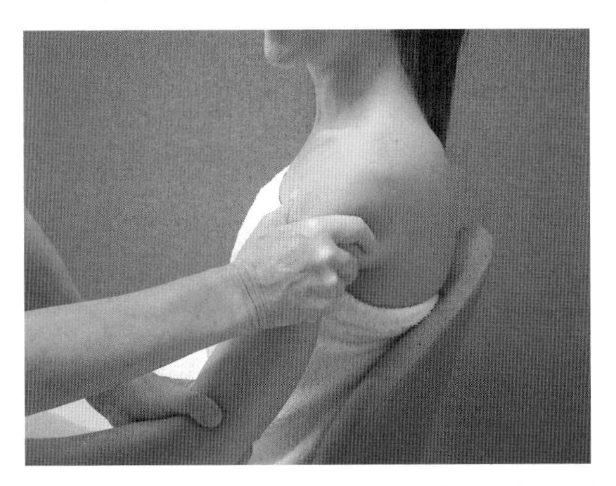

Figure 7.13 Picking up to deltoid – note the 'C' shape of the hand.

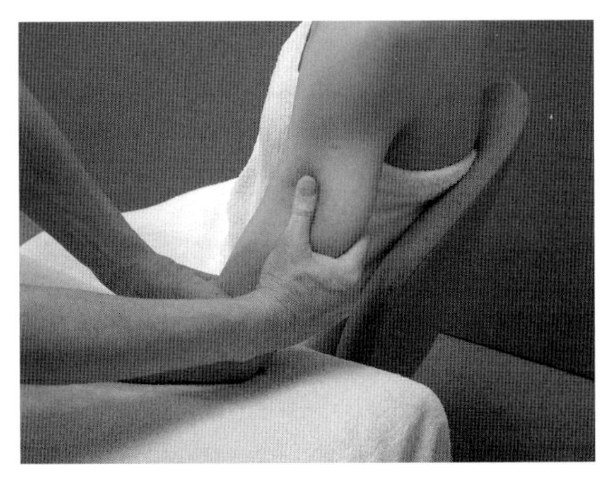

Figure 7.14 Picking up to triceps – note the practitioner's forearm is behind the model's arm and the hand is 'C' shaped.

The triceps

The triceps is treated by sliding your hand from the tendon of the deltoid to the back of the arm near the axilla, so that you encompass the triceps muscle belly (Fig. 7.14). Your finger tips should lie posterior to the medial border of the humerus, and the length of your thumb should be posterior to the lateral border of the humerus. Again, keep the whole of your palm in contact with the muscle belly, and your forearm low and parallel with that of the patient. Your stabilising hand should be on the biceps near the elbow.

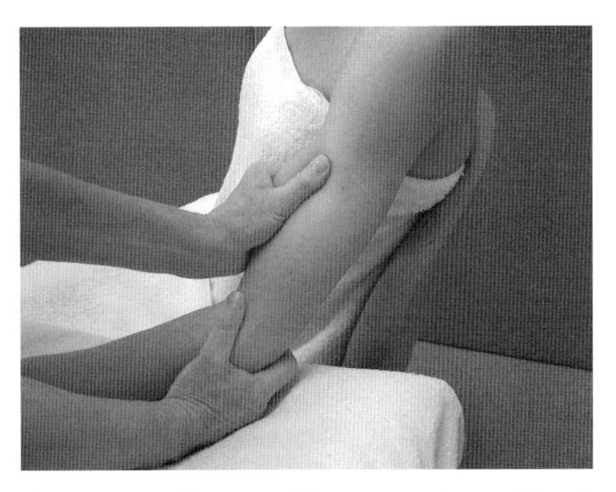

Figure 7.15 Picking up to biceps – note the practitioner's forearm is parallel with that of the model.

The biceps

As the triceps is completed, your other (stabilising) hand slides out of the way and up to the proximal part of the biceps. Again, your finger tips and length of your thumb lie in front of the adjacent bony borders of the humerus, with your palm in full contact (Fig. 7.15). As you work down the biceps muscle, your other hand should initially stabilise on the back of the elbow and move out of the way to the outside of the wrist which is lifted and the palm supinated, so that the working hand can continue to the tendon of insertion of the biceps, then slip medially to the forearm flexors.

Forearm flexors

These muscles are picked up using the 'V' formation of the hand with your fingers on the posteromedial aspect and your thumb on the anterolateral aspect. Again, maintain full palmar contact and narrow the 'V' as you proceed down the forearm to the wrist.

The brachioradialis

This requires the use of your outer hand to effect a smooth change by grasping and supporting at the wrist with the previously working hand, and sliding your outer hand up the length of the brachioradialis (Fig. 7.16). Keep the forearm lifted to relax the muscle, and pick up using a 'V' formation until you

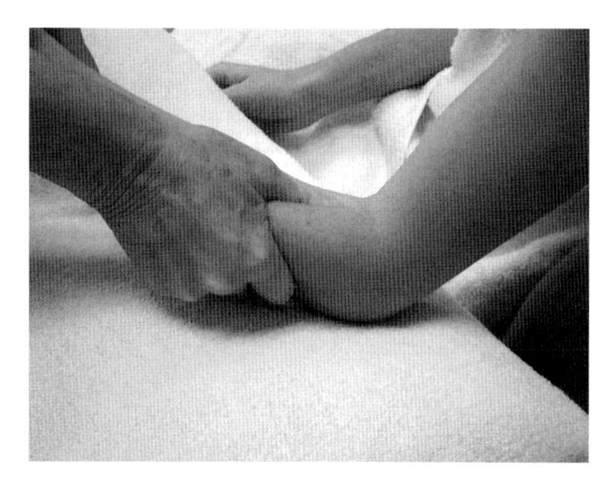

Figure 7.16 Picking up to brachioradialis – note the 'V' shape of the hand.

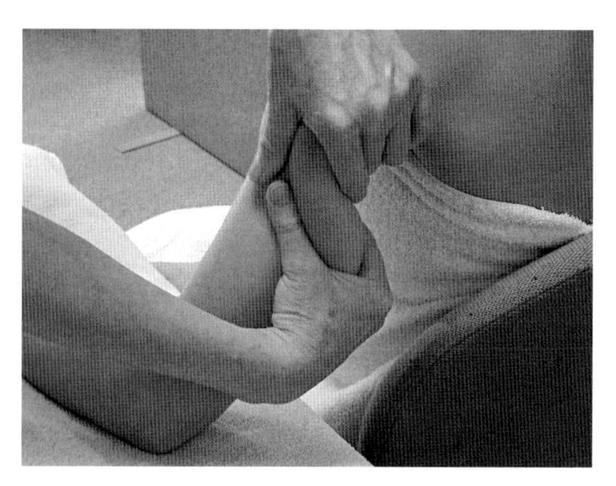

Figure 7.17 Wringing to the triceps.

reach the musculotendinous junction, which is two-thirds of the way down the forearm. Many people continue to perform a picking-up action as a squeeze on both aspects of the distal end of the forearm to preserve continuity of contact. At this point in a sequence on the arm, the forearm extensors are often thumb kneaded. Alternatively, you can return to the shoulder area to perform wringing.

Wringing

Wringing is most easily performed on the long muscles of the triceps and biceps brachii. It is possible to wring a flabby or very relaxed deltoid, but the muscle is so short that it presents difficulties in performance.

The deltoid and triceps

These can be wrung by pivoting your stance and body so that you are nearer to the patient and your nearest foot is between the model and the table. In both cases, your fingers should be on the back of the arm and your thumbs towards the front and medial side. Ensure that these components of your hands are not lying over the adjacent bony border – the bicipital groove in the case of the deltoid and the lateral border of the humerus in the case of the triceps (Fig. 7.17). The muscles should be grasped at their most proximal end and you should work to the distal end and perhaps return. Try to proceed in small stages so that your hands move about 2–4 cm (1–1.5 in) at a time and move constantly.

The biceps

For the biceps you will need to move your stance slightly to the outer side of the arm support and, again, use your fingers on the medial side anterior to the medial border of the humerus, and your thumbs on the lateral side anterior to the lateral border of the humerus. Again work from most proximal to the distal part of the muscle and perhaps return, and work in small stages similar to the triceps.

Be very careful in wringing these muscles not to drag on the skin, and to keep your hand changes of direction very smooth. Dry hands are a great help in ensuring smooth, non-dragging work.

The brachioradialis

The belly of the brachioradialis may be wrung using your thumb pads and the pads of your index, middle and sometimes ring fingers. The patient's forearm should be fully supported in mid-pronation and supination.

The hand

Tiny wringing manipulations done with the tips of your index fingers and sides of your thumb tips can be performed on the intrinsic muscles of the thenar and hypothenar eminences. The two abductor and two flexor muscles are more easily treated in this way.

Muscle shaking

The deltoid

The shorter deltoid muscle can be shaken using your outer hand. Take care not to bounce on the bicipital groove with your thumb.

The triceps

The triceps is shaken again using your outer hand and proceeding from near the axilla to the elbow (Fig. 7.18).

The biceps

The biceps is shaken using your inner hand, proceeding from near the axilla to the musculotendinous junction.

The brachioradialis

In the forearm, a bulky brachioradialis may be shaken using the thumb pad and the lateral side of the flexed phalanges of the index finger of your inner or outer hands.

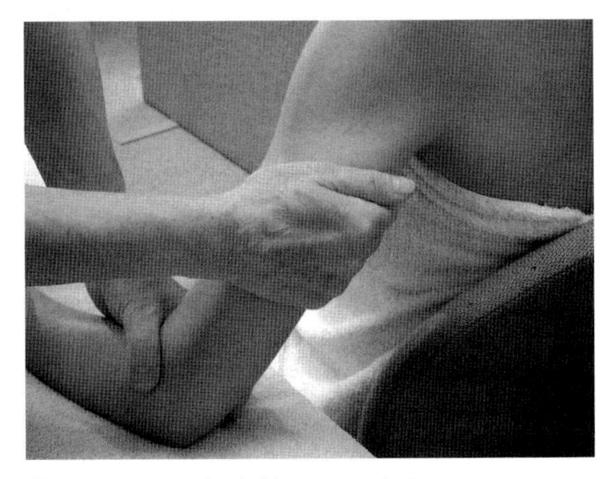

Figure 7.18 Muscle shaking – note the loose grasp.

The hand

In the hand you may be able to shake the bulk of both the hypothenar and thenar eminences and, in some subjects, to select and shake the abductor brevis pollicis and abductor digiti minimi using the tips of your thumb and index finger.

Muscle rolling

Muscle rolling can be performed on each of the upper limb muscles which can be picked up, and this manipulation is often easier to perform on the brachioradialis than either wringing or picking up.

Place your thumbs and fingers as though you intended to do wringing – as described above – and push the muscle belly gently first with both of your thumbs while your fingers relax but stay in contact, then pull with the distal phalanges of all your fingers while your thumbs relax but stay in contact. Proceed along the length of each muscle working down, then up, with this rocking action. Work fairly quickly and with a slight pressure inward towards the mid-line of the limb so that the muscle rolls from side to side.

Muscle rolling can also be performed with the thumb and finger tips on the two flexor and two abductor muscles of the thenar and hypothenar eminences. This manipulation can also be used to roll or 'rock' scars and adherent tissue.

Hacking and clapping

Hacking and clapping are usually performed successively to first one aspect of the upper limb, then to the other, so that the limb is moved only once.

With the patient's forearm pronated, start at the posterior axilla and work down the posterior part of the deltoid, triceps (reach round to the back of the arm to do so) and then on to the forearm extensors. You may need to stop the hacking at mid forearm in bony subjects, but should be able to clap on to the dorsum of the hand. Stand nearer the patient for this work.

Turn the forearm to supination and lift the elbow medially, so that the limb rests comfortably on the

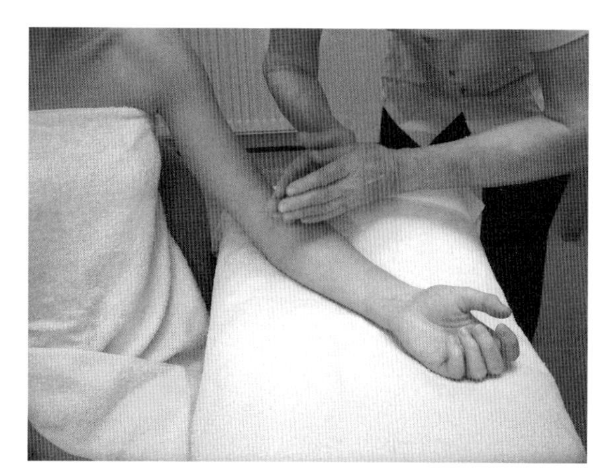

Figure 7.19 Hacking to the forearm flexors.

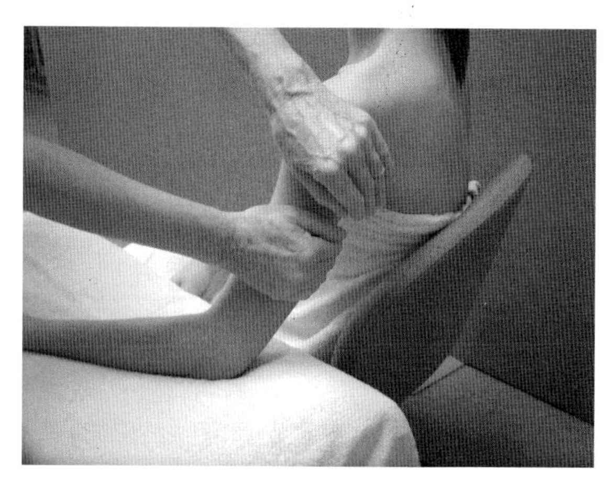

Figure 7.20 Clapping to the upper arm.

support. Either stand on the outer side of the support or step nearer to the patient's feet, and starting at the axilla work down the front of the deltoid, biceps, the forearm flexors (Fig. 7.19) and the palm of the hand, and reverse up the limb.

By working in this way you will strike the muscle fibres across their longitudinal axis. In both lines of work you should:

- Work in a zigzag fashion on each muscle if it is bulky or wide enough.
- Avoid bony prominences and large tendons and jump over them.

Clapping is performed in a similar pattern using a more cupped hand on the more slender parts of the limb (Fig. 7.20).

8 Massage to the lower limb

Margaret Hollis and Elisabeth Jones

Preparation of the patient

Ask the patient to remove all clothing below the waist except briefs or pants. Check that the feet are clean and not malodorous. If necessary wipe with surgical spirit or cologne, saying that it is freshening to the feet.

Preparation of the treatment couch

Cover the couch with an underblanket and towels. Provide two pillows for the patient's head, and either one large pillow to go under both knees or two small pillows to go under each knee.

Treatment of the lower limb with the patient supine

If possible the patient should lie flat, but some people prefer or some patients may need to have the elevating head end of the couch raised so that half lying is the position used. Avoid an angle of elevation of the backrest of more than 45° so that drainage is not impeded. Cover the legs with towels and provide a second small cover for the upper part of the body. If the lower limb needs elevation for the treatment of oedema, then it should be supported by pillows or by raising the end of the couch by no more than 45°. In this case, the trunk must not be raised 45° as well. Provide additional head pillows instead of elevating the head end of the couch.

When working on an elevated lower limb, it may be necessary either to lower an adjustable couch or, if the couch is of fixed height, for you to stand on a low platform in order to reach.

Treatment of the lower limb with the patient prone

(To gain access to the posterior aspect of the lower limb.)

The patient lies prone, with head and abdomen supported. Place one pillow under both ankles to allow a little flexion at both knees, and sufficient pillows under the calf of the limb to be treated so that the knee is flexed no more than 45°. Ensure that the ankle is supported in some plantar flexion. This position is suitable for treatment of the hamstrings and/or the calf. If insufficient pillows are available, the patient's ankle can rest on your shoulder, but arrange yourself carefully so that if possible you can half sit (perch) on the edge of the couch, as the calf can feel very heavy by the end of the treatment and more so if you stand to work and support the limb.

Before starting work always uncover the whole limb in order to examine it and especially observe the state of the skin for:

- Dryness
- Callosities
- Abrasions
- The presence of any varicose veins
- The posture of the joints, which may need extra supports.

Then palpate – run your hand down the length of each aspect of the limb – and note:

- Temperature
- Tenderness
- Muscle tone.

Ensure there is only light pressure over bony prominences.

Effleurage

To the whole limb

Stand in lunge standing with your rear foot distal to the patient's foot, and your forward foot level with the patient's calf. Both hands usually work together: your nearside hand on the sole of the foot and more medial aspect of the limb, and your more lateral hand on the dorsum of the foot and the more lateral aspect of the limb.

There are two methods of working on the foot:

- Each hand starts with the fingers over the toes; then on to the dorsum (Fig. 8.1a) with one hand moving to the anterolateral side of the ankle. The other hand moves to the plantar aspect, then passes under the instep to the anteromedial side of the ankle (Fig. 8.1a).
- The alternative method of working on the foot is only different for the hand on the dorsum. For each stroke, one hand starts initially passing over the toes, then over the dorsum of the foot. The heel of this hand moves near to the lateral malleolus. The stroke with this hand is initiated by pivoting it with some depth on the dorsum of the foot, so that your fingers turn to lie on the outer side of the foot and then proceed as described above (Fig. 8.1b). This method is useful where there is a painful ankle joint or foot as the counterpressures of the hands prevent unwanted ankle plantar flexion which can be inadvertently caused by the latter method.

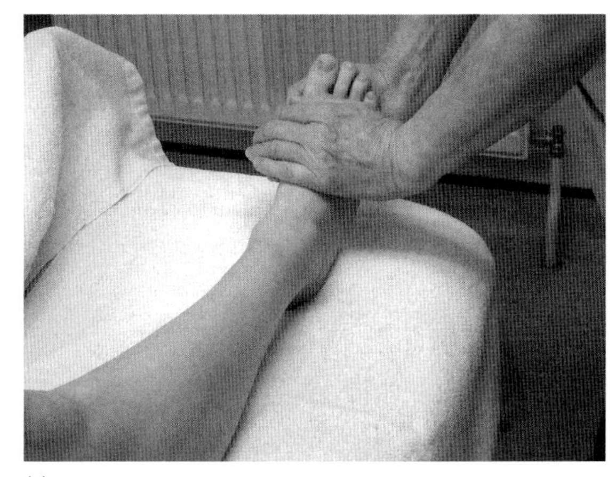

(a)

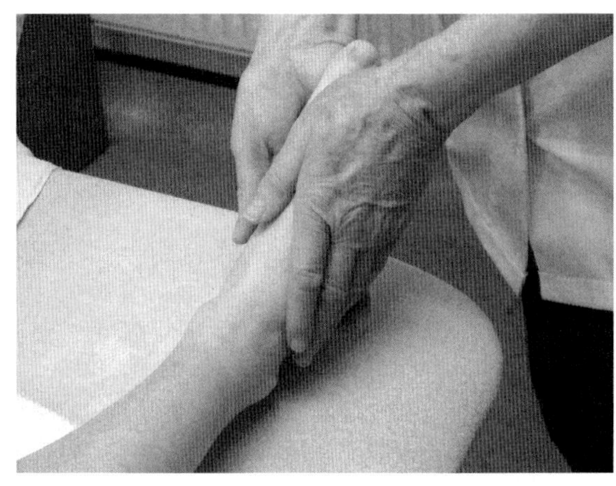

(b)

Figure 8.1 Optional starting positions (a, b) of the hands on the foot, for effleurage to the lower limb.

Whichever method you have used you must now abduct and extend your thumbs so that your hands span first the sides (Fig. 8.2), then the front of the ankle and proceed almost up the front of the leg (Fig. 8.3) over the knee and thigh to the femoral triangle where you should increase your pressure and pause briefly. Throughout this part of the

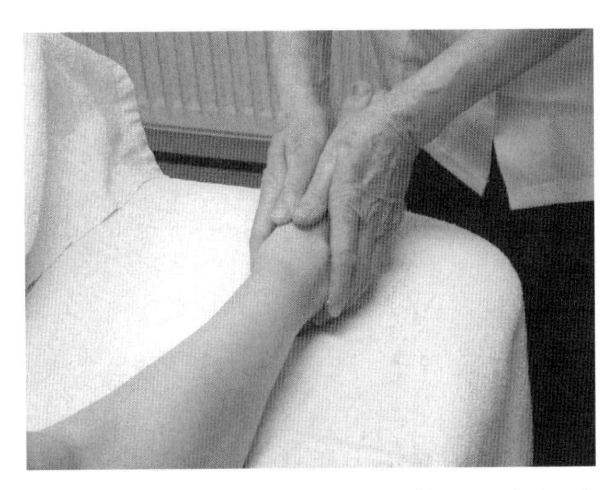

Figure 8.2 Effleurage continues at the ankle. Note the hands moulding to the part.

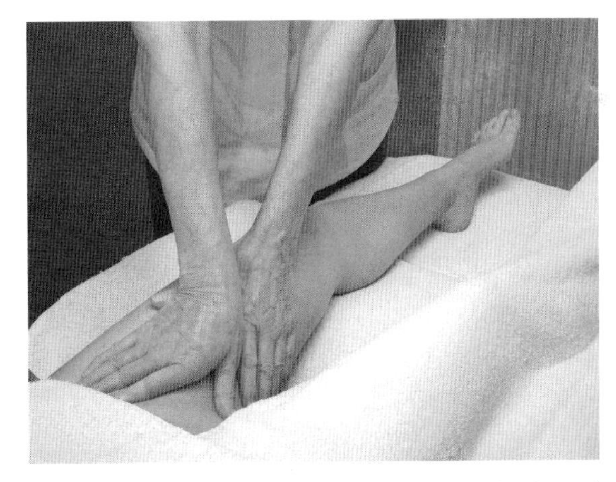

Figure 8.4 The finish of an effleurage stroke at the femoral triangle.

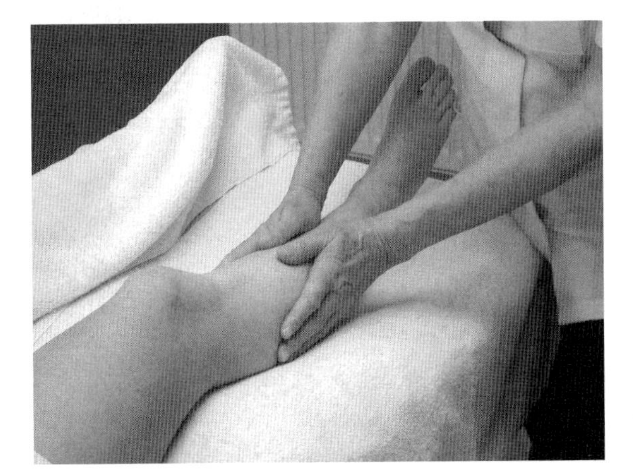

Figure 8.3 Stroke 1 – effleurage to the front of the leg.

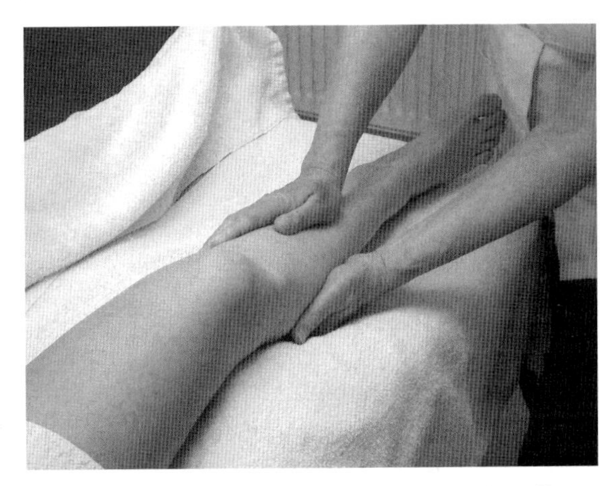

Figure 8.5 Stroke 2 – effleurage to the sides of the calf continues up the sides of the thigh.

stroke your hands fit together (Fig. 8.4) with the thumb of your outer hand lying alongside the index finger of your inner hand. For each successive stroke your hands should fit together in this way as they come round to the front of the thigh and continue to the femoral triangle, where overpressure is given with a slight pause. The next stroke starts in the same way, but your fingers pass behind the malleoli so that your hands can continue up the medial and lateral aspects of the limb (Fig. 8.5). Your outer hand should, again, be slightly in advance of your medial hand and both move more anteriorly at the junction of the upper and middle third of the thigh so that they encompass the femoral triangle.

The third stroke starts like the second stroke, but at the malleoli your fingers pass the tendocalcaneus and proceed up the posterior aspect of the limb (Fig. 8.6) with your outer hand slightly in front of your inner hand. You will have to extend your back and lift the patient's limb very slightly to proceed under the thigh from the back of the knee. At the upper third of the thigh, your hands circumnavigate to the front to finish at the femoral triangle. Pressure has to be varied to allow for the smaller ankle, bulky muscular calf, more bony knee and bulky muscular thigh. This can be best controlled by adjusting your foot position and ensuring your arms start to 'reach' before your body moves. You should feel your shoulder girdle protracting to assist the reaching process. At no time should you bend either your hips or your back.

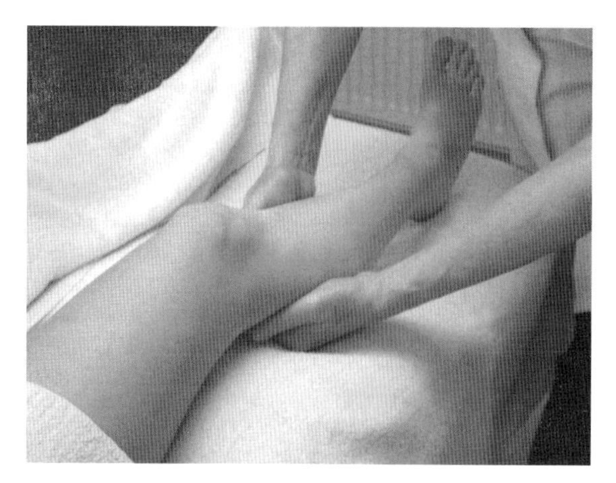

Figure 8.6 Stroke 3 – effleurage to the back of the calf continues up the back of the thigh.

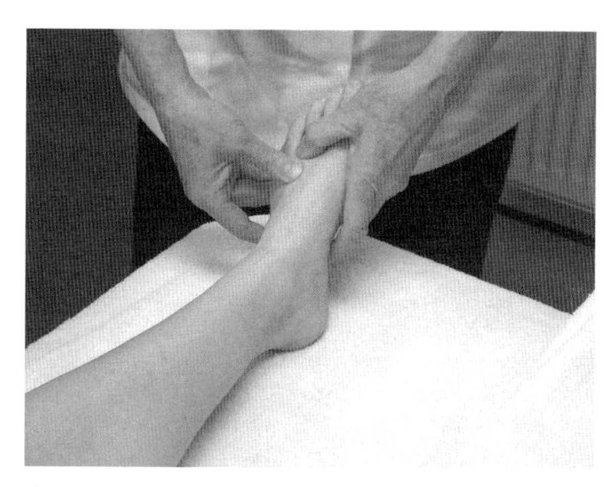

Figure 8.8 Position of the hands for either an effleurage stroke or kneading to the interosseous spaces of the foot.

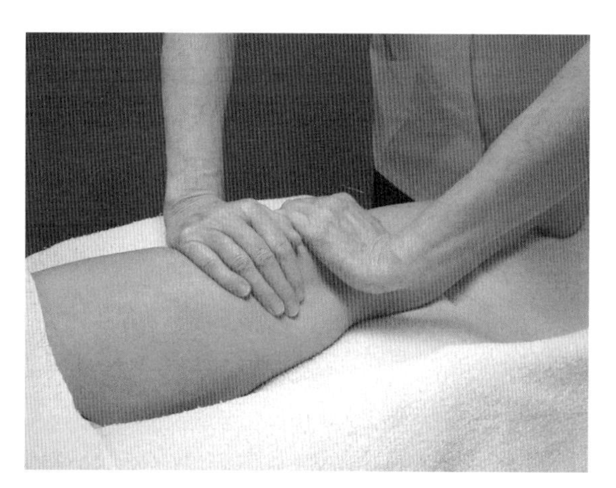

Figure 8.7 Start of effleurage to the knee.

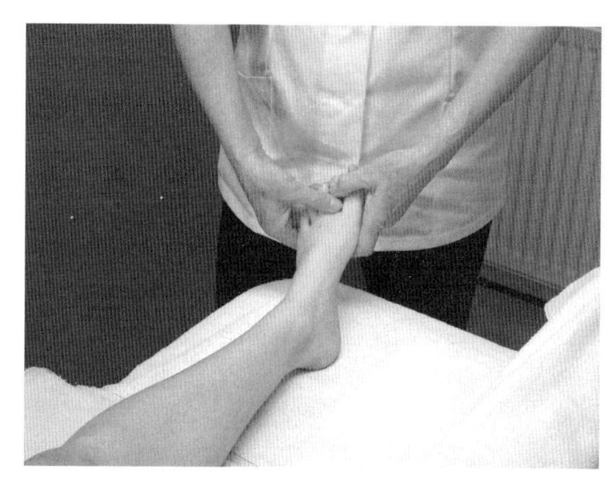

Figure 8.9 Position of the hands for either an effleurage stroke or kneading to the toes.

Part strokes

The **thigh** can be effleuraged alone if the patterns of strokes previously described start at the knee and proceed to the femoral triangle. The posterior stroke is started by sliding the hands from each side to underneath the knee.

The **knee** is effleuraged by crossing your hands above the patella (Fig. 8.7), drawing them backwards on each side of it until the heels of your hands meet below the patella, then turning your hands to allow your fingers to pass behind the knee over the popliteal fossa.

The **leg** is effleuraged from the foot or ankle to the popliteal fossa, following the lines of work for the whole lower limb.

The **foot** is effleuraged by starting in one of the two described ways and finishing at the ankle.

The **interosseous spaces** are effleuraged using the sides of your thumbs, meantime supporting the plantar aspect of the foot with your fingers (Fig. 8.8).

The **toes** are effleuraged by supporting the tip of each toe on the tip of your middle finger, and your thumbs stroke up (Fig. 8.9).

Take care to follow the basic rules for effleurage, especially ensuring you do not give maximum pressure with the leading edge of your hands. To continue working on the thigh, cover the leg and foot with part of the covering.

Kneading

All the kneading manipulations on the lower limb are performed using the circling technique described in Fig. 6.4b, with modifications for the size of the area under treatment. Ensure you are working on muscle or soft tissue and avoid deep, moving pressure over bony ridges and prominences. The pressure of all the manipulations should be inwards to the centre of the limb with an upward inclination so that you can envisage assisting venous blood and lymph flow from distal to proximal.

The thigh

The thigh is usually treated with double-handed, alternate kneading dealing with the medial and lateral aspects together, and the anterior and posterior aspects together. Consider the anatomy: the hamstrings extend from the ischial tuberosity to the tibia, and the rectus femoris extends from the ilium to the patella. Two groups extend the whole length of the thigh so, except on the medial aspect, the manipulations start as high as your hands can be placed and continue to the knee.

The adductor group occupies most of the upper medial half of the thigh, and the vastus medialis the lower half. On the lateral side is the vastus lateralis, covered by the strong fascia lata and extending most of the length of that side. Thus there is a long length on the lateral side and less than half that length on the medial aspect.

Stand in lunge standing at the level of the lower calf with your outer foot forward. For the lateral and medial lines of work, the lateral hand initiates the kneading at half tempo and works down the thigh until it is opposite the medial hand, which is resting ready on the middle of the medial aspect. This hand now works alternately with the other hand to continue down to the knee (Fig. 8.10). For

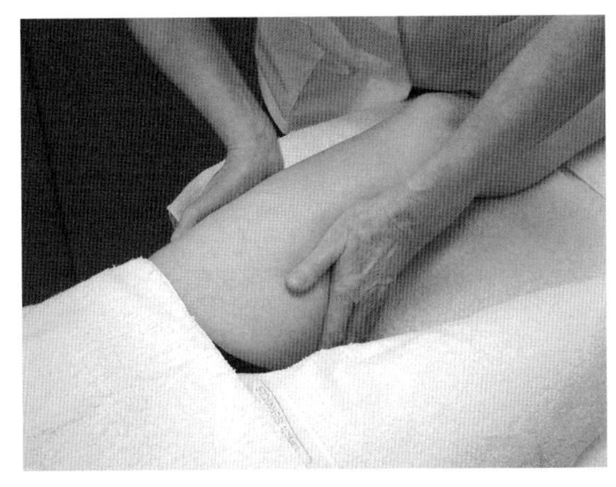

Figure 8.10 Kneading the thigh: medial and lateral aspects.

the anterior and posterior lines of work, the anterior and posterior muscles are kneaded:

- *Either* by remaining in the same posture as for the lateral/medial aspects and inserting your nearer (medial) hand under the thigh from the inside to work on the hamstrings, while your outer hand works on the anterior aspect
- *Or* by turning your body more to face across the thigh, you then insert your hand nearest to the patient's hip (outer hand) under the thigh from the outside, and the further, formerly medial hand works on the anterior aspect.

In order to work deeply on these great muscle masses you must lean forward with a straight back, working always with your hands in front of the level of your shoulders. As your hands proceed down the thigh, transfer your weight from your forward to your rear foot, but your weight must also be transferred constantly from one foot to the other by pivoting your pelvis. Your weight should be more on the forward foot when kneading with the outer hand, and more on the rear foot when kneading with the inner hand.

When you work on the thigh muscles keep the anatomy constantly in mind and envisage straight lines down the length of the centres of the muscles you are working upon. Keep the middle of your hand along this line so that you do not work across two muscles or muscle groups at once, which is much harder work for you as well as less effective and less comfortable for the patient.

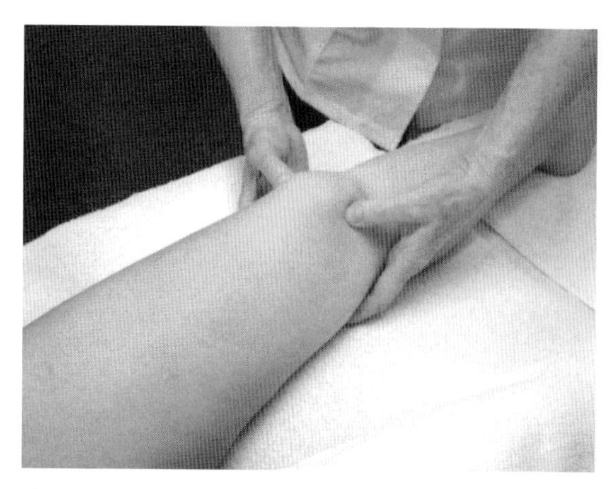

Figure 8.11 Thumb kneading to the knee.

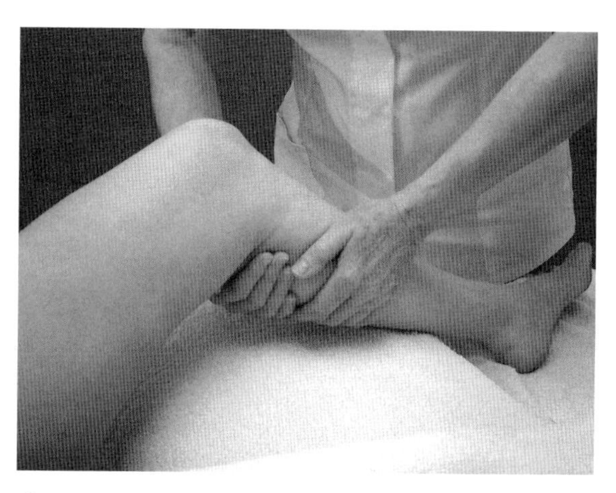

Figure 8.12 Kneading the calf muscles. The knee has been flexed for the photograph.

Round the knee

Whole-handed kneading round the knee should extend from just above the superior margin of the synovial membrane to a hand-width below the flexure of the knee so that you encompass all the structures in the region. Start with both hands on the anterior aspect with the heels of the hands touching above the patella. Work down, letting the heels of your hands divide round the patella to avoid working over it. Let the heels of your hands meet again below the patella. Next, insert each hand from opposite sides under the lower thigh until your fingers overlap. Now work down on this aspect, covering the same level as in the previous line of work.

Thumb kneading round the patella

Use your thumbs and work with your thumbs one on each side of the patella, i.e. starting near each other and dividing round the bone margin (Fig. 8.11).

Finger kneading the knee

Use your fingertips to work on each side of the bony areas of the knee with your thumbs resting on an adjacent area. Place your fingertips in a linear formation, first one side, then the other side of the tendons of the hamstrings at the knee so that one hand is on the biceps femoris and the other is on the semimembranosus and semitendonosus tendons.

If you are practising the kneading manipulations to increase your skill, continue on to the leg and foot – in which case, cover the thigh and uncover the leg and foot and continue as described below. If you are working on each area to give treatment, then complete all the manipulations for the thigh, in which case turn to Chapter 6 for the petrissage manipulations and tapôtement manipulations.

The calf muscles

Stand in lunge standing distal to the patient's feet. The lower limb may be flexed with the foot resting almost flat on the couch to give better access, but it is feasible to perform double-handed kneading with the limb flat, although you should push the knee pillow higher under the thigh so that the lower edge is at the level of the knee flexure. Insert one of your hands from each side under the calf so that your palms clasp the calf muscles. On the medial side, the heel of your hand must be behind the medial border of the tibia, and the heel of your hand on the lateral side must be behind the line of the fibula.

As you knead, ensure your fingers stay beside each other. Your hands should overlap more as the manipulation proceeds down the limb so that eventually one is superimposed on the other (Fig. 8.12).

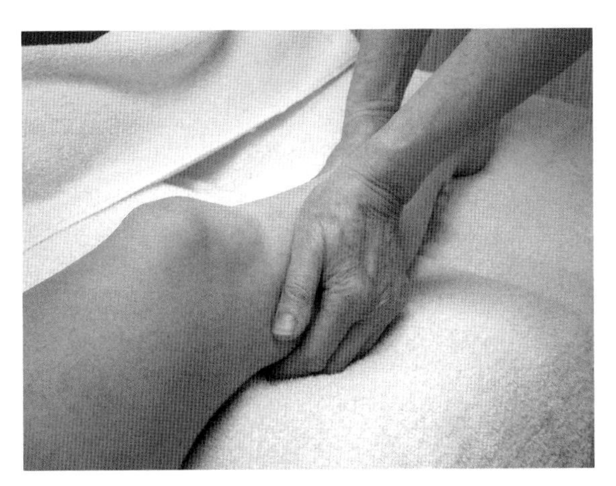

Figure 8.13 Palmar kneading to the anterior tibial muscles.

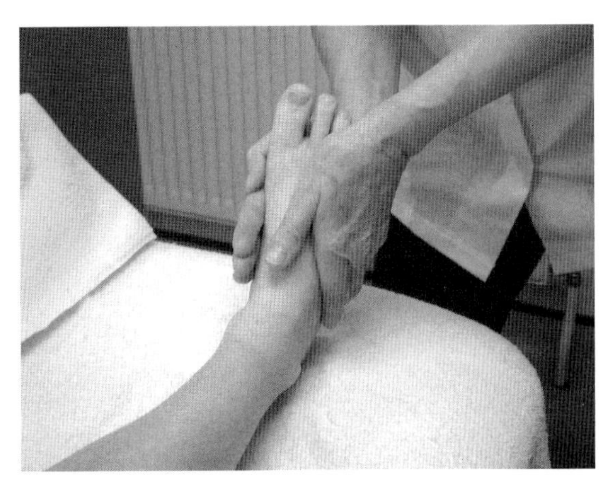

Figure 8.14 Kneading the foot.

Palmar kneading the anterior tibial muscles

Place the heel of your palm, thumb close to it, over the upper extremities of the anterior tibial group with your fingers slightly off-contact. Stabilise the limb with your other hand (Fig. 8.13). Work down the muscle, coming more to the front of the limb as the muscle bulk diminishes, and continue on to the dorsum of the foot to the insertions of the muscles on the medial aspect of the foot, and on the toes.

Palmar kneading the peronei

Place the heel of the palm of your hand, thumb closed to it and fingers slightly off-contact, on the upper limit of the peronei and work down the lateral aspect of the calf to above the lateral malleolus.

The foot

Place your outer hand on the dorsum of the foot, with your fingers lying laterally (Fig. 8.14). Place your other hand on the sole of the foot, with your thenar eminence fitted into the medial longitudinal arch, fingers on the lateral side.

Work down the foot with a kneading manipulation which should also squeeze. You will find that you must always maintain some pressure with both hands all the time, or the foot will rock back and forth.

Thumb kneading the anterior tibial muscles

Medially rotate the whole limb slightly, and place both thumbs as flat as possible on the upper extremity of the bulk of the anterior tibial muscles. The remainder of your hands should rest round the calf, so that the palms are slightly off-contact but the fingers are supporting the limb. Carry out a kneading manipulation so that the thumbs work throughout their length and, by bypassing one another, the whole width of the muscle group is treated (Fig. 8.15). As you work down the part, move your line of work anteriorly so that your thumbs finish on the front of the ankle and can proceed if desired over the tendons to their distal attachments on the tarsus and phalanges.

Thumb kneading the peroneal muscles

Medially rotate the whole limb and bend yourself a little sideways, so that you can place both thumb pads on the upper extremity of the peronei. The remainder of your hands rest round the calf as described above. Using only the thumb pads, work

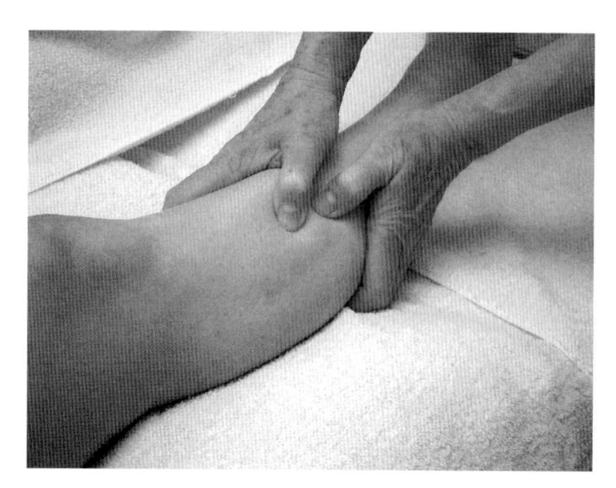

Figure 8.15 Thumb kneading to the anterior tibial muscles.

down the length of the muscles and on to the tendons as they lie behind the lateral malleolus.

Thumb kneading the dorsum of the foot

Palpate the muscle belly of the extensor digitorum brevis just anterior to the lateral malleolus. Place both thumb pads over the muscle belly and, with your fingers firmly supporting the sole of the foot, work along the dorsum using an increasing amount of the length of your thumbs until you are working over the dorsum of the four medial toes.

Thumb kneading the sole of the foot

Lean over to put your thumbs over the medial aspect of the foot, to treat the abductor hallucis and plantar aspect in mid-line. Turn to put your thumbs over the lateral aspect of the foot, to treat the abductor digiti minimi. Palpate the line of the abductor hallucis muscle belly and, using your thumb pads, work from the heel to the base of the big toe with your finger tips resting on the outer side of the foot.

Next, lean further over and work under the middle of the plantar aspect from the heel to the transverse arch.

Turn your body and palpate the line of abductor digiti minimi and, using your thumb pads, knead along the muscle to the little toe. Avoid tickling by using considerable depth.

Thumb kneading the interosseous spaces

Palpate two alternate spaces, either one and three or two and four, and place the sides of your thumb pads in two spaces at the proximal end. Work simultaneously with both thumbs with a narrow oval manoeuvre along the length of the space. Your fingers should be giving counterpressure on the plantar aspect of the foot (Fig. 8.8). Repeat for the other two spaces.

Thumb and finger kneading the toes

The big toe is kneaded by using your medial hand, with your thumb on the dorsum and your index finger curved round the medial, plantar and lateral aspects of the big toe. The manipulation is a squeeze knead performed from proximal to distal.

The four small toes are kneaded by holding each of them between your thumb tip and the tip of your index finger, and working along the length of the dorsal and plantar aspects (Fig. 8.9). You may need to hold each toe by its tip and work on that one toe alone, or to work on two alternate toes at once, depending on their state of flexion and rigidity.

Picking up

The thigh

Picking up may be performed on the vastus medialis, rectus femoris and vastus intermedius, and on the vastus lateralis with the patient supine. The hamstrings can be most easily treated with the patient prone, but from the supine position access may be obtained by flexing the knee a little and rolling the thigh laterally. To perform picking up on these muscles individually, single-handed work is practised first.

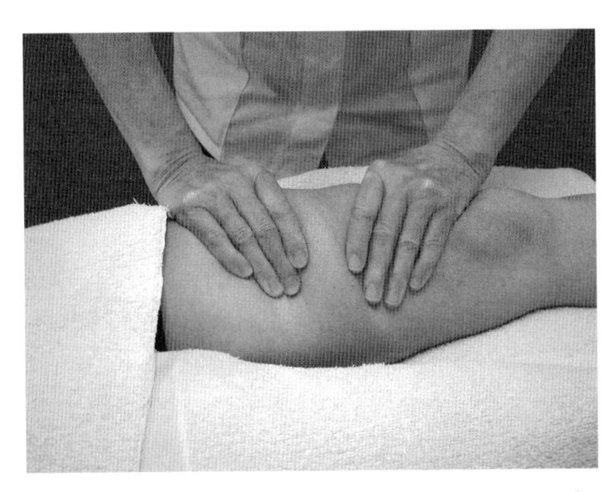

Figure 8.16 Picking up – double-handed alternate – on the anterior thigh muscles.

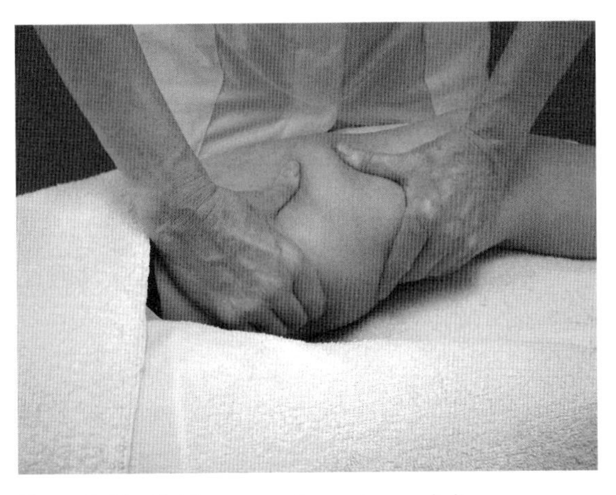

Figure 8.17 Picking up on the vastus medialis.

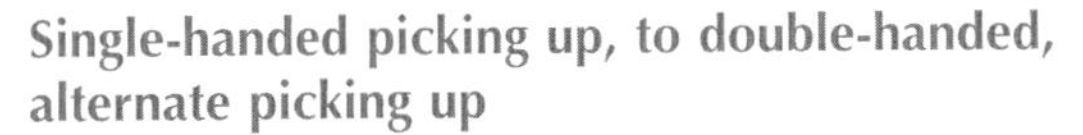

Single-handed picking up, to double-handed, alternate picking up

It is wiser initially to work on an accessible muscle group, and the anterior muscles are those of choice. Stand in walk standing opposite the thigh and facing the couch.

Place your hand which is nearer the patient's foot on the proximal end of the rectus femoris, and practise the technique, working until your hand reaches the patella. Keep your other hand in contact with the upper thigh. Change hands and work with the hand nearer the patient's head from just above the patella to the groin. Each hand thus travels backwards.

When you have worked enough to control your hand and body movements, then start to move forwards with each hand. This means that on the release your hand slides forward instead of backwards, before reimposing pressure on the part.

Skill in working in either direction can then be combined in working backwards with one hand and forwards with the other, thus passing the lifted tissues from hand to hand (Fig. 8.16).

The same procedure should then be practised on the vastus medialis (Fig. 8.17), but in order to do so you must lean forward with a straight back, so that your shoulders are parallel with and over the medial side of the thigh. Start the line of work either at the mid-thigh or at the level of the knee flexure. For the lateral aspect of the thigh, you will have to take a half pace back with your rear foot and bend both knees and hips to allow your forearms to be level with the outer side of the thigh. Start the line of work at the level of the knee flexure, or just below the great trochanter of the femur.

Heavier 'on' pressure will be necessary to gain any effect through the tough, lateral fascial structures, and in some cases no movement may be possible. For treatment, give extra kneading to this area.

Access to the hamstrings is effected by flexing the patient's knee and lifting the thigh into lateral rotation. By using flexion at your hips and some flexion of your upper back, you can reach round the medial side of the thigh and work on the hamstrings from either the knee flexure or proximally as high as it is possible to reach under the thigh.

Double-handed, simultaneous picking up

Double-handed, simultaneous picking up may also be performed on the anterior quadriceps (see Fig. 6.16).

If the patient lies prone, with one or two pillows under the calf to flex the knee a little, the hamstrings can also be picked up as described for the vastus intermedius and rectus femoris. If the muscle bellies are very bulky, use two lines of work, one for the biceps femoris and one for the semimembranosus and semitendonosus. The extent of work is from just below the ischial tuberosity to the knee flexure.

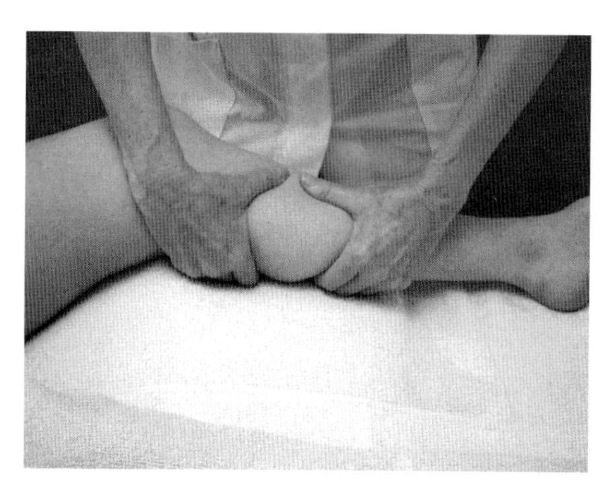

Figure 8.18 Picking up – double-handed alternate – on the calf muscles.

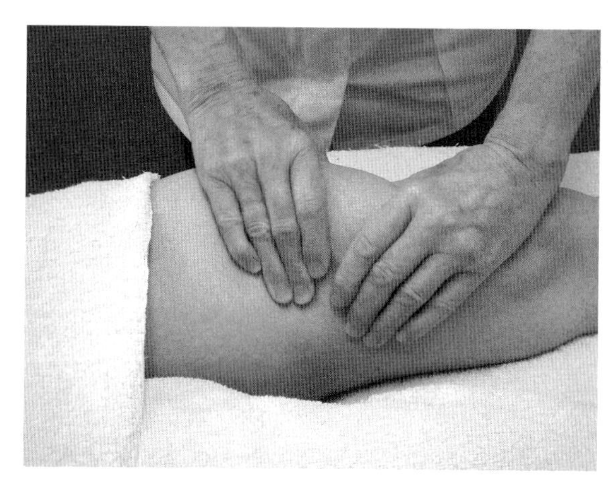

Figure 8.19 Wringing the anterior thigh muscles.

The calf

The calf muscles can also be picked up with the patient either supine or in prone lying. Only the muscle bulk can be picked up, but the tendocalcaneus is usually wrung.

Stand in walk standing, level with the calf. With the patient supine the best access is gained by rolling the whole lower limb laterally, and working from the knee flexure to the musculotendinous junction (Fig. 8.18). If the muscle is very bulky, it is sometimes possible to work from the lateral aspect as well, in which case the lower limb should be rolled medially.

With the patient in prone lying, and the foot and calf supported on one or two pillows, the calf muscles will be relaxed at the knee and ankle, and the upper two-thirds of the calf can be picked up from the knee flexure to the musculotendinous junction.

Wringing

The thigh

Stand in walk standing. Each of the thigh muscles can be treated by wringing. Your starting position, the lines of work and length of muscle treated are the same as for picking up, with the greatest effects being achieved on the anterior, medial and posterior muscle groups, in that order (Fig. 8.19). The manipulation can be difficult on the lateral aspect. Do ensure that you have lifted the muscle and are not just wringing the skin and subcutaneous tissues. The patient may be supine or in prone lying for wringing the hamstrings.

The calf

In exactly the same way as for the thigh, the calf can be treated by wringing. With the patient supine, the medial half of the calf can easily be lifted and have wringing performed on it; the lateral side can be treated only with difficulty. It is very important to be careful about both 'drag' and severe compression, with your finger and thumb tips only over superficial veins which may be becoming varicose. See Fig. 8.18 for the hand positions.

The tendocalcaneus can be wrung using the thumb pads and the pads of the index and middle fingers (Fig. 8.20). The basic, alternating pressures are performed on the tendon, being careful not to slip into the coulisse (the hollows between the tendon and the malleoli) on each side.

Muscle shaking

The thigh

Stand in lunge standing. The rectus femoris and vastus intermedius can be shaken throughout their length by placing your nearest hand on the proximal end of the muscles, and working down to the

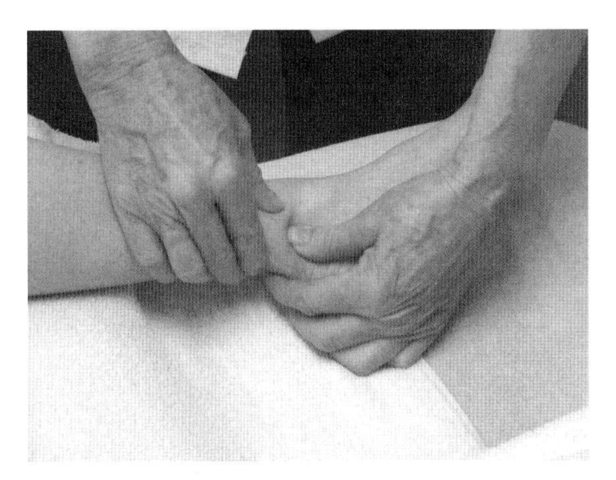

Figure 8.20 Wringing the tendocalcaneus.

level of the upper margin of the synovial pouch of the knee (Fig. 8.21a). The vastus medialis can be shaken from the mid-point on the medial aspect of the thigh, working down to just above the knee.

With the patient in prone lying, the hamstrings may be shaken together in the more slender subject, but in two lines of work when the muscles are bulky. For the biceps femoris, your thumb should be carefully placed to the lateral margin of the muscle and your finger tips equally carefully placed on the medial margins of the semimembranosus and semitendonosus.

The calf

The whole of the calf muscle bellies may be shaken, either by flexing the knee a little and rolling the lower limb laterally, then using your inside hand (Fig. 8.21b), or by turning the patient into prone lying, supporting the lower leg and foot on pillows and, again, using your inside hand to perform the shaking manipulation.

Skin rolling and skin wringing

The knee

Skin rolling over a small range may be performed, and is useful, on the tissues round the knee. The basic manipulation is adapted to be performed with the index and middle fingers on one side and the flat thumbs on the other. It is uncomfortable when performed with too great a depth or over too great a distance. It is, however, a most useful manipulation when disease or trauma has caused the structures round the knee to thicken.

Skin wringing may also be performed for similar reasons, and may be more tolerable if small areas of skin are lifted and wrung.

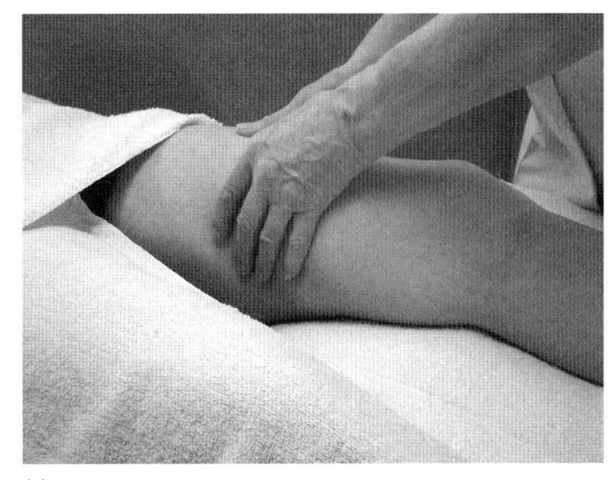

(a)

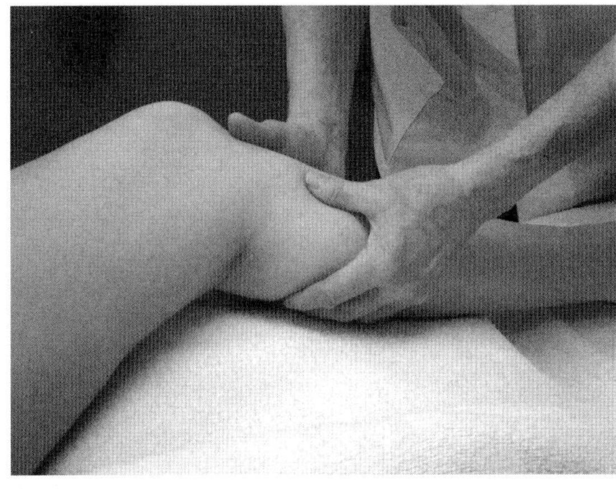

(b)

Figure 8.21 Muscle shaking – note the fingers and thumb are in contact and the palm is off contact: (a) the thigh; (b) the calf.

Hacking and clapping

Stand in adapted walk standing. Hacking and clapping on the lower limb are usually performed regionally. Both manipulations can be completed on the thigh before proceeding to the calf; follow

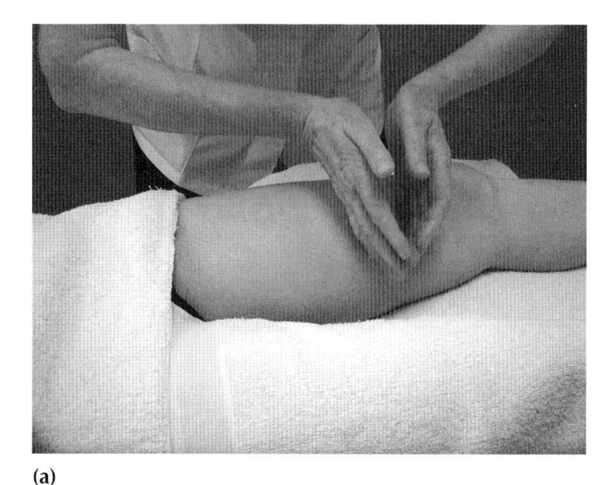

(a)

(b)

Figure 8.22 (a) Hacking and (b) clapping the thigh.

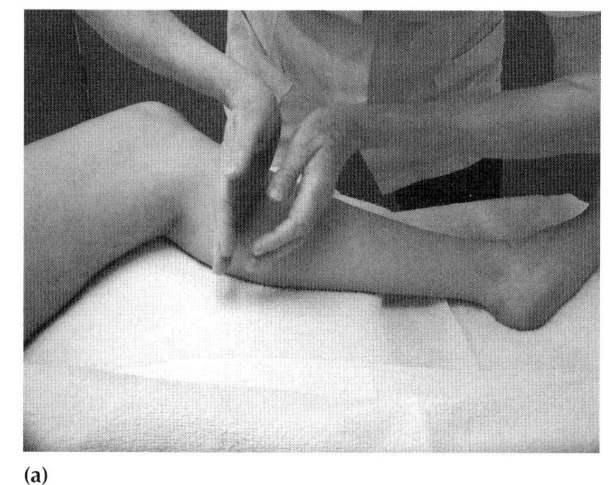

(a)

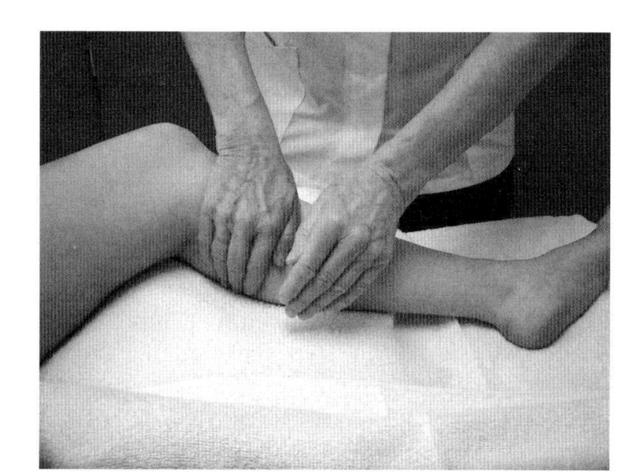

(b)

Figure 8.23 (a) Hacking and (b) clapping the calf.

the petrissage to the thigh before kneading is practised on the calf.

The lines of work should go up and down the limb, with the hands striking the muscles across their length and so across the long axis of the muscle fibres.

The thigh

For the quadriceps, start at mid-thigh on the medial side and work down the vastus medialis to the knee, work to the front and continue up the rectus femoris to the groin. Then move laterally to work down the vastus lateralis by bending your hips and knees, after taking one pace back to get better access; then reverse along these lines (Fig. 8.22).

The bony point to avoid is the adductor tubercle, and bulky muscles may need zigzag lines of hacking to effect complete cover.

The hamstrings are more accessible with the model in prone lying as for the petrissage manipulations. Medial and lateral lines of work may be necessary, working down and up the semimembranosus and semitendonosus together and then the biceps femoris, in each case stopping before reaching the myotendinous junctions when hacking.

The calf

The calf muscles are usually hacked and clapped by turning the whole lower limb into lateral rotation and slightly bending the knee. Work only on the muscle bulk and avoid the tendocalcaneus. Take care when hacking to avoid any varicosed vessels (Fig. 8.23).

The anterior tibial and peroneal muscles

The anterior tibial and peroneal muscles are best treated by medially rotating the whole limb, more so for the peronei, when you may also need to step further back with one leg and bend your hips and knees to allow your forearms to be parallel with the limb. Work down to just above the level of the lateral malleolus in each case, and more lightly as the muscle bulk diminishes.

9 Massage to the back, gluteal region and neck

Margaret Hollis and Elisabeth Jones

The back and neck may be conveniently divided for treatment. The lumbar and thoracic regions are usually treated together as the 'back', but the cervical region is usually included with them for sedative treatments. The gluteal region is usually treated alone, but the lumbar region may be included with it. For treatment of the neck, the area exposed usually extends from the occiput to the lower thoracic region, so that the whole of the trapezius may be included in the treated area.

THE THORACOLUMBAR REGION

Preparation of the patient

Ask the patient to remove all clothing except briefs/pants and, in the case of the female, the bra.

Preparation of the treatment couch

Cover the couch with an underblanket and towel. If the couch has a nose piece, retain it; if not place two pillows or rolls of towel crossing one another at right angles at the head of the couch, so that the patient's nose can rest at the crossing when in prone lying. Provide a small pillow to go under the abdomen and possibly one to go under the ankles. Have ready a towel to cover the body and one large one for the trunk and legs.

Treatment of the patient in prone lying

Check by observation the state of the skin, the bony points and posture; especially check that the axilla and groin are accessible. Ensure there is only light pressure on the bony prominences; avoid the throat area of the neck, and the thyroid gland.

Effleurage

The back can be divided into three overlapping areas for effleurage (Fig. 9.1). Neck effleurage is directed to the supraclavicular and axillary spaces, thoracic effleurage to the axillary space, and lumbar effleurage to the groin. Avoid the throat and thyroid gland. It is more usual to work bilaterally and simultaneously. Stand in lunge standing at the level of the patient's lower thighs and lean your trunk sideways so that you can exert equal hand pressure.

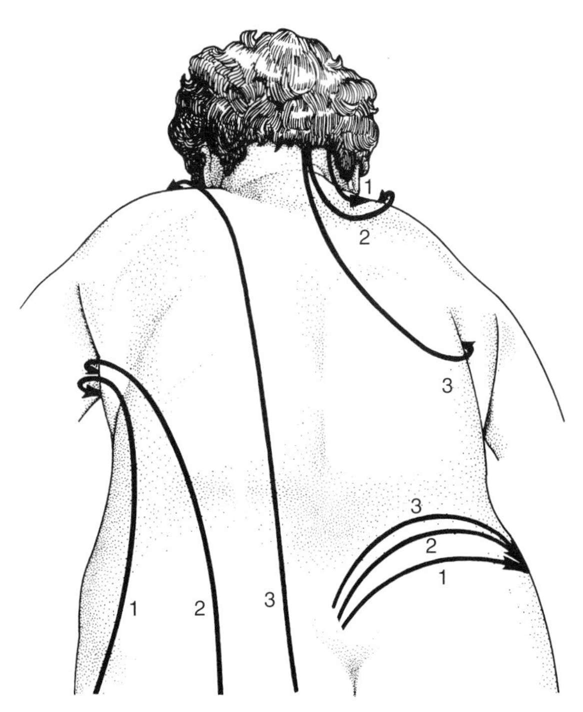

Figure 9.1 The lines of effleurage for the lumbar, thoraco-lumbar and neck region.

Your shoulders should be parallel with the patient's shoulders.

The **lumbar strokes** start with your hands on the middle of the lumbar region at its lowest point and finish at the groin, with your fingers inserted into the space by their full length. About three strokes should be made, each with an upward curve so that the whole lumbar region is treated (Fig. 9.1).

The **back strokes** also start with your hands in the lumbar region. The first stroke at the sides goes to the axilla (Fig. 9.2 a and b). The second stroke goes from the more central area also to the axilla (Fig. 9.3a and b). In both cases your fingers should go into the space by their full length. The third stroke proceeds up the middle of the back to the supraclavicular area, curving over the middle of the upper fibres of the trapezius (Fig. 9.4).

In all cases, ensure your hands lie obliquely on the back until the appropriate space is reached, when the stroke is terminated with the fingers leading. If you lead the strokes up the back with your finger tips your hands will be prevented from conforming to the hollows and humps of the back and may also stick and make jumpy strokes. Each stroke finishes with overpressure and a slight pause at the space.

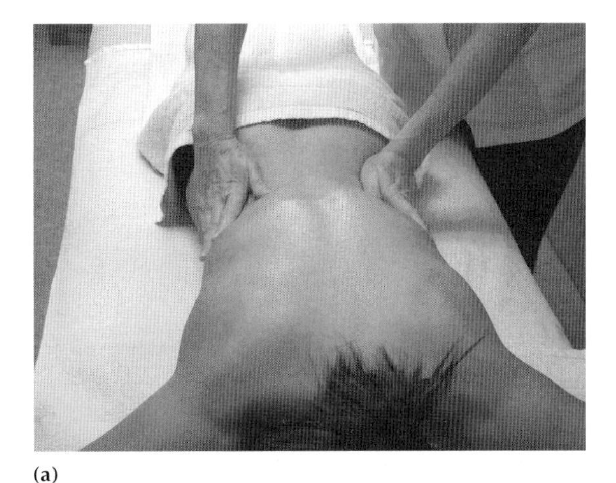

(a)

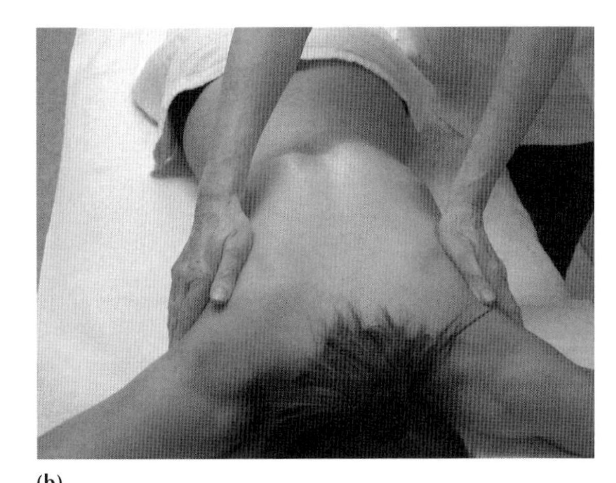

(b)

Figure 9.2 Back massage: (a) the start of the most lateral stroke of effleurage; (b) the finish of the most lateral stroke of effleurage.

Kneading

Stand in lunge standing. Kneading the back involves keeping your hands much flatter than on the limbs, yet they must curve to the part. The pressure is directed towards the axilla on the main part of the back in an upward and outward direction (Fig. 9.5). Take care that your pressure is such that the depth treats the soft tissues. Poor direction of pressure can cause either uncomfortable compression of

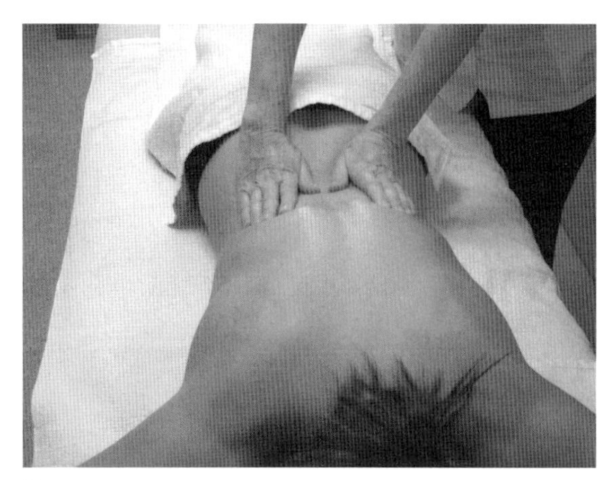

(a)

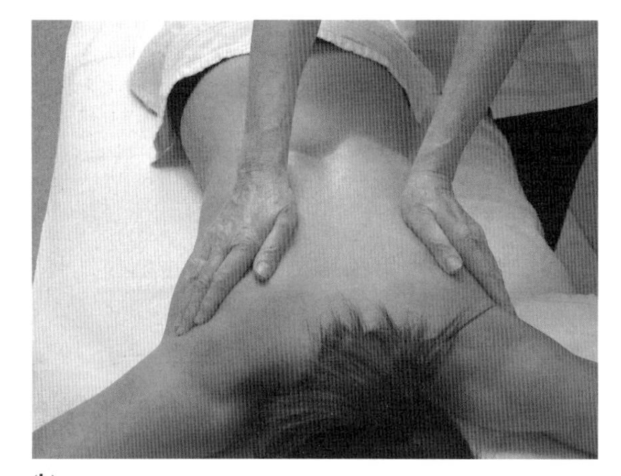

(b)

Figure 9.3 Back massage: (a) the start of the two medial strokes of effleurage; (b) the finish of the second stroke of effleurage.

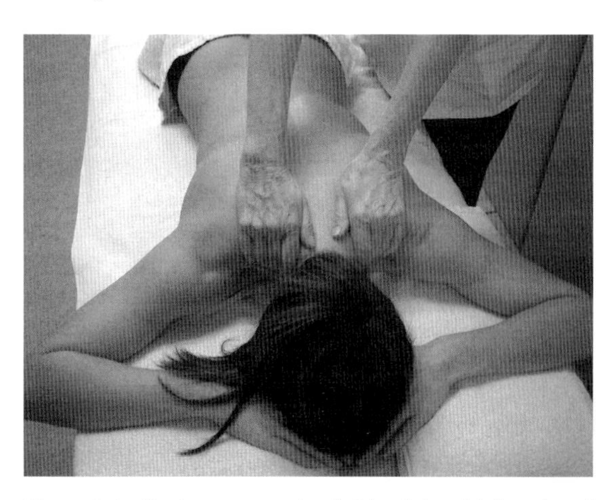

Figure 9.4 Back massage: the finish of the third stroke of effleurage.

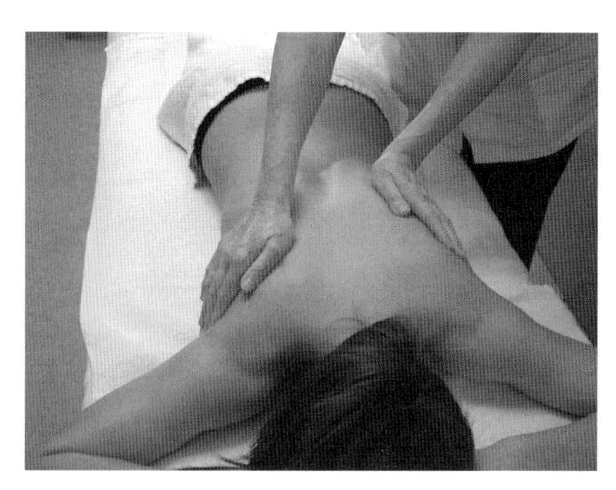

Figure 9.5 Kneading the back. Note the obliquity of the hands and the size of the circle. The two hands are at the maximum points of their circles from each other.

the trunk or equally uncomfortable movement of the body either up and down or from side to side on the support.

Alternate, double-handed kneading

The lines of work proceed downwards from:

- Just below the axilla to the outside of the buttocks.
- Over the scapula to the buttocks.
- Over the superior angle of the scapula to the buttocks.

Work in three straight lines. A narrow back will be adequately treated with two lines of work and, obviously, a broad back may need four lines of work. Each line should overlap that adjacent by half a hand width.

Your own standing position should be lunge standing, with the outer leg forward and your inner hip against the couch at about the level of the patient's thighs or knees. As you work down the back, you should transfer your weight from your forward to your rear leg by gradually easing your touching thigh down the couch. In order to use your hands with even weight, lean your trunk sideways across the bed (Fig. 9.5).

As you perform the kneading, you will find that it is necessary to start with your hands slightly oblique to the long axis of the back, and to increase the obliquity as you proceed down the back so that on the lumbar region your hands may lie almost horizontally. This change in hand position is essential for maintaining full hand contact (Fig. 9.5), and to allow you to work more deeply on the lumbar area. It is more usual to work with alternate hands, but more depth or more sedative work may be performed using both hands simultaneously; take care, however, not to cause the patient's body to move up and down on the couch.

Do not be tempted to work at the upper back with straight elbows – this causes the whole model to move up and down on the couch.

Single-handed kneading

Single-handed kneading can be performed on any area of the back. It is usual to stand in adapted lunge standing facing across the couch, and either hand may be used. Keep your other hand in firm contact, ready to change hands as you tire or as you work on another area.

Superimposed kneading

Superimposed kneading is performed for a greater depth effect than single-handed work. One hand is placed over the other as in Figs 9.6 and 9.7, and the under hand maintains the contact and pressure up and out towards the axilla, but both hands provide the depth which is transmitted from your feet.

Stand in adapted walk standing facing across the back to treat the opposite side (Fig. 9.6), and in adapted lunge standing obliquely to the couch to treat the nearside (Fig. 9.7). On the opposite side the fingers of both your hands point laterally (Fig. 9.6) and circle clockwise. On the near side your deeper hand should point laterally reinforced by your other hand (Fig. 9.7), and circle counterclockwise. The lines of work are usually from:

- The axilla to the buttock.
- Over the scapula to the buttock.

Some people prefer always to work from proximal to distal, sliding the hands up the back to restart. Others work in a continuous line which starts under the far axilla, goes down to the far buttock, slips medially and goes up to the far scapula, slides across the mid-line and reverses the direction of work down to the adjacent nearside buttock and up the nearside from buttock to axilla. When this type of work is performed, difficulty may be experienced with progressing up the back without dragging on the second and fourth lines. The trick is to perform the circle and pressure, then release your pressure, allowing the skin and subcutaneous tissues you have moved upwards to slide down under your hands as you start the next circle and reapply pressure.

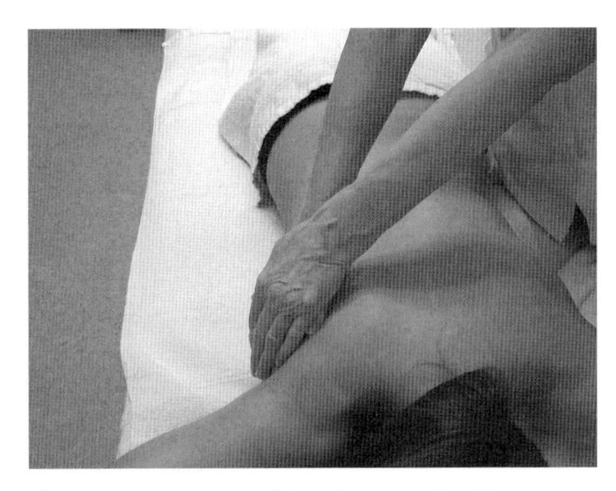

Figure 9.6 Superimposed kneading – the far side.

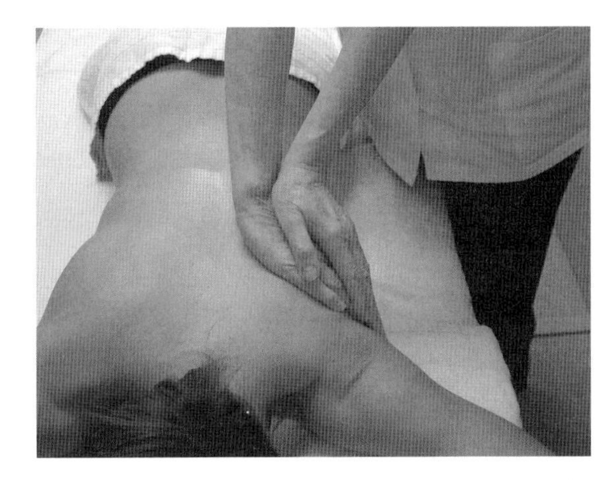

Figure 9.7 Superimposed kneading – the near side. Note the practitioner's total change of position of feet, body and hands.

Thumb kneading

Stand in walk standing facing the head of the couch. Single- or double-handed, alternate thumb knead-

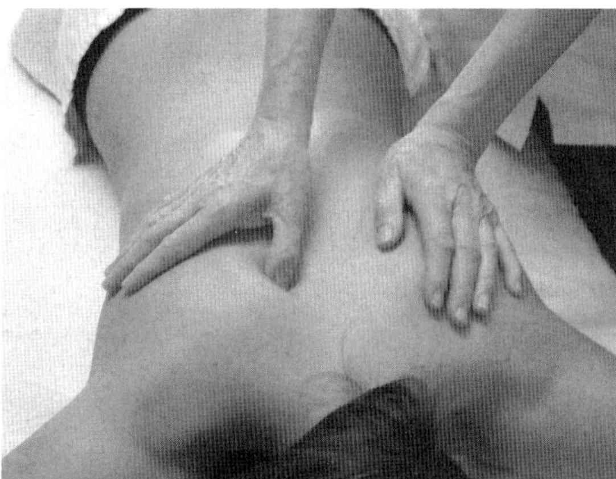

Figure 9.8 Thumb kneading on the sacrospinalis – right thumb working and left relaxing. Note their obliquity and the bulge of tissue on the outer side of the right thumb.

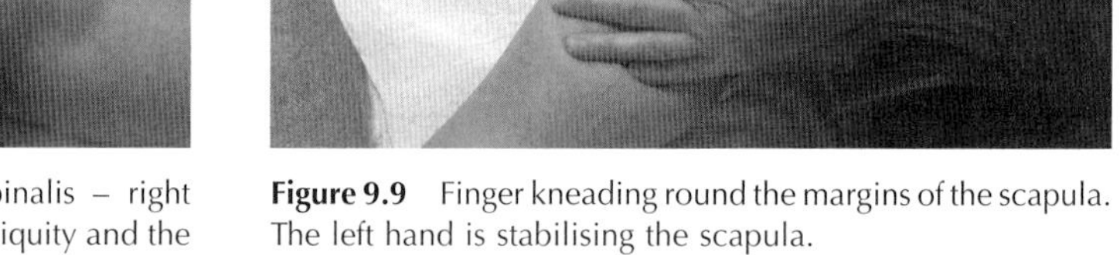

Figure 9.9 Finger kneading round the margins of the scapula. The left hand is stabilising the scapula.

ing may be performed locally to any area of the back. Your thumbs are used as flat as possible, and your finger tips should rest on the back to act as a pivot but not at a depth to perform work (Fig. 9.8).

The area most often given thumb kneading is the length of the sacrospinalis. One thumb works on each side of the spinous processes, and the thumbs should circle round one another (not be lifted off) to move onwards. Again, use a proximal to distal sequence, starting at midscapular level and continuing to upper sacral level. Reach forward to start and transfer your weight backwards as in alternate-handed kneading.

Finger kneading

Stand in adapted walk standing facing the direction of work. Finger kneading is, again, more usually performed on the sacrospinalis, with the fingers of each hand on each side of the spinous processes. The finger pads are used, and greater depth is achieved if you tuck your thumbs into your palms rather than using them for support.

Localised finger pad kneading may be performed to any area such as the margins of the scapula or specific muscles in the second layer of the back, e.g. the rhomboids or the levator scapulae. In this case, always work from the margins of the muscle inwards towards its main muscle bulk (Fig. 9.9), and change direction of your stance as needed.

Skin rolling

Stand in adapted walk standing facing across the couch. Deal with the back one side at a time (Figs 6.18–6.20). The lines of work are the same on each side except that on the side further away from you, work from the mid-line to the side, and on the near side you may roll the skin from the side towards the midline, but some people prefer to perform the manipulation by pulling from the mid-line to the sides by lifting the skin with the thumbs, and thus reversing the performance.

The lines of each rolling of the skin start from the lateral end of the spinous process of the scapula and proceed to below the axilla. The lower lines of work are horizontal from the mid-line to the side. On the near side you work from the side to the mid-line in straight lines, until the area below the axilla is reached when the lines spread towards the spine of the scapula. Thus on the far side you work down the back, and up the back on the near side.

In a similar way short lines of work can be used over the shoulders from near the acromion of the scapula to the base of the neck, working forwards from the scapular spine and from the mid-line to the front and sides on each side of the neck. However, if there is considerable subcutaneous fat, the model/patient may find skin rolling in this area somewhat uncomfortable. The lines of work should be close enough together to achieve an effect on all the skin, not just on a few lines of skin.

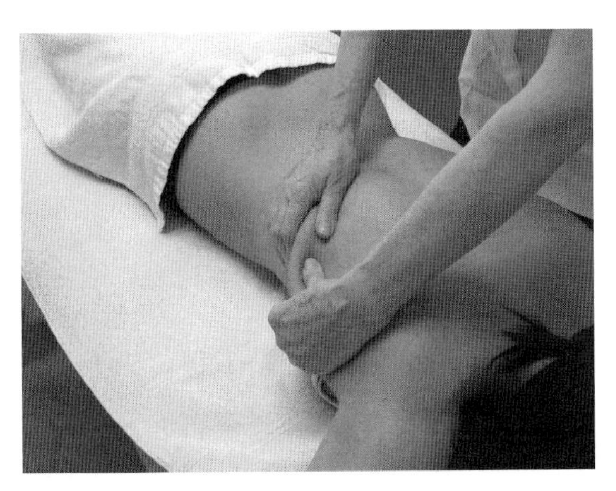

Figure 9.10 Skin wringing.

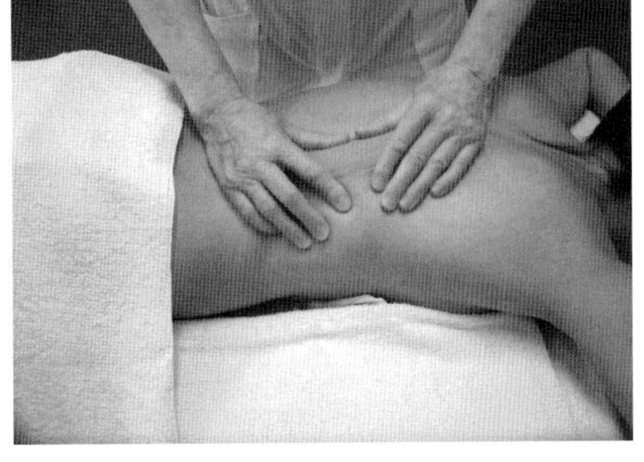

Figure 9.11 Muscle rolling on the sacrospinalis – push compression with the length of the thumbs.

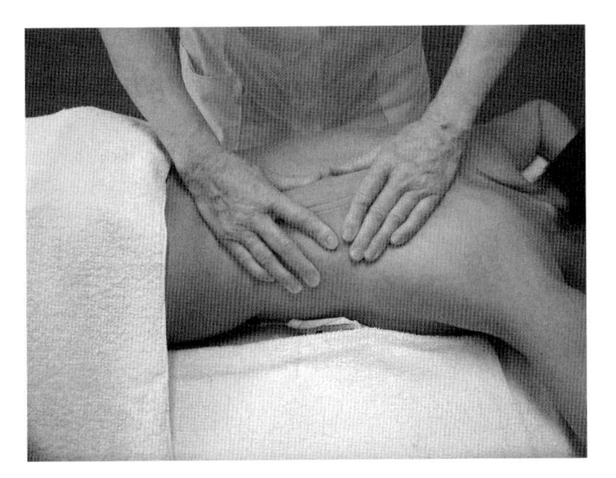

Figure 9.12 Muscle rolling on the sacrospinalis – pull compression with the fingers.

Wringing

Stand in adapted walk standing facing across the couch. Wringing is not an alternative manipulation to skin rolling. It is less conducive to production of a good erythema. Use it for a more mobilising effect.

The lines of work are as those for reinforced/superimposed kneading, i.e. down and up each side of the back. The tissues are lifted up by placing your hands flat on the surface, then exerting pressure with the flat fingers of one hand towards the flat thumb of the other hand (Fig. 9.10). Do not allow your hands to slide on the skin and you should obtain a roll of tissue between your hands. Continuous reversal of the opposite compressing components of the hands will cause a wringing action. Do not try to work too deeply. The object is to lift and wring the tissues. Some people convert this manipulation into picking up, but the author believes that the back muscles are, on the whole, too flat to respond to such a manipulation.

Muscle rolling

Stand in adapted walk standing facing across the couch. Rolling of the sacrospinalis is performed one side at a time. Your two thumbs form a straight line and on the far side are placed to exert pressure outwards from between the vertebral spinous process and the medial margin of the far-side sacrospinalis. All your fingertips in a straight line should be ready to exert pressure on the margin of the sacrospinalis adjacent to the rib angles/lateral processes of the vertebrae. Now, alternately push outwards with depth with your thumbs (Fig. 9.11) and then press inwards and medially with your fingertips (Fig. 9.12) and then release the pressure with each set of hand components as the other set exerts pressure, and move them on to the adjacent area so that you proceed down and then up the muscle.

On the near side of the back your fingertips will work on the medial margin of the sacrospinalis, and your thumb lengths on the lateral margin of the muscle. The lines can proceed from the mid-scapular to the sacral region on the back.

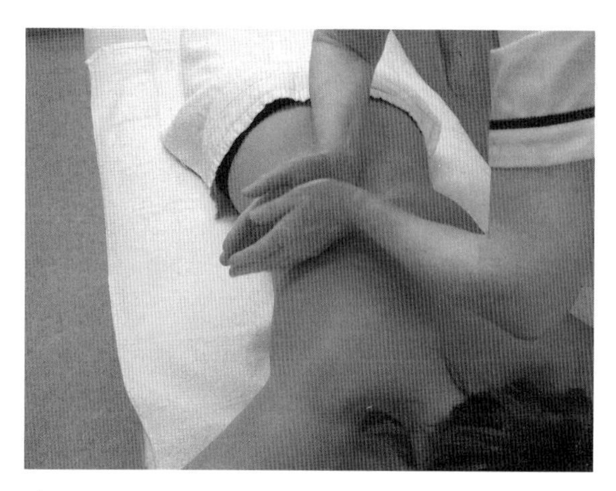

Figure 9.13 Hacking on the back – across the fibres of the latissimus dorsi.

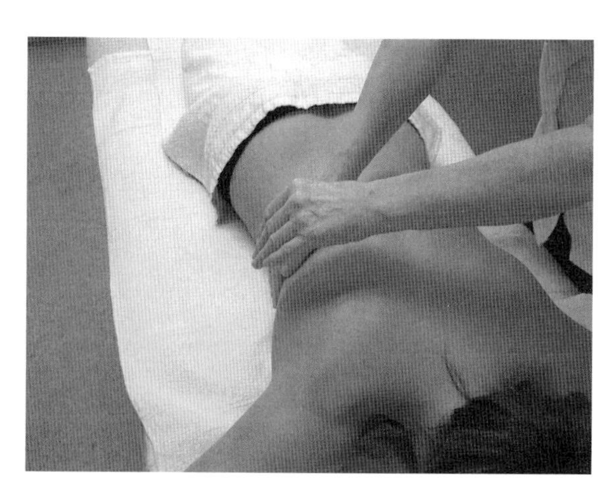

Figure 9.14 Clapping on the back.

You may be able to roll the margins of the latissimus dorsi, and by careful palpation to identify and roll levator scapulae. This latter muscle is, however, more likely to need treatment with a neck condition.

Hacking and clapping

Stand in walk standing facing across the couch. Hacking and clapping on the back is done in the four lines described for kneading, i.e. two each side of the mid-line, and is started under the more distant axilla.

Work down the far side to the lumbar area and move medially and work up to below the spine of the scapula (Fig. 9.13). Avoid the spine by jumping your hands across the mid-line by slightly lifting (and, in the case of hacking, pronating them more), stepping one pace backwards to do so, and continue down the medial line on the nearside of the back, then up again to the axilla.

If you wish to include the neck in the lines of work, start on the far side of the neck and work down the upper fibres of the trapezius, making a little hop over the lateral part of the spine of the scapula to continue to the axilla, and on down the back. At the near side, when you reach the axilla you must turn your body towards the patient's head and hop your hands over the spine of the near-side scapula to work up the near side of the neck.

Clapping on the back should have a similar depth over all areas, but be lighter on the neck (Fig. 9.14). Hacking should vary in depth so that the more bony areas have lighter treatment than those that have more soft tissue bulk, where the work should be deeper.

THE GLUTEAL REGION

Some practitioners treat both buttocks at once, but the patient may suffer discomfort as bilateral work tends to separate the gluteal cleft. Much deeper work is also feasible if one side is treated at a time.

Preparation of the patient

A similar arrangement to that for the back is used. To expose only one buttock, stand on the opposite side of the prone patient, grasp the towels with both hands, one each at the upper and lower levels of the buttock and lift them towards you, turning the central part between your hands over as you do so. In this way, an oblong area is uncovered with the covers pleated on each side of the exposed area.

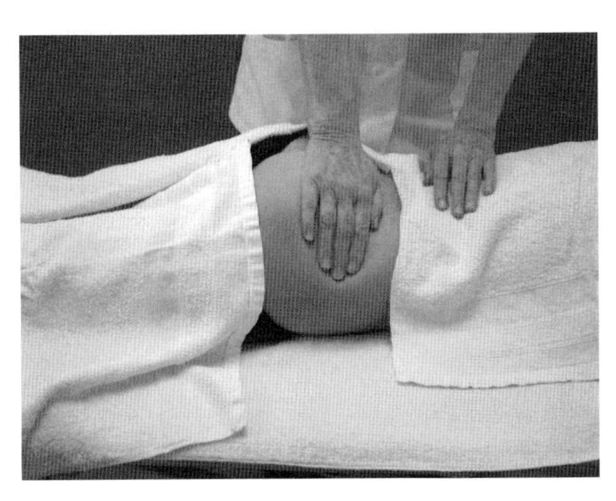

Figure 9.15 The glutei – effleurage starting position. The thumb is on the cross marking the posterior superior iliac spine and is pivoting to stroke along the iliac crest.

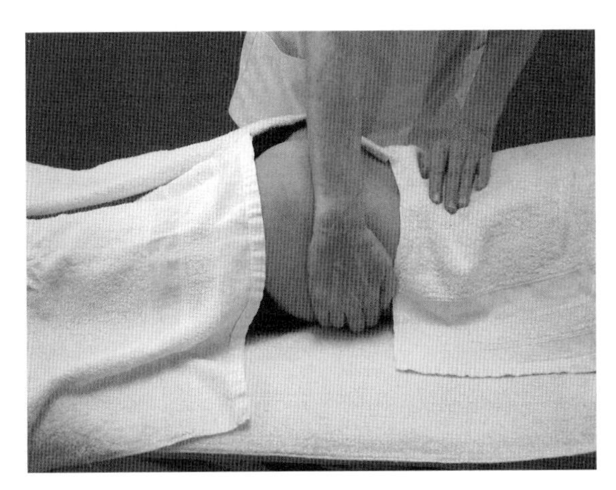

Figure 9.16 The glutei – effleurage: the finish of all the strokes.

Effleurage

Stand in walk standing. Three effleurage strokes are usually performed, each finishing at the groin. It is very important not to pull the buttocks apart, which is uncomfortable, and this is avoided by making every effleurage stroke curve. The first stroke is started with your hand nearest the patient's feet on the middle of the buttock and your thumb on the posterior, superior, iliac spine – marked by the dimple (Fig. 9.15). Pivot your hand so that your thumb strokes round the whole iliac crest, then adduct it to meet your palm and continue to stroke down and out until the fingers can curve under the body to above the groin (Fig. 9.16). The next two strokes curve, respectively, with an upward arc and a downward arc, from the same mid-point of the buttock to the same point above the groin. When the patient is lying with a pillow under the abdomen, there is a triangular gap formed by the upper thigh, the lower abdomen and the support. This is the groin – immediately above the superior border of the femoral triangle.

Kneading

Stand in walk standing. As in performing effleurage, it is more usual to treat each side of the gluteal region separately. Kneading this region is performed in walk standing facing the couch. The opposite buttock is treated.

Start by thinking of two or three lines of work which follow the lines of the main muscle fibres from above medially to below laterally. Place one hand, usually that nearest the feet, so that it lies across the muscle fibres and over the gluteus minimus and gluteus medius and work down and out towards their insertions on the upper extremity of the femur. Next, move your hand, still oblique, to the origin of the gluteus maximus on the iliac crest and work down and out to the fascia lata. Repeat if necessary for a third, more medial line of work.

Superimposed kneading

Superimposed kneading should be used when the muscle bulk is great, using exactly the same lines of work. The kneading manipulation, in both single-handed and superimposed work, is done in such a manner that the pressure is on to and through the glutei, and with great depth in the second and third lines of work, but on the more lateral line the pressure is directed inwards as though pulling towards yourself (Fig. 9.17).

Frictions

Circular frictions

Stand in adapted lunge standing. Circular frictions can be performed on selected areas to achieve local,

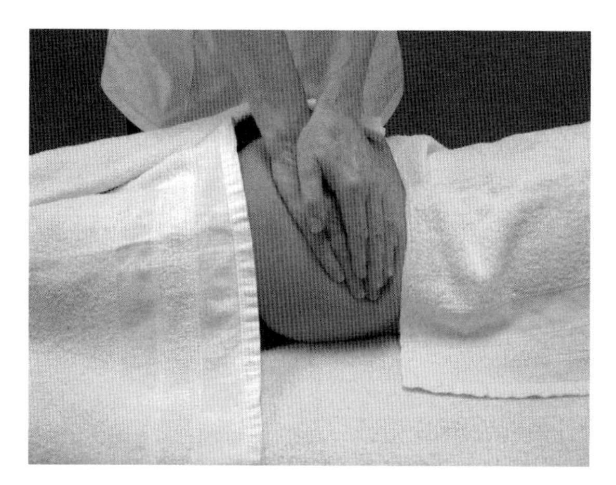

Figure 9.17 The glutei – superimposed kneading: note the contact hand lies across the muscle fibres.

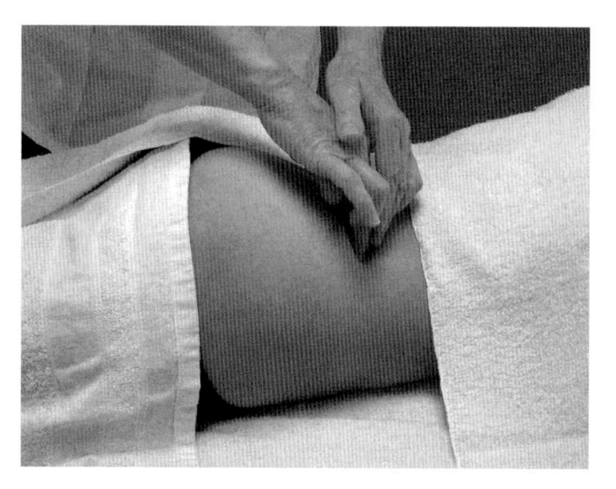

Figure 9.18 Circular frictions to the attachments on the iliac crest.

deep effects. The margin of the iliac crest over aponeuritic structures giving rise to the muscles is an area sometimes needing attention. Use your unsupported thumb or fingers and gradually encroach inwards to the area of discomfort (Fig. 9.18).

Picking up

Work in the same lines along the length of the muscle fibres as used for kneading. Stand in walk standing, using your body weight by transferring

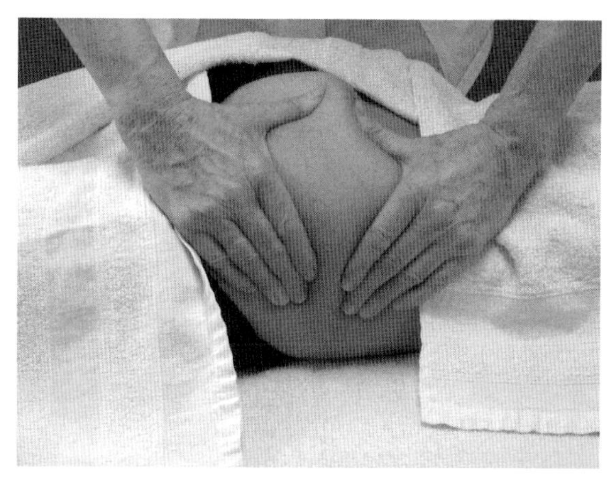

Figure 9.19 The glutei – picking up: along the muscle fibres.

your weight forwards and backwards to exert deep pressure on the pressure phase of the picking-up manipulation. Your hands will thus also have a maximum span, so that the muscles can be lifted and squeezed more easily (Fig. 9.19). The lines of work are short, and you can work up and down the muscles using single-handed, alternate picking up.

Wringing

Wringing may be feasible on some subjects. Your position and lines of work are as for picking up, but the muscle bulk is passed between your hands once it has been lifted by exerting pressure with all the fingers of one hand and the thumb and thenar eminence of the other hand at the same time.

Hacking and clapping

Stand in walk standing. The lines of work are as for kneading. Hacking and clapping (Figs 9.20 and 9.21) can both have considerable depth, but very bulky tissues may need beating or pounding, which can be very deep without stinging and which are less uncomfortable for the operator to perform.

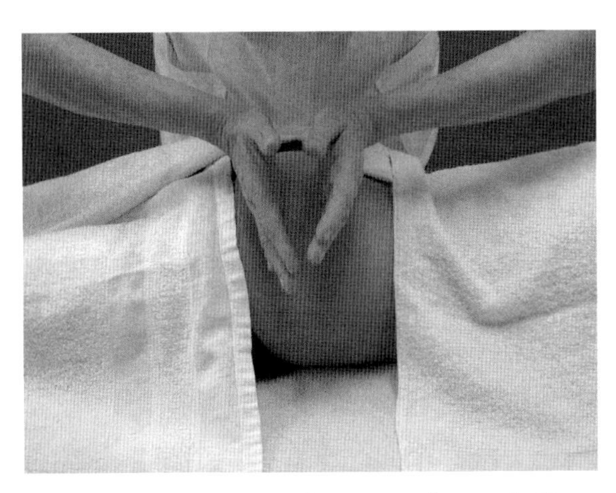

Figure 9.20 The glutei – hacking: across the muscle fibres.

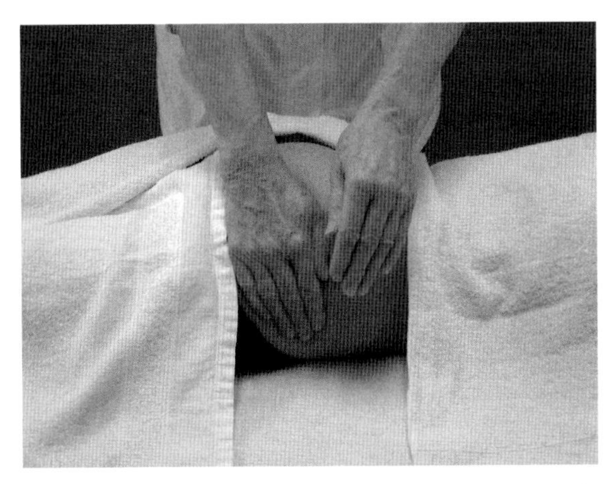

Figure 9.21 The glutei – clapping: across the muscle fibres.

THE NECK

There are four positions for neck massage.

Client in prone lying

A similar arrangement to that for the back is used, but the towel is turned back to the level of the upper lumbar region. For work in this position, stand level with the patient's hips and in lunge standing. Lean sideways towards the patient.

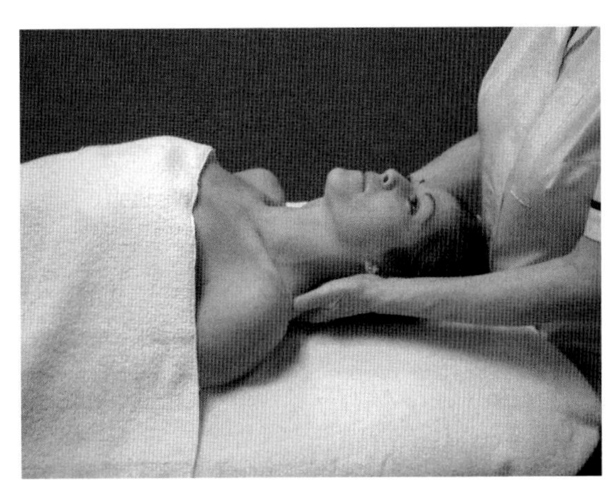

Figure 9.22 The position of the model and practitioner for treatment of the neck when it is very painful. Effleurage – neck to axilla.

Client in lying

The patient lies supine with one or no pillows under the head. The therapist sits at the head of the couch (Fig. 9.22). This is an excellent position in which to massage a very painful neck with much protective spasm.

Client in side lying

The position of side lying, with two head pillows and a pillow at the front of the patient to support the upper arm, can be used for unilateral work. The large towel should be arranged to leave the upper side of the neck and the scapular region free to be massaged (Fig. 9.23). Stand behind the patient in walk standing at about the level of his or her waist.

Client in forward lean sitting

Arrange the couch or a table against a wall and place on it a pile of pillows against which the patient can lean with full support of his or her upper trunk, arms and head. Ask the patient to sit in front of the table or couch, preferably on a stool or a chair with

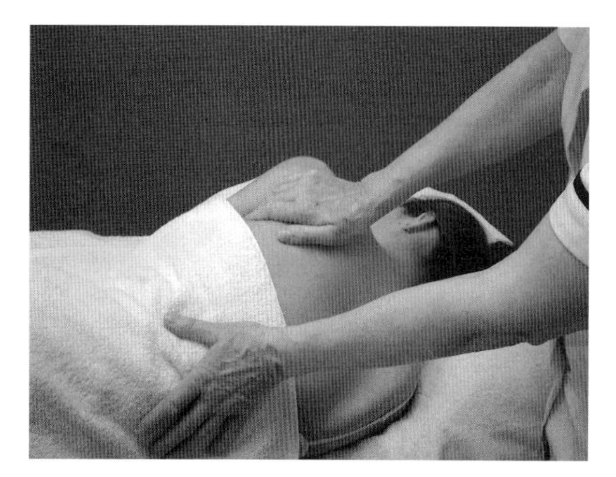

Figure 9.23 The position of the model in side lying for treatment of one side of the neck in side lying. Effleurage – neck to axilla.

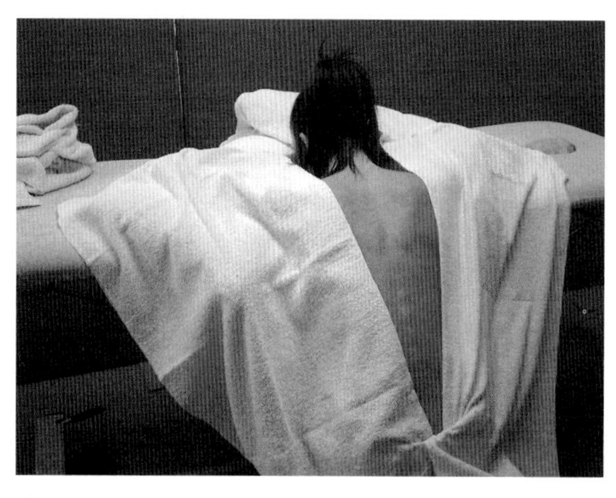

Figure 9.24 Lean forward sitting position of the model for neck massage.

a very low back (Fig. 9.24). Remove the top pillow and spread a large towel on top of the pillow pile and in front of the model. The patient should be already undressed except for the bra in the case of a female. Ask him or her to place both arms on the pillow and towel pile, leaning forward with a straight back and neck. The upper corners of the towel are then lifted, pulled across the patient's arms and tucked into the patient's waistband at the centre back (Fig. 9.24). In the case of a female, the bra can then be undone and slipped off the arms. Replace the top pillow on the pile and ask the patient to lean his or her head against it. If necessary, two top pillows may be crossed as in prone lying, to accommodate the nose. Check that the forward lean is still with a straight back and neck. Stand in walk standing behind the patient, and be prepared to transfer your weight forwards and backwards, and also possibly to bend your hips and knees to gain comfortable access to the thoracic region. You may, additionally, need to take a side step to each side in turn, to gain full access or better pressure for some manipulations. Ensure there is only light pressure on bony prominences and avoid the throat and thyroid gland areas.

Effleurage

The neck strokes are performed with the flat of the fingers starting on the sides of the neck and going to the supraclavicular glands. A second stroke down the back of the neck goes to the same glands, and a third stroke if necessary may go down the back and sides of the neck with more of the hand in contact, and in side lying, turning over the area of the medial angle of the scapula to continue to the axilla (Figs 9.22 and 9.23).

Similar strokes to those performed on the back should also be performed when the patient is in prone lying or lean-forward sitting.

When the patient is in lying or side lying the lines of work are devised to follow the above patterns, bearing in mind the need for maximum hand contact and a comfortable and effective stroke, finishing at a group of lymph glands with slight overpressure and a pause.

Kneading

The neck is a difficult area as it is so confined and may be very short in some subjects. If it is treated with the patient in prone lying, then kneading may start on the neck and proceed down to whole-handed work on the wider part of the back (Fig. 9.25). As much of your hand as possible should be used for kneading, whatever the position used for the patient.

The finger pads are used on the posterior aspect from the occiput (Fig. 9.25) down to where the

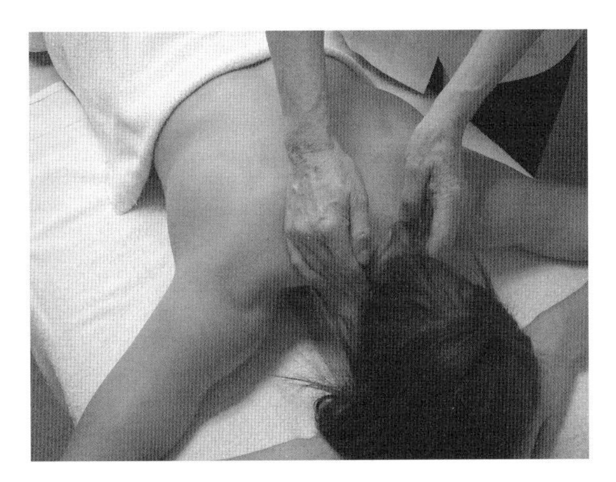

Figure 9.25 Neck massage – kneading.

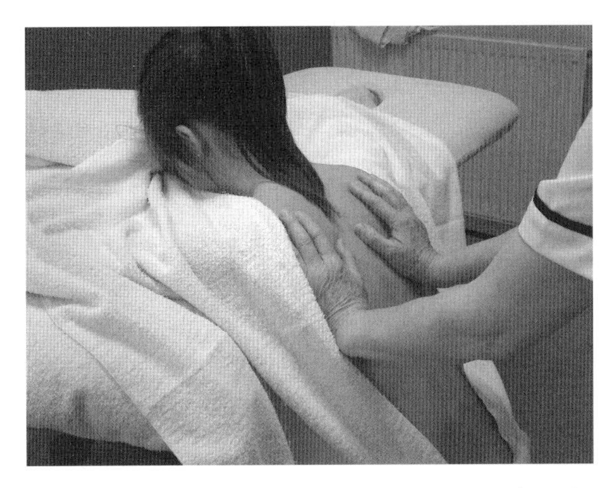

Figure 9.26 Neck muscles – kneading continued to the middle and lower fibres of the trapezius.

neck widens, and then the hands are flattened, possibly overlapped, and continue on the interscapular area. On the lateral aspect of the neck, the fronts of the two distal phalanges of all four fingers are used until the swell of the trapezius allows your whole hand to be in contact, using your palm at the back and your fingers at the front on the upper fibres of the trapezius. A squeeze knead is now performed. Flat-handed kneading is performed on the upper thoracic area in a line from the interscapular area towards the axilla (Fig. 9.26). When using your fingers, the pressure should always avoid contact with bone (the spinous and transverse processes of the upper cervical vertebrae) and should be upwards and inwards on the muscle bulk lying between the processes.

With careful adaptation of your hand the neck muscles may be treated if required from occipital to mid-scapular levels, and so may the upper and also middle and lower fibres of the trapezius throughout their length by turning the patient into side lying (Fig. 9.27). With the patient supine, flat finger kneading can be performed on the upper trapezius muscles (Fig. 9.28).

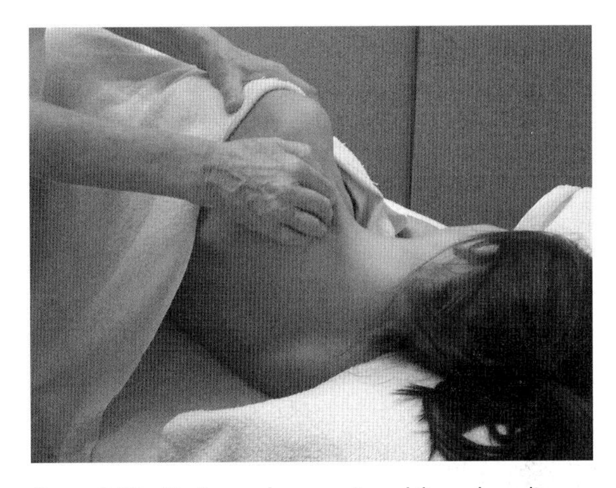

Figure 9.27 Neck muscles – continued finger kneading on the trapezius with the model in side lying.

Picking up

Place one hand round the whole posterior aspect of the neck and perform a single-handed picking-up manipulation which can evolve into simultaneous work done on the lower part of the upper fibres of

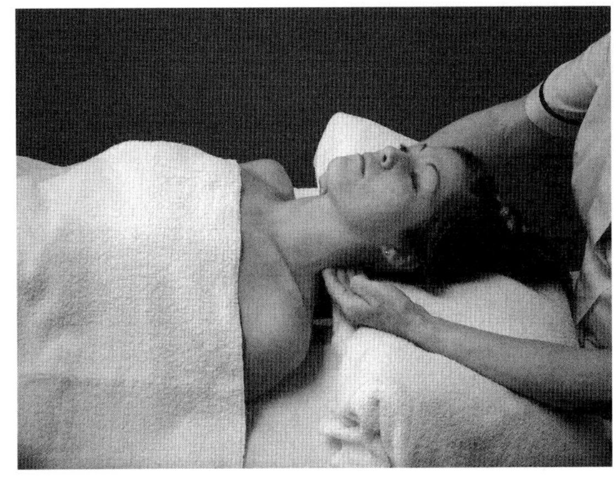

Figure 9.28 Neck finger kneading to the posterior muscles with the model supine.

the trapezius with one of your hands on each side of the neck. Your fingers should be over the front of the muscle and your palms and thumbs at the back. The change from one- to two-handed work must be smooth.

Muscle rolling

The posterior column of the neck muscles on each side may be rolled by placing your fingers just behind the transverse processes and your thumbs alongside the spinous processes and on the same side as your fingers (as on the sacrospinalis). Work on each side in turn.

The sternocleidomastoid can be rolled in a similar manner (be very careful to exert sideways pressure only) if the patient is in a suitable position, but you may find it more feasible to put your index and ring finger tips one on each side of the muscle, and roll it by small supination and pronation movements.

Hacking and clapping

Hacking and clapping may be performed on the neck alone, with the lines of work starting near the occiput and proceeding to the lateral part of the shoulder. Two lines may be used – one more lateral and one more posterior on the neck. The more lateral line would continue on the anterosuperior part of the upper fibres of the trapezius, while the more posterior line would continue on the posterior part of the same muscle fibres. Lines of work extending on to the upper thoracic region follow the lines described earlier.

In clapping the neck it may be necessary to work mainly with the flat fingers, and be careful not to sting. (Listen for stinging – the sound is sharp.)

10 Massage to the face and scalp

Margaret Hollis and Elisabeth Jones

Facial massage is usually given with the patient in supine lying, and he or she should be given a pillow under the knees, as well as a pillow under the head at the end of the couch. The practitioner sits at the head of the bed (Fig. 10.1). Check constantly as you work that as the patient relaxes, the head does not 'sink' into the pillow causing the neck to extend and the face to tilt.

Preparation of the patient

Ask the patient to remove outer clothing from the neck and shoulders and to remove shoulder straps. Necklaces and earrings should be removed as should make-up, which can become smudged. Obviously, spectacles must be removed, but discuss the removal of contact lenses with the patient. They must be removed if using essential oils. If the hair is long or likely to obstruct, it can be restrained by a headband.

Ask the patient to lie down, and cover the body up to the subclavicular level if he or she so wishes.

FACE MASSAGE

Most of the manipulations are performed with the fingers or finger pads, and it is important to control the position of the rest of your hand, including the thumb, so that you do not rest on the patient's face. Ensure there is only medium to light pressure, and avoid the throat and thyroid area.

The manipulations that may be used are:

- Effleurage.
- Finger tip kneading.
- Wringing.
- Plucking.
- Tapping.
- Vibrations to the exit foramina of the trigeminal nerve.
- Vibrations over the sinuses.
- Occipitofrontalis stretching to obtain scalp movement.
- Clapping to the area of platysma.

Effleurage

Effleurage is directed from the mid-line of the face to just below the ear (subauricular glands), taking care that as you effleurage you do not constantly move the ear lobe. The pressure should be moderate to light.

As much of the palmar surface of the hand as possible is used to start the effleurages. The finish is always with the finger pads, as the palms lift to

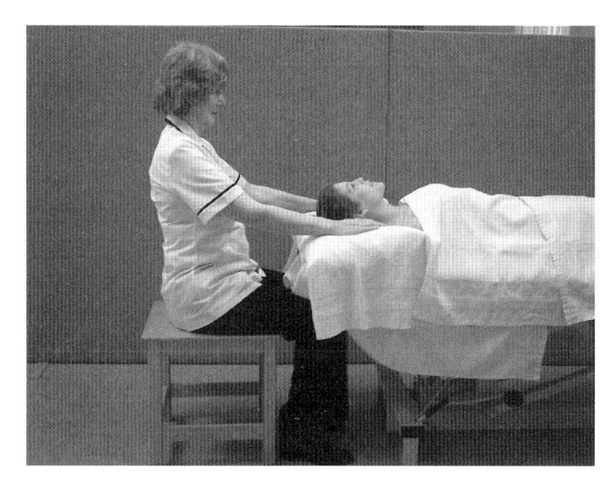

Figure 10.1 Starting position.

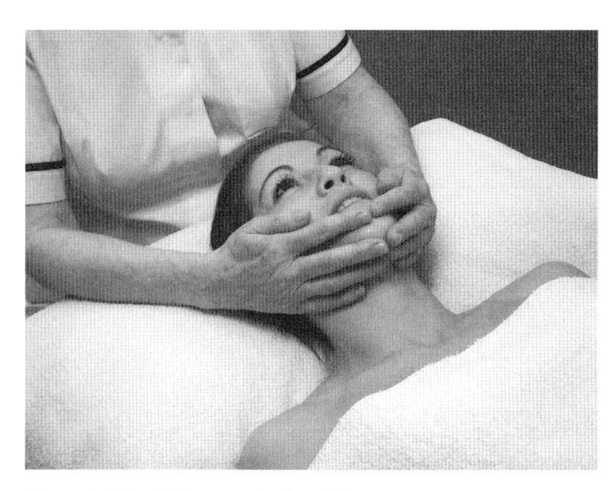

Figure 10.3 Effleurage to the chin.

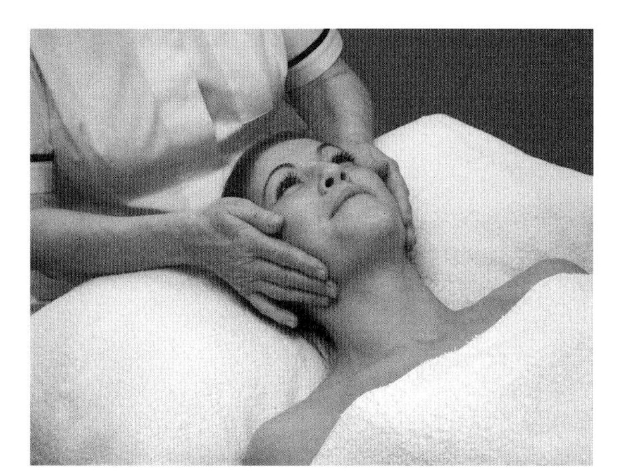

Figure 10.2 Effleurage – finishing position for all three strokes shown in Figs 10.3, 10.4 and 10.5.

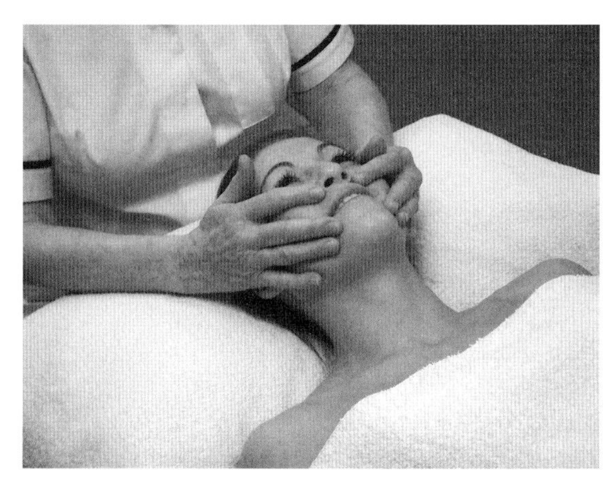

Figure 10.4 Effleurage to the cheeks.

clear the ear (Fig. 10.2). After each effleurage, stroke back gently to the next starting position.

The **first** effleurage goes from under the chin – use your full hands (Fig. 10.3).

The **second** effleurage starts with the fingers spread above and below the mouth – use your full hand. The **third** effleurage starts at the nose – use your finger tips to start, then your full hands (Fig. 10.4). On a small face, the **second** and **third** effleurages are often combined.

The **fourth** effleurage starts in the mid-line of the forehead and curves downwards – use your full hands, and repeat for a **fifth** effleurage if the forehead is high (Fig. 10.5).

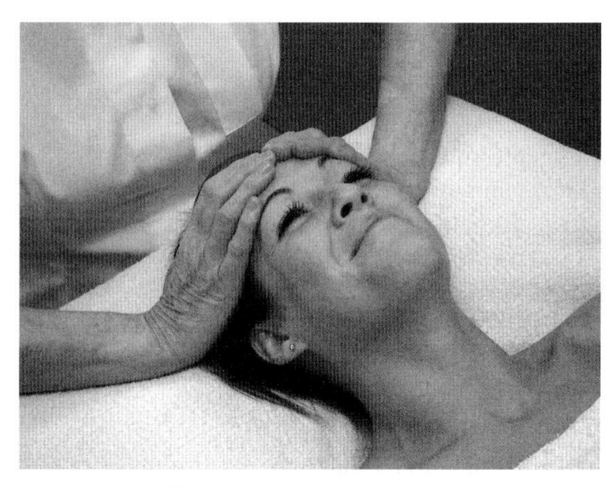

Figure 10.5 Effleurage to the forehead.

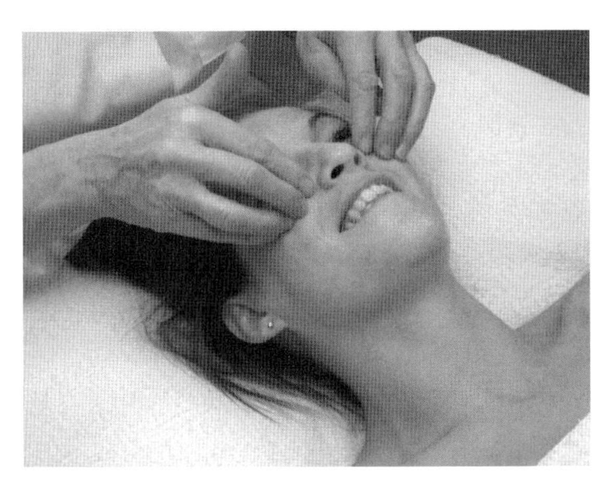

Figure 10.6 Kneading the cheeks.

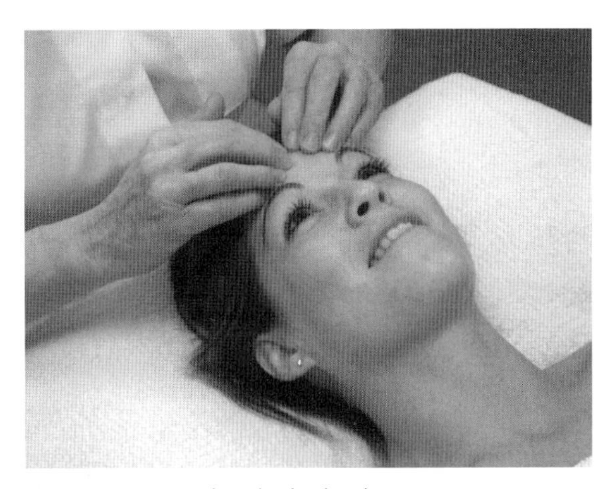

Figure 10.7 Kneading the forehead.

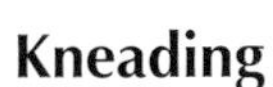

Kneading

The lines of work are similar to those for effleurage, proceeding from the mid-line to the subauricular area with moderate pressure, returning to the next position with a gentle stroke:

- The first line under the chin is done with the flat of the fingers, which are also used on the cheeks to finish the next three movements (Fig. 10.6).
- Then the chin to ear line is started with the two distal phalanges.
- Next the upper lip to ear line is started with one finger pad.
- The nose to ear line is done with one or two finger pads.
- On the forehead two or three lines are performed with two, three or four finger pads (Fig. 10.7).

All the manipulations are performed with a lifting pressure upwards and inwards so that the delicate muscles are not dragged.

Wringing

This is a finger tip wringing performed between the finger pads of the index fingers and thumbs. It is a very small manipulation. Start at the corner of the mouth and work out to the ear, then across the chin

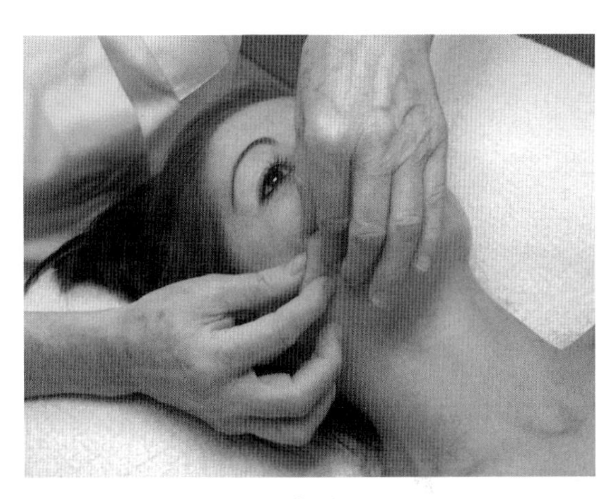

Figure 10.8 Wringing the cheeks.

to the other ear. Now work back to the mouth, out to the ear from the nose on one cheek (Fig. 10.8) and across the forehead in three lines to the opposite ear, in to the nose and you are back at the start (Fig. 10.9).

Some people consider that this manipulation should be avoided when treating facial palsy, in case the muscles are overstretched, but if the depth is light and the speed is fast, there is little reason to omit it.

Plucking

Plucking is a stimulating manipulation performed by the tips of the thumb and index finger, in which

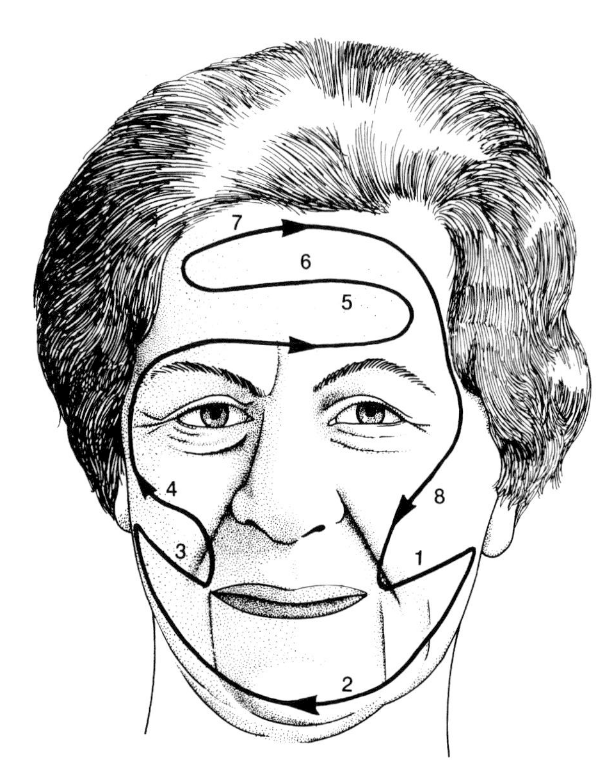

Figure 10.9 The lines of work for wringing.

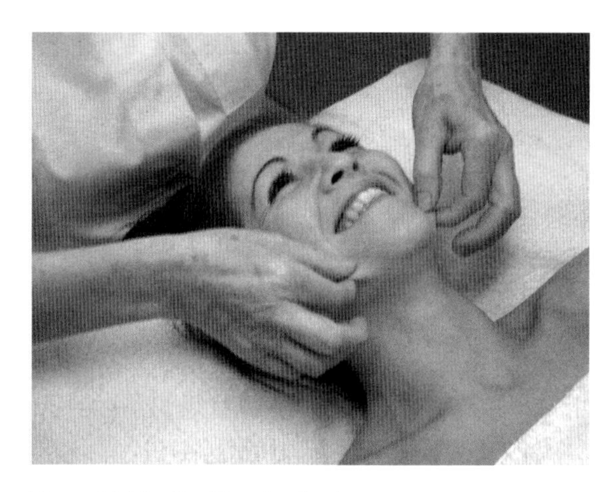

Figure 10.10 Plucking the cheeks.

the tissues are literally 'plucked', i.e. grasped and let go very quickly (Fig. 10.10). If the tissues were held longer you would be pinching. Plucking may be performed with one or both hands simultaneously, in similar work lines to kneading.

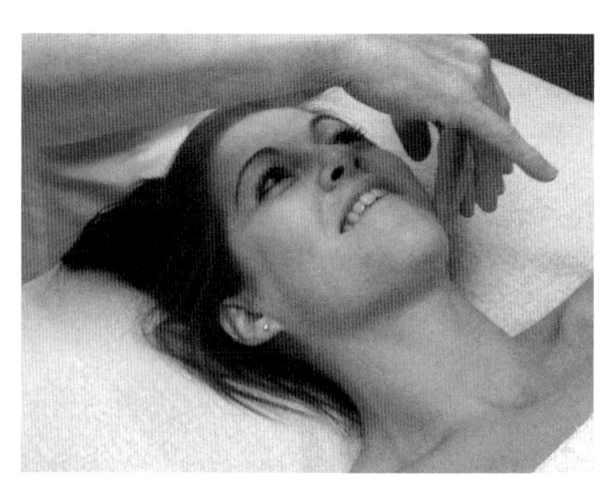

Figure 10.11 Tapping the cheeks.

Tapping

Tapping is performed with the fingertips (Fig. 10.11). Either one, two or three finger tips are used according to the size of the area of the face being treated. If two or more fingers are used, they may tap simultaneously, or in rapid succession as in striking two or three adjacent piano keys. The light tap should be firm enough to cause slight indentation of the skin at each tap. Note that the simultaneous use of two or more fingers is likely to be heavier than sequence tapping. The lines of work are those used in effleurage. The work may be performed on both sides of the face simultaneously, or one side of the face at a time.

Vibrations

Exit foramina of the trigeminal nerve

Finger tip vibrations may be performed using either the index or the middle finger tip over the points of exit of the ophthalmic, maxillary and mandibular divisions of the trigeminal nerve. They emerge respectively from the supraorbital notch and the infraorbital and mental foramina. The finger tip should rest lightly over the exit, and constant vibrations of a small dimension are performed until discomfort diminishes. This technique is used in the treatment of both trigeminal neuralgia and tension headaches.

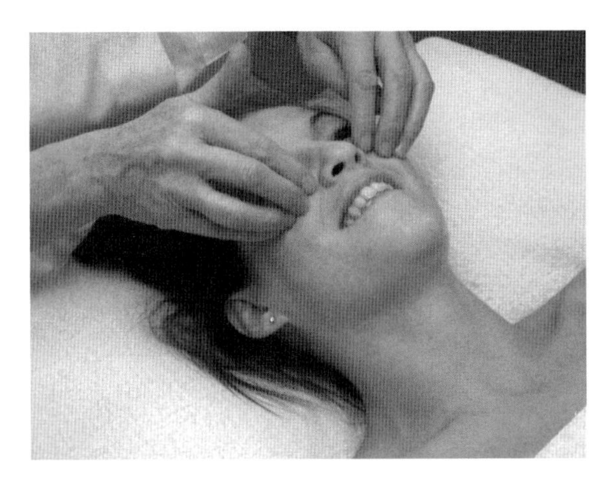

Figure 10.12 Vibrations with all the finger tips over the maxillary sinus.

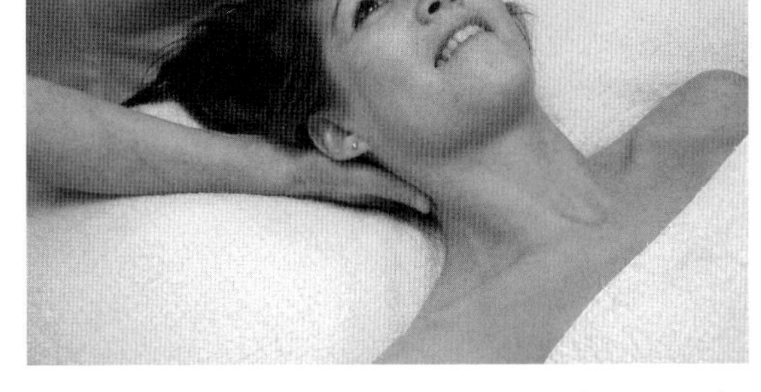

Figure 10.13 One hand over the anterior and one over the posterior belly of the occipitofrontalis to rock the muscle and scalp.

Over the sinuses

If the tips of your fingers and thumbs are held bunched together, and your hand is raised so that the ends of the tips rest on the skin, vibrations can be performed over a circular area (Fig. 10.12). The fingertips can be placed over the area of the frontal sinus and of the maxillary sinus, and static vibrations performed to encourage a mechanical effect on the sinuses when they are congested and perhaps blocked. The patient can be taught to perform this manipulation, and may find that the frontal sinuses are cleared best when he or she is upright and the maxillary sinuses are in the side lying position. The right sinus is drained in left side lying and vice versa.

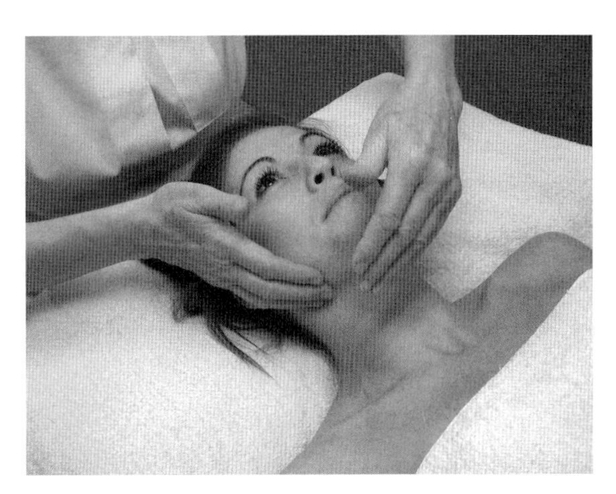

Figure 10.14 Clapping the platysma.

Muscle stretching

Occipitofrontalis

Place the palmar surface of one hand on the forehead and the palmar surface of the other hand under the occiput. Move them simultaneously so that the hand on the forehead takes the front of the scalp downwards towards the eyebrows, and the hand on the occiput takes the back of the scalp upwards (Fig. 10.13). The movement should be smooth and slow and reversed equally smoothly. The scalp will be felt to move forwards and backwards. This stretching movement is of great use in severe headache when the two bellies of the occipitofrontalis often remain in painful spasm.

Clapping

To the platysma

The area below the chin can be clapped using the cupped fingers (Fig. 10.14). Your hands must circle round one another in such a manner that the 'strike' is in a forward and upward direction. Be careful

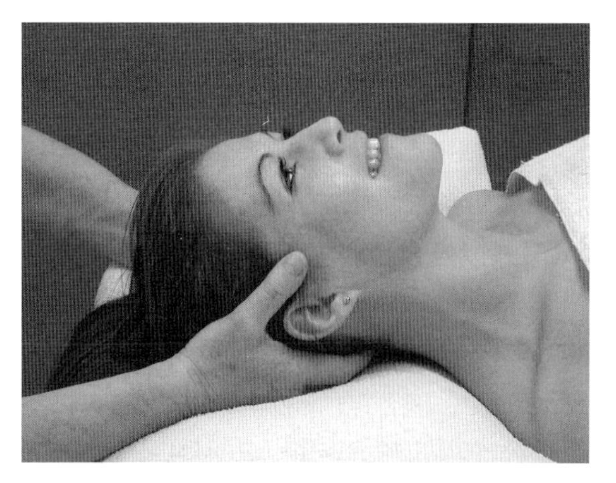

Figure 10.15 Effleurage stroking to the scalp.

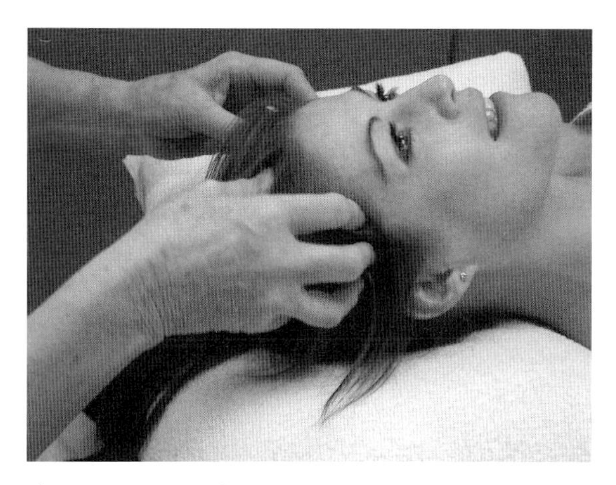

Figure 10.16 Kneading to the scalp.

not to touch the front of the throat, and work at a brisk speed. The patient may learn to do this himself or herself, using the backs of the fingers.

SCALP MASSAGE

Scalp massage is given usually following facial massage with the patient in the supine lying position (the therapist sitting behind as in Fig. 10.1). Scalp massage helps ease tension in the underlying tissues and aids relaxation of the neck, shoulders and whole body.

Effleurage/stroking

The therapist places her hands either side of the patient's temporal region and cups the head in her hands, drawing her hands round the parietal and occipital region of the head and then gently off the head (Fig. 10.15).

Kneading

Kneading of the entire scalp is performed over the same area as for effleurage/stroking ensuring there is definite movement of the galea occipitofrontalis over the cranium underneath. This helps particularly to relieve tension headaches (Fig. 10.16).

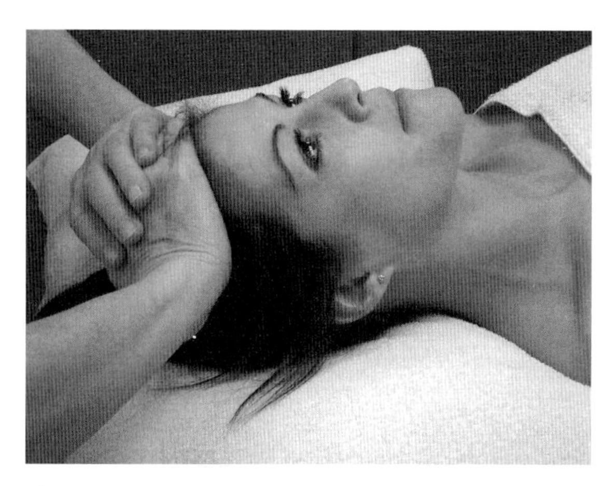

Figure 10.17 Vibrations to the scalp.

Vibrations

Particular attention should be given to the occipital, temporal and frontal attachments of the muscle where there are tight areas. Vibrations are given again over the same area as for effleurage/stroking. Again this facilitates easing of tension in the scalp and helps relieve tension headaches and has a general relaxant effect throughout the whole body (Fig. 10.17).

11 Massage to the abdomen

Margaret Hollis and Elisabeth Jones

The abdomen is usually massaged for one of two specific purposes. The inflated abdomen needs treatment to assist the removal of flatus and the constipated person needs treatment to stimulate the passage of faeces.

Preparation of the patient

Ask the patient to remove all covering of the area so that up to the lower rib case is bared as is the area to the level of the anterior superior spines. Heavy clothing on the chest and pelvis should be removed so that there is no obstruction to access by a roll of clothing. The patient should wear pants or briefs and a vest or bra.

The patient should lie supine on a treatment couch prepared with a towel, with pillow(s) under the knees to keep the lower limbs in a low crook position. Small size pillows which just fit under the knees are less obstructive than full size pillows. A low raise should be applied to the head of the treatment couch; use one to two head pillows.

Cover the upper chest with a towel and the lower limbs with a large bath towel. Stand on the right of the patient for all procedures.

Palpation

The state of the abdomen must be ascertained first. Place your relaxed right hand flat over the area of the umbilicus and exert gentle pressure. This will tell you if there is any tension. Let your hand remain there as you question the patient with regard to painful areas – moving to these areas in turn and gently but firmly using flat fingers to increase the depth of the palpation. If the indication is of no specific area of pain then the following sequence can be used:

(1) Run your hand over the lower ribs from left to right.
(2) Palpate below the left costal margin then the right costal margin, taking particular note of the crossing of the right lateral margin of the rectus abdominus with the costal margin for the gall bladder.
(3) Now use both hands superimposed to palpate more deeply, starting in the right iliac area and paying particular attention to McBurney's point (one-third of the distance from the umbilicus to the anterior superior iliac spine) and the potential content of the ascending colon. Faeces present as firm rouleaux or as a mass.

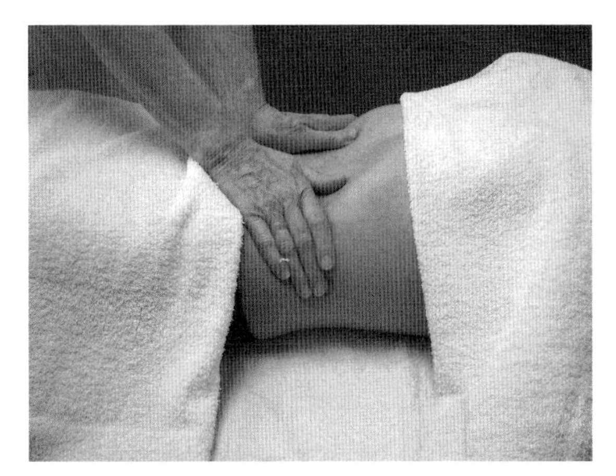

Figure 11.1 Effleurage – the stroke is from the waist to the symphysis pubis.

Continue to the costal margin then move to the right costal margin and palpate down the line of the descending colon to the left iliac area. On slender subjects the depth can be moderate but on obese subjects considerable depth has to be attained before the abdominal content can be palpated.

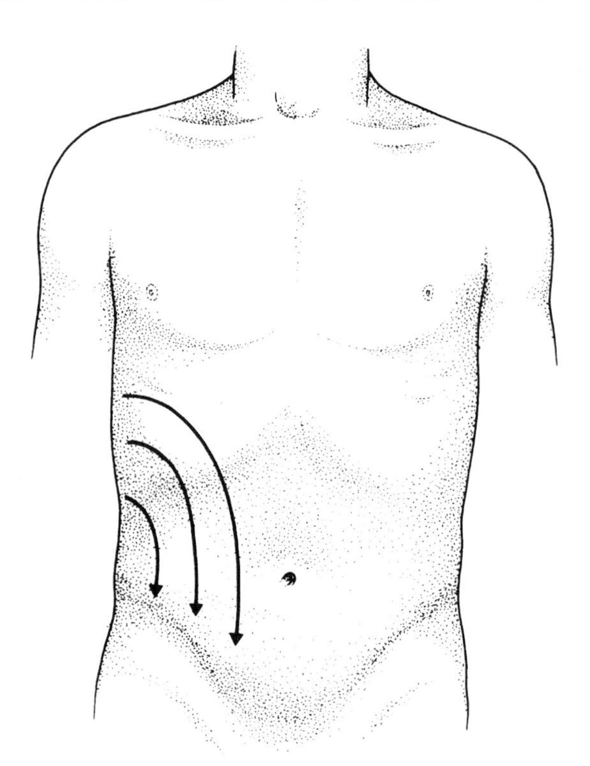

Figure 11.2 The lines of work for effleurage and kneading.

Effleurage

Stand in adapted lunge standing below the level of the patient's hips and lean slightly to your own right to place your right hand on the side of the upper buttock and with your left hand on the left side. Start with a curved stroke going towards the midline ending just above the groin. The second and third strokes each start higher at the side so that the third stroke comes from over the lower ribs (Figs 11.1 and 11.2).

Kneading

The same lines of work as in effleurage may be used and the hands should simultaneously do the same thing. Do not do alternate work with your hands or the patient will rock from side to side (Fig. 11.3a and b).

Vibrations

Vibrations can be performed in several ways.

In walk standing facing across the patient:

(1) With flat hands over the area of the umbilicus, perform stationary vibrations initially of small range and getting larger and deeper (i.e. of bigger amplitude) (Fig. 6.28).
(2) With flat hands following one another across the abdominal area work in the same lines as stroking. This again can start gently and the amplitude can increase.

Brisk lift stroking and shaking

Stand in walk standing facing the patient. Place the hands one each side on the waist in a similar position to the start of vibrations. Stroke deeply and very briskly inwards to the midline. Repeat several

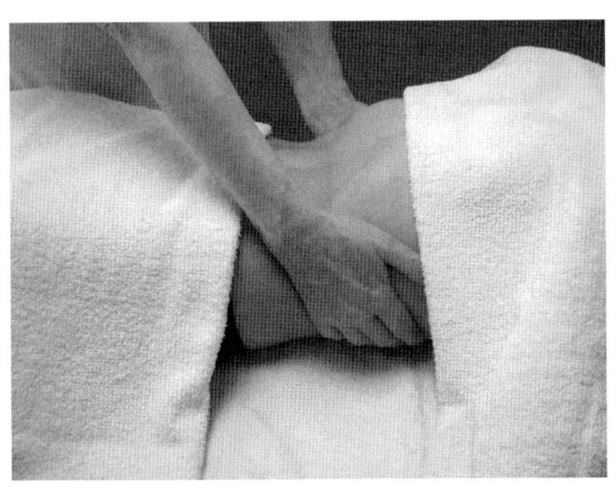

(a)

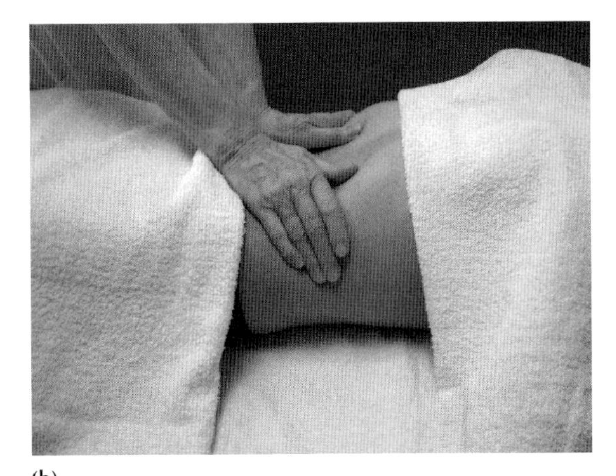

(b)

Figure 11.3 Kneading the abdominal wall: (a) start at the waist; (b) finish over the groin.

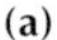

times or intersperse with coarse vibrations done with brisk strokes (Fig. 6.28).

Stroking

The ascending colon

Cup the back of the right hand in the palm of the left hand and place the back of the left forearm near the elbow in the left iliac fossa. Stroke with the backs of the left then right forearm upwards and outwards in the direction of the position of the ascending colon (Fig. 11.4).

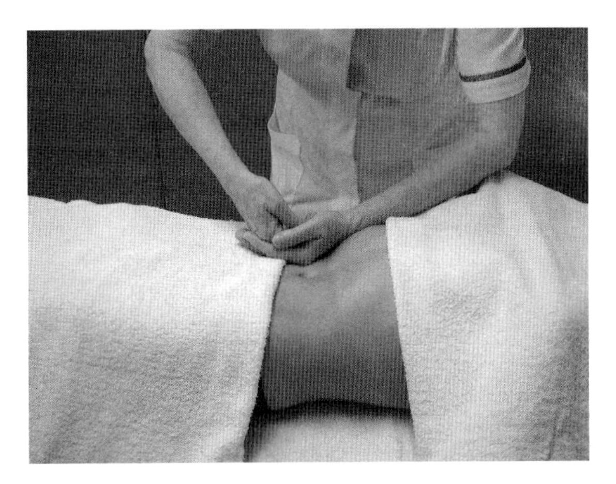

Figure 11.4 Stroking to the colon: start with the ascending colon.

The transverse colon

As you will not know where the transverse colon lies, its position being dependent on the contents and gravity, this is a continuation stroke to take the hands to the left side of the abdomen. As the hands leave the body after the ascending stroke and only the right forearm is in contact on the. ascending stroke, the hands are changed over so that the back of the left hand lies in the right palm. The right wrist leads the way across the abdomen to the left waist (Fig. 11.5a).

The descending colon

The hands are one on top of the other, palm down with the right hand underneath. A deep stroke is performed from the left waist to the left iliac fossa. Greater depth is obtained if the thumb of the underneath (right) hand is adducted and opposed so that it lies in the palm with the tip of the thumb over the proximal phalanx of the third and fourth digits (Fig. 11.5b).

Kneading

The ascending colon

Start in the right iliac fossa and work towards the waist using the right hand cupped so that the fingers

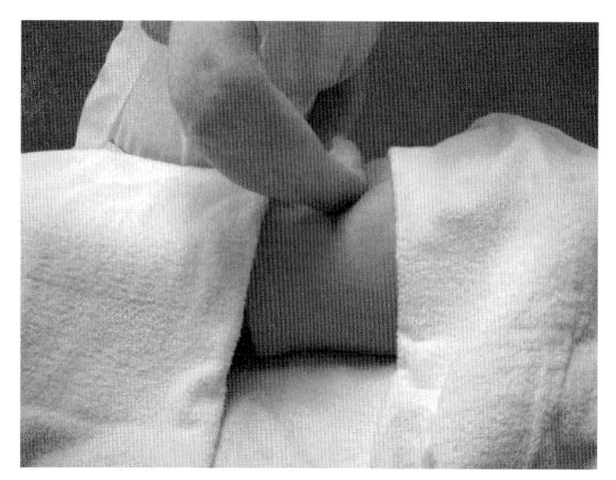

(a)

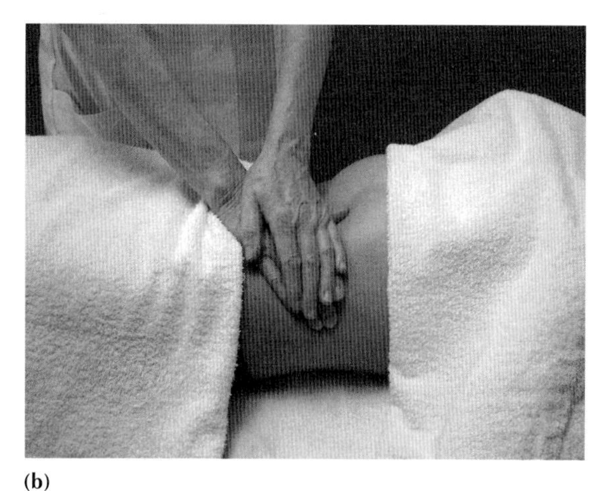

(b)

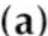

Figure 11.5 Stroking to the colon: (a) the transverse colon – note the hands have changed over; (b) hands turned ready to work down the descending colon.

are slightly elevated from the skin and the kneading is done with the palm. An upward and outward pressure is exerted while retaining the depth.

The descending colon

Start at the left waist and work towards the left iliac fossa using the right hand. Narrow the hand by adducting and opposing the thumb into the palm. Exert downward and medial pressure while retaining the depth and finish with flat fingers as the palm has to be lifted to avoid the pubic area.

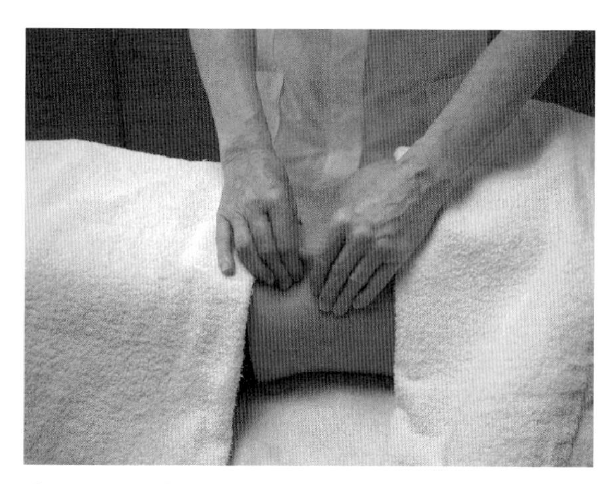

Figure 11.6 Skin wringing to the abdomen.

Rolling

This manipulation can be performed if the content of the colon can be palpated as a sausage-like mass. The rolling is performed as in muscle rolling described in Chapter 6, but the area will be more circumscribed. Use the finger pads of both hands in line on one side of the mass and the thumbs in line on the other side of the mass. Roll gently forth and back and move on after a few manipulations. This manipulation can be used on both the descending and ascending colons.

Skin wringing

This manipulation is performed by laying your hands on the abdomen and lifting the skin into your hands by pressure from both thumbs lying flat and tip to tip, and from the fingers lying with all four pads in line (Fig. 11.6). Once the skin is lifted, a wringing manipulation is performed by bringing the fingers of one hand towards the thumb of the other hand.

Points to be observed

Abdominal massage can be performed at considerable depth once the patient is used to your hands.

So always start more lightly and quickly work up to greater depth. Remember, the contents of the abdomen are soft and can be moved by deep manipulations, except where they are tied down to other organs as in the two fossae and at the flexures of the colon.

If the treatment is for constipation, the sequence of manipulations is:

- Palpation.
- Whole abdomen stroking.
- Whole abdomen kneading.
- Stroking to the colon – starting with the descending colon.
- Kneading to the colon – starting with the descending colon and possibly at the iliac fossa and working upwards to the splenic flexure. Then deal with the ascending colon, possibly starting at the hepatic flexure and working down to the iliac fossa.
- Rolling of the colon contents is done on the descending colon first, from below upwards, and then the ascending colon from above downwards.
- Colon stroking is done again.
- Finish with brisk lift stroking.
- If the abdominal wall is flabby, hacking may be performed in a pattern of vertical lines.

12 Uses of classical massage in some health care settings: an overview

Elisabeth Jones

This chapter gives a very general picture of the health care settings and types of classical massage manipulations that may be useful for the therapeutic treatment of patients within the client groups described. For best practice it is important to train in each setting with an experienced tutor who has nationally recognised qualifications. The aims behind each manipulation are outlined in Chapter 6. The evidence-based effects, risk-awareness and contraindications are outlined in Chapters 3 and 4.

Stress

The endocrine and autonomic nervous systems are brought into play when there are stress symptoms in an individual. (See Chapter 2 for the relevant anatomy and physiology of each of these systems.) This is because there is an 'alarm' response of fear, pain or strong emotion to any perceived threat. The 'fight or flight ' syndrome, as described by Selye, occurs. The consequent results among other symptoms can be increased blood pressure, heart rate and muscle tone.

A normal individual can cope with 'temporary' stress, causing short-term feelings of tension, fatigue and poor sleep, but in a 'chronic' stress situation, long-term health problems may evolve. Pain and fatigue often accompany the main stress reactions. Sometimes individuals with 'chronic' stress may need prescribed medication and medical advice on managing and coping with their situation.

Massage, which has a sedative effect on the nervous system and helps to reduce muscle tension, can be useful in helping to relax those patients who are suffering 'stress' in one form or another. This then may alleviate the symptoms described above and provides a means of returning to a balanced state mentally and physically.

Some useful massage manipulations are:

- Effleurage/stroking
- Petrissage/kneading

The movements should be performed slowly, rhythmically and with gentle pressure.

Locally the head, neck, shoulders, lower back, hands and feet often need massage as stress frequently manifests itself in these areas. Generally a whole body massage may be appropriate if there is a feeling of tension throughout the patient's being.

Essential oils such as lavender and sandalwood could be incorporated in the massage medium (see Chapter 15 on Aromatherapy) for their relaxing effect, provided there are no contraindications.

The position of choice accords with the patient's condition. The environment needs to be peaceful and, if the patient wishes, soothing background music could be played.

Depression

Most people feel anxious and/or depressed when faced with severe life traumas such as major illness, divorce, bereavement or financial problems. The 'adaptation' processes develop in a healthy individual, but if the natural 'low' feeling becomes deeper and does not seem to lift, then 'clinical' depression sets in.

'Clinical' depression can manifest itself in many ways depending on its severity, for instance, a feeling of isolation and 'emptiness', loss of concentration, sleep disturbance, emotional imbalance, apathy and eating disorders. Suicidal thoughts can be a characteristic of severe depression. Again, prescribed medicines and medical advice may be required to help the patient through this situation. Massage which is at first sedative, then more stimulating will help to uplift the mood of the depressed patient.

Some useful massage manipulations are:

- Effleurage/stroking
- Petrissage/kneading

The movements should be performed at a slow, then brisker speed with moderate pressure and rhythm.

Generally speaking, a depressed patient will find a total body treatment more therapeutic than a localised one. Essential oils such as lemon, grapefruit, bergamot, lavender and clary sage can offer a revitalising effect (see Chapter 15).

The environment should be peaceful, fresh and well lighted. Suitable mood-enhancing music may be played in the background if the patient wishes.

Anxiety

Anxiety may accompany 'clinical' depression and/or severe life trauma. Depending on the severity of the condition there may be considerable chronic apprehension about all and everything, fearful thoughts and phobias. Panic attacks may occur if fearfulness becomes overwhelming. Other symptoms that are common are shortness of breath, hyperventilation, heart palpitations, dizziness and trembling.

Pain and fatigue, sleeplessness, headaches, depression, irritable bowel syndrome and painful muscle trigger points may be other symptoms. Medical intervention is often required as well as different therapies appropriate to the syndrome.

Some useful massage manipulations are listed under the section on 'Stress'.

Occupational situations

When people have a physical or mental overload in their workplace, there may be symptoms of 'occupational stress'. Work-related upper limb disorders (WRULDs) are common. Repetitive strain injury (RSI) is particularly noticeable in those who are performing the same task, hour after hour, day after day; e.g. sitting and working at computers particularly if they have poor posture and if they do not take frequent breaks.

Headaches, pain and tension in the neck, shoulders and wrists as well as lower back are common symptoms. Other examples of occupational stress are neck, shoulder and back problems which are common in gardeners, nurses, physiotherapists and carers, particularly if they do not lift well, do not keep good posture and fail to give themselves adequate rest between physical activity. Fatigue and pain will often ensue. As can be seen, such symptoms manifested are aligned to the occupation.

Some useful massage manipulations are:

- Effleurage/stroking
- Petrissage/kneading, wringing, muscle rolling
- Deep frictions

Locally, the movements should be slow, rhythmical and with deep pressure, particularly over 'trigger' points. Generally, a total body massage will help relaxation, in which all massage techniques (see Chapter 6 on massage manipulations) may be utilised as appropriate.

'On-site' massage may be called for, in which treatment may be given in the workplace. Neck and shoulder as well as back massage may be given through clothes. The position will usually be in sitting, head on pillows on a table, or with a portable head rest on a table or couch. Offered by many organisations and companies during short breaks and in lunch times, this can aid relaxation and therefore enable personnel to work with increased efficiency. Essential oils (see Chapter 15) may be utilised.

The environment, if possible, needs to be peaceful and calming in a room separate from the workplace. If the patient enjoys it, soothing music can be played in the background.

Pre natal, labour and post natal

Pregnancy is a time of great physical and emotional change, often accompanied by emotional changes. Backache and mood swings (caused often by mechanical and hormonal influences) as well as fatigue may occur.

In labour contractions of the uterus can be painful and there may be apprehension of the birth process. Post pregnancy, the new mother may still have residual backache, anxiety, fatigue and sometimes post-natal depression. Learning to cope with a complete change of lifestyle can be very daunting. It is important for the therapist to have specific training in this field. In some countries, permission from the doctor in charge needs to be given.

Massage can be immensely helpful in all the above situations. Not only may it be helpful by soothing pain, but also 'touch' may provide reassurance, remove a sense of isolation and create a feeling of being cared for.

Some useful massage manipulations are:

- Effleurage/stroking
- Petrissage/kneading

Locally a light, slow rhythmical stroking over the abdomen in pregnancy will feel soothing and help reduce the sense of 'stretch'. Light effleurage and gentle kneading on the lower back will help relieve aching in that area, both in pregnancy and during labour.

Generally speaking, in pregnancy a full body massage can promote a feeling of well being and later, when the new mother is managing her baby, she will benefit from the relaxation it can offer. (In the latter situation, avoid the abdomen until after a 6-week check-up with the GP.)

Essential oils may be used, but be aware of contraindications (see Chapter 15).

The position in pregnancy will be three-quarters side lying, using pillows under the head, the upper limb and a pillow between the lower limbs. As the pregnancy time progresses the patient may well wish to be almost completely in side lying. The height of the couch needs to be adjusted accordingly to enable the therapist to accomplish the massage successfully.

The position in labour will be in accord with the wishes of the mother-to-be, and the midwife.

The position for the new mother after childbirth will be 'as normal' for the areas to be treated (see Chapter 6). The environment should if possible be peaceful, and appropriate music if enjoyed by the patient may be played.

Babies

In some cultures mothers use massage routinely to promote nurturing and bonding with their baby. Baby massage classes and groups are now being set up, run by health professionals, with the intention of providing similar benefits to the mother and infant. These can usually have anywhere from two to twenty mothers and their babies. The therapist, who should have specific training, and doctor's permission in some countries, can show the mothers how to give a gentle massage which may be applied daily when at home. Mothers are encouraged to watch and listen to their babies and enjoy touching and cuddling them.

Mothers can enjoy chatting over mutual experiences and feel supported by the therapist and the group. This is likely to help mothers to be more relaxed, which is good for their babies. Sometimes a mother may wish to have a therapist come to her home and a few friends may join her. The principles of massage will be the same as for the group.

Useful massage manipulation are:

- Stroking

Generally this should be very gentle, slow and rhythmical. The mother should have short nails and remove her watch and jewellery. The baby usually sits on the mother's lap and has eye contact with her, first in supine and then in a prone position.

Stroking can be given to the head, the trunk and the limbs. Massage should not be given for more than 10 minutes for babies under 10 months old and the time may be increased gradually as the baby increases in age, and if he/she enjoys it.

The environment needs to be a relaxing one, with soothing music if desired by the mothers.

Children

Massage for children may be much the same as the classical massage manipulations for adults. It, however, must to be adapted to the child's temperament, possible medical condition and age group. As children tend to have a shorter attention span than adults it is wise to work for short periods and no longer than half an hour. Specific training is necessary, and in some countries a doctor's permission is required before treatment.

Generally, children like to be massaged. Physical and emotional growing pains may be eased, particularly in adolescence. It is important to have a parent or guardian present and it is useful to show them techniques that they can use at home for the child's benefit. Massage through clothing may be a preferred treatment.

Some useful massage manipulations are:

- Effleurage/stroking
- Petrissage/kneading, muscle rolling
- Frictions

The techniques need to be applied slowly, lightly and rhythmically, with deeper pressure for young people.

Locally, if there are 'trigger points' associated with the 'growing pains' of adolescence, frictions may be applied as well as effleurage/stroking and petrissage/kneading /muscle rolling techniques.

A general total massage is sometimes useful in helping to relax a child who is tense, anxious or even depressed (see sections above on 'Stress', 'Depression' and 'Anxiety').

The environment needs to be peaceful and calming. Children usually like music. It is worth offering them a selection to choose from.

The older population

The term 'old' is a difficult one to apply to any particular age group these days. However, it is considered that, at this time, people of 60 years and onwards present definite aging signs. Connective tissue in general becomes affected. Skin becomes thinner, bones more fragile and joints less supple. Cartilage becomes worn, osteoarthritis is more evident and fractures more likely. Muscle tissue diminishes and circulation, particularly in the hands and feet, becomes less efficient.

Fluid in the body cells is reduced and gravity has a more pronounced effect on the skeletal framework, pulling the head and shoulders forward because of muscle weakness. Pains and aches and fatigue are often evident. Youthful activity may be impaired.

Many elderly people feel isolated due to the death of their partner and lack of interest from busy offspring, who may also live far away. Some may be in residential homes. All this can lead to loneliness, inactivity and lack of comforting touch which may then in turn precipitate depression. Some may have dementia, and their GP and relatives' permission for massage may be required before treatment.

Massage can be helpful as the use of touch may bring back a sense of worth, a feeling of being cared for and a reduction in an elderly person's sense of 'aloneness'. Massage may also help to keep tissues hydrated, increase blood and lymph flow and improve muscle tone.

Some useful massage manipulations are:

- Effleurage/stroking
- Petrissage/finger kneading

The movements should be gentle (due to skin fragility), slow and rhythmical.

Because of problems associated with mobility it is often better to massage a local area. Massage is often given through the clothes, in a sitting position. A total massage is likely to be too strenuous and therefore neck, shoulders, hands and feet are commonly treated instead. Essential oils are useful if there are no contraindications (see Chapter 15). The environment should if possible be cheerful and uplifting with suitable music if the patient wishes.

Learning disabilities

People who find it difficult to process sensory input can be helped by massage. It can help to develop sensory awareness which in turn builds self-esteem and improved social interaction. The patient must agree to having treatment and the therapist should ensure that she/he feels there is a relationship of trust and support.

Some useful massage manipulations are:

- Effleurage/stroking
- Petrissage/kneading

Massage can be done by the therapist or by the patient to her/himself (self-massage). There can also be reciprocal massage between the therapist and the patient. The massage environment should be relaxing and if the patient wishes there may be soothing background music.

Mental health

If one is giving massage in mental health settings it is extremely important to obtain 'informed consent'. The therapist should work with a mental health support team as the massage will be part of a total care plan. Most patients find hand massage acceptable as it does not appear to feel invasive. Self massage can be taught. Sometimes massage may be given through clothing, which is particularly useful if a patient feels very vulnerable.

If body image has become disturbed or even lost, massage may help to retrieve it.

'Stress' massage techniques and the environment are the most useful, done locally or generally and adapted to both the patient's condition and his/her acceptance of the therapy (see the section on 'Stress' above).

Physical disabilities

Physical disabilities are broken down into neuromuscular-skeletal conditions or neurological conditions. Physical disability can be short term or long term. See Chapter 3 regarding the effects of massage and Chapter 4 regarding examination and assessment.

Neuromuscular-skeletal conditions

These may arise for many different reasons, for example as a result of:

- Mechanopostural defects
- Traumatic/surgical factors
- Disease

The environment for neuromuscular-skeletal conditions should be calm and relaxing, with soothing music if the patient desires playing in the background.

Mechanopostural defects

These can be caused be disease or occupational and lifestyle situations. Common problems are headaches with neck and shoulder pain, and low back pain. Some muscles will shorten, others will overstretch, if the body is habitually contorted into unbalanced postures. Connective tissue will lose length and flexibility. Joints will eventually be affected. Inflammation and adhesions may result. Pain and muscle spasm will become evident.

Some useful massage manipulations are:

- Effleurage/stroking
- Petrissage/all kinds
- Frictions

Effleurage/stroking is useful for relaxation of muscle tension and/or spasm and for increased circulation in the area. Petrissage/all kinds – wringing, kneading, muscle rolling and picking up – are useful as appropriate to the situation, for relaxation of muscle tension and increased circulation in the area. Frictions may be used to release adhesions and reduce tension in and around trigger points.

Traumatic/surgical factors

Ligament and muscle strains and sprains, depending on whether they are minor or major, will create minimal to severe inflammation, oedema and adhesions in the area. Joint mobility may therefore be affected to a lesser or greater degree. Among some common problems found in the upper limb are 'rotator cuff' lesions, 'tennis' elbow, 'golfers' elbow and carpal tunnel syndrome.

In the lower limb, piriformis syndrome and lesions of knee ligaments and tendons, foot ligaments and tendons are conditions often seen.

If surgery is indicated, a joint if immobilised may show stiffening due to adhesions with shortening of connective tissue elements and muscle weakness. These will be most apparent when the splinting is removed. Massage can, together with other modalities, be employed to help restore the structures to normal activity.

Some useful massage manipulations are:

- Effleurage/stroking
- Petrissage/kneading, skin rolling, muscle rolling, wringing
- Frictions

Effleurage/stroking will help relax muscles and improve blood circulation and the lymphatic flow. Petrissage/kneading, particularly finger kneading, will be useful for helping to reduce oedema and soften adhesions, and return soft tissue to its original length. Skin rolling and muscle rolling will increase mobility of the structures.

Wringing will stretch tight tissues. Frictions including the Cyriax type will help loosen adhesions (Cyriax and Cyriax 1993).

Disease

Arthritis (inflammation of the joints) can come in many forms. Osteoarthritis (degenerative) and rheumatoid arthritis (inflammatory) are the types most often encountered by the therapist.

Overall massage helps people with physical disability, short or long term, to relax, counter fatigue and improve blood and lymphatic circulations and sleep. Acute and active phases of disease are a contraindication to massage.

Some useful massage manipulations are:

- Effleurage/stroking
- Petrissage/kneading

Light effleurage and gentle kneading can be useful in helping to improve circulation and reduce pain and spasm.

Neurological conditions

Those with neurological conditions such as multiple sclerosis, Parkinson's disease and hemiplegia (stroke), and so on, will often request massage and it can be useful, provided the therapist has a full knowledge of the condition. It is vital that great caution is used to avoid exacerbating abnormal muscle tone, e.g. some types of reflex spasticity may be triggered by certain forms of touch, particularly when stroking the ball of the foot or palm of the hand, if a patient has flexor spasticity.

Useful massage manipulations are:

- Effleurage/stroking

Slow stroking over the posterior primary rami area may help to reduce abnormal muscle tone and also help the brain reconnect to a limb which may have been ignored, due to altered body image.

Cancer care

One in three persons may develop cancer. Fortunately with great advances in cancer therapy a significant number of people survive. Having cancer may create not only physical problems but also psychological problems such as anxiety and depression.

It is a treatment area that requires the therapist to learn specialist techniques from a tutor with nationally recognised qualifications in this field.

Contraindications/precautions

See Chapters 3 and 4 and sections on 'Stress', 'Anxiety' and 'Depression' in this chapter.

Do not give massage if it is contraindicated by the patient's cancer specialist. Some consultants are happy for the patient to have massage, others are not. However, if the cancer specialist recommends massage as a therapy, the following techniques can be applied:

- Effleurage/stroking

Effleurage/stroking should be of light pressure, the main stroke being no deeper than the usual light return stroke. The manipulation needs to be slow and rhythmical and the therapist must be aware of skin sensitivity.

It is usual to do a lot of holding where it is anatomically comfortable (i.e. allowing the hand to fit the natural curves, e.g. the shoulders, curves by the ribs, elbows, hands, knees and feet).

Lymph nodes should be avoided and pressure points should not be used.

Do not pass comment on any areas that are felt to be different from 'normal', but ask the patient's permission to give an update on treatment to the doctor-in-charge, who may investigate further.

Essential oils may be useful (see Chapter 15). However, citrus oils are contraindicated in massage for clients receiving chemotherapy or radiotherapy as these treatments increase photosensitivity which would be further stimulated by the aforementioned types of essential oils. Some specialists contraindicate the use of all essential oils in massage until chemotherapy and radiotherapy have terminated.

If massage is contraindicated, the use of essential oils in other ways can be beneficial. Lavender and Roman chamomile in particular are considered by aromatherapists to have relaxing effects, helping with anxiety and depression and aiding a good night's sleep. Inhalation of these oils through the use of vaporisers, through baths (if allowed by the consultant) or by 1 or 2 drops on a tissue are the methods of choice.

It is important to acknowledge the effect that a patient's illness may have on the carer or relative who is looking after him/her. Massage given by carers/relatives to the patient can help make them feel they are doing something constructive. If they are interested in helping in this way they can be taught to give gentle hand or feet stroking to the client.

Carers and relatives will also benefit from massage to ease their stresses and this can be carried out as in normal practice.

Manual lymph drainage (MLD) may be used as an effective treatment for lymphoedema associated with cancer (provided it is recommended for the patient by the consultant).

HIV/AIDS

The therapist needs to have specialist training in this area of massage treatment. Those people who are infected with the human immune deficiency virus (HIV) often have symptoms of acquired immune deficiency syndrome (AIDS). Quality of life may become severely diminished. Painful muscles, skin sensitivity, infections, loss of mobility, and digestive, respiratory and neurological disorders are frequently encountered. These symptoms may bring about a deep sense of isolation, depression and anxiety, particularly if the patient suffers from a loss of touch.

Massage can help to relieve these feelings of stress which in turn may help the functions of the immune system.

Essential oils can be added to the 'medium' (see Chapter 15), but the therapist must be aware of allergic reaction and needs to check the possibility with the patient, as the immune system is compromised in this illness.

If the patient is at the terminal stage of the illness ensure that as a therapist one works in co-ordination with other health care professionals and the patient is willing to have treatment.

Useful massage manipulation are:

- Stroking

Stroking needs to be slow, rhythmical and light in pressure (taking account of skin sensitivity). Avoid skin lesions and body fluids. Keep strict hygiene precautions. Wear gloves if helping with general care of patients and always wash hands before and after massage.

Consider offering foot and/or hand massage (provided these parts are clear of infection) if there are skin problems elsewhere. Length of time of treatment will depend on the patient's condition. The environment should be calm and uplifting.

Pain

Pain is a symptom of a wide range of pathological conditions. Classical massage undoubtedly can help to alleviate this symptom. Different manipulations may be used according to the presenting situation (see this chapter and also Chapters 2, 3 and 4).

Respiratory conditions

Unlike in the past when tapôtement (percussion) massage together with postural drainage was commonly used for respiratory problems (requiring the elimination of secretions), such treatment is given less often these days. However, in intubated and ventilated patients, therapists do continue to aid the removal of secretions in this way when appropriate. Manual hyperinflation and suction will also be included in a treatment session when secretions are particularly difficult to clear.

In the cystic fibrosis patient group more emphasis is being placed on moving away from 'passive' sessions and allowing more self-directed treatments. This includes the use of hand-held positive pressure and vibratory devices, to aid clearance of secretions and the use of 'autogenic' breathing techniques.

Tapôtement may still be the treatment of choice with some patients, especially during a chest infection requiring admission to hospital for intravenous antibiotics. In such circumstances secretions may be especially difficult to clear and the addition of manual techniques may aid expectoration.

Some useful massage manipulations are:

- Tapôtement
- Vibration
- Shaking

Note: as always, care must be taken to ensure the correct patient groups are treated with the above, being aware of any contraindications expressed by the patient's consultant.

For those patients who suffer from musculoskeletal pain associated with tension in the respiratory muscles (typically in the thoracic area and often in the neck and shoulders), massage that helps to relax these muscles can be usefully employed.

Those people who suffer from anxiety due to 'breathlessness' may be helped by 'stress' massage techniques described earlier in this chapter.

Some useful massage manipulations are described in the section on 'Stress'.

See sections on 'Stress' and 'Physical disabilities' in this chapter.

Reconstructive surgery

Massage is used as part of treatment following trauma/reconstructive surgery to the body. It has a particularly important role in therapy following hand injury.

It has three main uses:

- Scar management
  - for tethering
  - for hypertrophic scars
  - for desensitisation
- Desensitisation
- Oedema management

Some useful massage manipulations are described below.

Scar management

Massage may be used on scar tissue. It is usually started 2 weeks or more following suture removal or over soluble sutures when the wound has healed.

Tethering

The thumb can be applied gliding deeply over the tissues. The patient is then taught how to do this technique three or four times daily. This will help not only to untether a scar but also to prevent further adherence and improve blood supply to the area. Creams must not be coloured or perfumed, to prevent allergic reaction. E45 cream is an example of a cream often used.

Hypertrophic scars

A more superficial thumb pressure is used with an E45-type cream. The cream may then be removed and a deeper thumb kneading applied. Silicone gel and compression are also utilised.

Desensitisation

Any scar that is not massaged can become hypersensitive. Gentle thumb pressure may be applied early and may be very effective in helping to desensitise the scar area, in particular those areas following limb or finger amputation or after nerve injury.

Oedema management

Post-traumatic and surgical oedema is a problem that needs to be treated early, namely in the first 2–3 weeks following injury. Thereafter its presence prolongs the inflammatory stage of healing, leading possibly to chronic fibrotic oedema. Massage is given with thumb pressure distal to proximal with the use of an E45-type cream. This is then followed with compression, active exercises and elevation.

Reference

Cyriax, J.H. and Cyriax, P.J. (1993) *Cyriax's Illustrated Manual of Orthopaedic Medicine*, 2nd edn. Butterworth Heinemann, Oxford.

Further reading

Auckett, A.D. (2004) *Baby Massage: Parent–Child Bonding Through Touch*. Newmarket Press, New York.

Charman, R.A. (2000) (ed.) *Complementary Therapies for Physical Therapists*. Butterworth Heinemann, Oxford.

Field, T. (2006) *Massage Therapy Research*. Churchill Livingstone, Edinburgh.

Fritz, S. (2004) *Fundamentals of Therapeutic Massage*, 3rd edn. Mosby, St Louis.

Hess, D.R. (2002) Evidence for secretion clearance techniques. *Cardiopulmonary Physical Therapy Journal*, December.

Holey, E. and Cook, E. (2003) *Evidence Based Therapeutic Massage and Practical Guide for Therapists*, 2nd edn. Churchill Livingstone, Edinburgh.

Hollis, M. (1998) *Massage for Therapists*, 2nd edn. Blackwell Science, Oxford.

Lewis, M. and Johnson, M.I. (2006) The clinical effectiveness of therapeutic massage for musculo-skeletal pain; a systemic review. *Physiotherapy*, **92**, 146–58.

McNamara, P. (2004) *Massage for People with Cancer* (ed. V. Speechley). Cancer Research Centre, London.

Mustoe, T.A., Cooter, D., Gold, M.H., et al. (2002) International clinical recommendations on scar management. *Plastic and Reconstructive Surgery*, **110**(2), 560–71.

Price, S. and Price, L. (1995) *Aromatherapy for Health Professionals*. Churchill Livingstone, Edinburgh.

Tappan, F.M. and Benjamin, P.J. (2004) *Tappan's Handbook of Healing Massage Techniques; Classic, Holistic and Emerging Methods*. Prentice-Hall, New Jersey.

Thomson, A., Skinner, A. and Peircey, J. (1991) *Tidy's Physiotherapy*, 12th edn. Butterworth Heinemann, Oxford.

Vickers, A. (1996) *Massage and Aromatherapy, a Guide for Health Professionals*. Chapman and Hall, London.

III Some specialised techniques

13 Some types of massage and soft tissue therapies

Elisabeth Jones

This chapter gives a brief overview of the wide variety of massage types that may be used in therapy. Each method, if it is to be safe and effective, needs to be learnt from a competent and experienced tutor who has attained well-recognised qualifications. Do not work in these fields without such training.

The descriptions in this chapter are a 'taster' of the different ways in which the 'laying on of hands' can help to promote healing. The subsequent chapters give a fuller explanation of some of the specialised techniques that have a particularly wide use.

Active release technique (ART)

Developed and patented by P. Micheal Leary DC, CCSP, this is a state-of-the-art soft tissue system/movement-based massage technique that treats muscles, tendons, ligaments, fascia and nerves. There are over 50 specific moves, unique to ART. Headaches, back pain, carpal tunnel syndrome, shin splints, shoulder pain, plantar fascilitis, knee problems and tennis elbow are just a few of the many conditions that may be helped by ART. They have got one thing in common, namely they are often the result of overused muscles.

Acupressure

Acupressure incorporates the concept of energy pathways and specific points, as in acupuncture, on parts of the body, but uses thumbs, fingers, sometimes even elbows, to apply pressure on the points instead of needles. Some sources consider this therapy to be older in origin than acupuncture, originating probably from China.

Other similar therapies such as tuina and shiatsu (see later) also come from the East. Stimulating such points may trigger the release of endorphins, the hormones that help to reduce pain and tension in the musculoskeletal system. Circulation and energy flow may also be improved.

Balance of activity throughout all the body systems is aimed for and this promotes a feeling of 'wellness'.

Animal massage

Unlike working in the human field, direct referrals are not permitted; the Veterinary Act requires that any person working on an animal must have obtained permission from the veterinary surgeon employed by the owner. Animals respond remarkably well to massage, and in 1984, when a specific interest group, the Association of Chartered Physiotherapists in Animal Therapy, was formed, the veterinary profession accepted the undoubted benefits of massage offered by professionals, particularly for small animals in post-operative situations.

The dog and cat can usually be persuaded to lie recumbent, and relaxation follows acceptance of a stranger's hands. The masseur/euse needs to adapt when working with horses, as the animal is neither recumbent nor relaxed due to effects from gravity, and because the stay system of the appendicular skeleton remains in a state of constant tension, to ensure the animal is in readiness to flee from a predator. The masseur/euse is working with the subject, not below but in front of the animal, and adaptation of the use of body weight and arm position is required.

A knowledge of surface anatomy is essential. Swedish massage techniques have proved the most beneficial when dealing with animals; effleurage, compression, skin rolling and cross fibre friction being those of choice.

Aromatherapy

Aromatherapy is a therapeutic procedure which utilises the fragrant components extracted from aromatic plants. The aromatic substances are those essential oils of certain plants that are considered to promote health and wellbeing. The combination of the beneficial effects of essential oils, together with the healing results of appropriate massage techniques, provides a 'natural' treatment of considerable value.

Aromatherapy massage probably creates the most diffuse therapeutic effect, if compared with other methods of use of essential oils. The oils are utilised not only by skin absorption, but also by olfaction and inhalation, when applied by massage.

Aromatherapy massage may be used for many client groups. Mental health settings; pre-natal, labour, and post-natal events; stressed, anxious and/or depressed individuals; musculoskeletal disorders; those in terminal care; and the elderly are a few examples of the situations in which aromatherapy massage can offer a valuable contribution towards 'wellbeing'.

Ayurvedic massage

Ayurvedic massage utilises the concepts of Ayurveda (an ancient practice from India which balances three life forces – energy, movement and digestion) together with warm oils and massage techniques on certain energy points. The aim is to create a sense of harmony of body and mind. It may be used for stress-related conditions to help achieve relaxation and increase vitality.

Bio-energy therapies

Massage is considered by many practitioners to be one of the bio-energy therapies, which are gaining greater credence following new research. Many scientists, including James Oschman PhD in the USA, consider that connective tissues which extend throughout the body form a semiconducting electronic network. Pressure from massage techniques may stimulate the conduction of 'piezo-electricity' through this energy system (see Chapter 2).

It is well known and accepted that humans have energy fields and the interaction of the practitioner's magnetic and electrical patterns with those of the patient may influence the treatment. Positive 'intention' may therefore create positive energy effects, which together with massage techniques gives beneficial outcomes.

Bowen therapy

The Bowen method, also known as Bowen therapy, is a gentle hands-on, soft tissue mobilisation technique. Light rolling moves of skin over underlying tissues are made at specific sites, grounded in an understanding of anatomy. This is followed by the therapist leaving the treatment room at intervals during the session. Specific conditions are not treated. However, there is no situation where it cannot be used safely. It has had beneficial effects on organic conditions and the whole range of musculoskeletal problems.

Classical massage

Classical massage is based on Swedish massage techniques, and comprises four main types of movement:

- Effleurage/stroking
- Petrissage
- Tapôtement/percussion
- Friction

It is the most frequently used technique, either in its own right or in combination with other techniques (see Chapter 6).

Connective tissue manipulation (CTM)

Connective tissue manipulation (CTM) is the German Bindegewebsmassage technique which was developed in the 1930s by Elisabeth Dicke. It is a highly specific technique which targets the interfaces within the skin and connective tissue. By working on connective tissue reflex zones (after the head), powerful autonomic reactions are induced through the somatovisceral reflexes.

Therapeutic effects include stimulation of the parasympathetic nervous system, inducing relaxation in sympathetic activity and the physical symptoms of anxiety. Enhanced peripheral circulation and autonomic and hormonal balance are also induced (Holey 1995).

Craniosacral therapy

Craniosacral therapy uses a light touch to uncover, evaluate and facilitate the release of subtle causes of ill health and dysfunction in the neuromuscular-skeletal and fascial systems. It addresses the entire physiology, right down to cellular level, embracing the emotional, energetic and spiritual dimensions of personality. The craniosacral system is composed of the membranes and cerebrospinal fluid that surround and protect the brain and spinal cord. There is a mild cranial pulse that can be felt at 8–12 beats per minute, which can vary in volume and range and variations in this pulse may signify restrictions in the body systems. The treatment is gentle and relaxing.

Heller work

Developed by Joseph Heller, the soft tissue manipulation and body movement re-education are similar to Rolfing (see later), yet acknowledge the relationship between body and mind, using guided verbal dialogue to address emotions that lock muscles and affect breathing. There are typically eleven sessions working to bring consciousness into the body, to bring choice and empowerment and awareness. There is a focus on balance at all levels, especially the deep core musculature.

Heller work can help: muscle pain, especially in the neck, shoulder and back; stress-related conditions; sports injuries; and conditions related to poor posture.

Indian head massage

Indian head massage has been practised among families in India for many centuries, mainly by women, with the use of oils to improve the condition of their hair. Known as 'champi' from which the word 'shampoo' is derived, it is still practised by barbers in India as part of their routine, and it is often carried out in public places.

The Western version includes not only the scalp but also the neck, shoulders and upper back, where we hold tension, using both soothing and invigorating strokes, as well as pressure on acupoints.

The use of oils on the scalp is optional, as the main benefit these days comes from relief of tension and pain in the muscles over which the hands are worked, and therefore a reduction of feelings of stress.

Lomi lomi

This is a type of Hawaiian technique, based on the Hawaiian Huna philosophy that there can be balance achieved between mind and body. It is an intuitive form of massage using the hands and arms of the healer on the person's physique, utilising long gliding strokes. A prayer may begin the session, and sometimes a number of healers may apply the massage at the same time.

Manual lymph drainage (MLD)

This is a massage technique used to treat lymphoedema, i.e. a condition of the lymphatic system which arises as a result of damage or disease. The swelling can affect the limbs, trunk and head. The lymph collects in the tissues under the skin, causing the skin to stretch and the tissues to become congested and painful, resulting in stiffness of the joints.

The massage is extremely gentle and is performed using the palm of the hand and the flat of the fingers, in direct contact with the skin, and is composed of small circular movements, working in the direction of the flow of the lymph.

The treatment session is in three parts:

(1) In order to improve the lymph flow through the body, the main groups of lymph nodes are stimulated; these are in the axilla, the groin and the base of the skull and neck. Gentle pressure is used on these nodes in the direction of the heart.
(2) The area of the trunk closest to the swelling is cleared, and the fluid is directed towards the cisterna chyli, thence to the thoracic duct, emptying into the left subclavian vein, and leaving space for the fluid to drain from the limb.
(3) Only then in the third phase is the affected limb touched. Treatment always starts at the top and progresses slowly down to include the fingers and toes, then up the trunk. The flat of the hand is used to guide the fluid up the limb; pressure is gentle and the skin is never dragged.

The technique should never produce pain, and a sound knowledge of the lymphatic system is essential.

Muscle energy technique (MET)

Muscle energy technique (MET) is an adaptation of another type of soft tissue manipulation called proprioceptive neuromuscular facilitation (see later), initially developed in the 1950s and which has seen a resurgence since the late 1970s, particularly in the osteopathy profession.

It is used to facilitate joint mobilisation and release of muscle shortness. It has been described as a 'highly sophisticated system of manipulative methods in which the patient uses her/his muscles, on request, from a precisely controlled position in a specific direction, against a distinctly executed counter force'.

There are all sorts of variations of this basic principle which involve post-isometric relaxation, reciprocal inhibition, variations in the effort of the patient, variations in the counterforce by the practitioner, subsequent stretch, variation in contraction, time of contraction, rhythm of contraction, and combination with pressure techniques. Often the variety of methods within MET are described as positional release techniques or strain counterstrain.

Myofascial release (MFR)

Myofascial release (MFR) techniques deal predominantly with the fascial (connective tissue) system, although muscle is implicated. The fascia supports and gives structural integrity and interconnectivity to all systems of the body. When there is emotional and physical trauma, the myofascial tissue may tighten in response, in certain areas. This can cause restricted movement and pain.

Torticollis, chronic muscle tension (e.g. upper fibres of the trapezius), fibrous scar tissue, adhesions, fibromyalgia and chronic fatigue syndrome are among some of the conditions that it is suggested may be helped by MFR.

After subtle palpation, gentle pressure and then gentle stretch are applied to the affected area which allows this restriction to elongate ('unwind') as a spontaneous release of myofascial tissue. Somatoemotional changes may happen and the patient will need to feel the therapist is supportive and that he/she is in a trusting environment. (See Chapter 17.)

Neuromuscular therapy

Neuromuscular therapy is sometimes called 'trigger point therapy' or 'myotherapy'. Local soft tissue dysfunction sometimes presents as local specific spots of pain or tenderness, often referred to as 'trigger points'. The pain produced in these areas of dysfunction often radiates away from the tender spot. Thumb and/or finger pressure is used to release spasms, interrupt the pain cycle and help return tissues to normal function.

Periosteal massage

Periosteal massage involves small circular movements which are often conducted with the therapist's knuckle on the superficial aspects of bone. It is thought to have a reflex effect, but can be rather uncomfortable, although it has been widely used in Europe. It is used to help reduce pain.

Pin and stretch

This is an American version of soft tissue release (STR) and specific stretch (SS) (see later). It relies on pressure being applied to an area of muscle and stretch being combined to produce change in the resting length of the muscle/group of muscles being worked upon. The aim is to 're-set' muscle fibres to their resting length.

Polarity therapy

Devised by Dr Randolph Stone, polarity therapy employs a blend of both Eastern and Western concepts of health, working with the human energy field. Using light touch, bodywork, diet, exercise and self awareness, the therapist aims to restore optimum energy flow, therefore enabling the body to heal itself naturally on emotional, mental and spiritual levels. Polarity therapy forms part of the foundation of craniosacral therapy and myofascial release.

Positional release

This non-invasive technique to release muscular contraction, tension or spasm was first discovered by Lawrence Jones, DO who found that placing a patient in a position of ease, for a period of time, released tension.

The method has been likened to untangling a knotted jewellery chain instead of pulling it apart; pushing the links together releases the chain very effectively. The practitioner achieves this by passively placing a person's body or body part into a position that brings the origin and insertion of the muscle or muscle group together. Fine tuning of position is administered until the patient is at his or her most comfy state. This position is held by the therapist for 90 seconds which facilitates muscle spindle resetting. The patient then must be slowly and passively returned to the neutral position.

All these methods are used to increase flexibility, to loosen muscles and to reduce pain in a muscle prior to deep massage and trigger point work, as may be used, for example, with sports problems or occupational stress.

Proprioceptive neuromuscular facilitation (PNF)

Proprioceptive stimuli are applied for processing in the spinal cord or brain, to modulate the output of motor neurones and recruitment of motor units. Activity of the motor neuromuscular system is altered for therapeutic effect.

Proprioceptive stimuli are applied as:

- Touch – manual contact (guiding strength of contraction and direction of movement).
- Verbal – explanation, commands, tone of voice.
- Visual – demonstration.
- Patterns of movement – functional combined movements.
- Compression/distraction of joint surfaces – stimulates mechanoreceptors.
- Pressure – recruits motor units to produce the appropriate response for the patient's therapeutic needs.

PNF techniques involve the patient actively contributing to the therapy. Developed in the USA in the 1950s, variations have evolved, but the fundamental principles remain the same. PNF may be used for relaxation/lengthening of muscles, regaining joint movement, rebalancing muscle activity, and restoring postural reflexes and stability.

Important philosophical principles are: a positive approach, no pain and achievable tasks set up for success (Adler *et al.* 2008).

Techniques of PNF used by chartered physiotherapists are: hold relax, repeated contractions, combining repeated contractions with soft tissue techniques, slow reversals and stabilisations.

Hold relax (HR) (contract relax)

HR aims to improve the range of movement at joints, limit factors of muscle spasm, increase tone and improve 'muscle tightness'. The patient moves the joint to resistance (motion barrier). The shortened muscles (antagonists to the movement to be gained) are held contracted isotonically against the therapist's manual pressure, followed by a relaxation phase. The patient is asked to move the joint into the new range gained by the lengthening effect on the shortened muscle.

Repetitions are carried out until no further movement is gained – typically 3–6 repetitions. There is no consensus in the literature regarding the length of time for HR phases – the minimum is 15 seconds and maximum 30 seconds. The relaxation phase is in the order of 15 seconds.

Auto hold relax

A patient may perform hold relax to lengthen muscles on his/her own. This requires special tuition to make sure that the exercise is performed correctly, but it is very much in keeping with the patient being involved actively in his/her rehabilitation from an early stage.

Repeated contractions (RC)

- To gain joint range – the joint is moved to the motion barrier. Manual pressure is applied to resist the agonists of the movement. An isometric hold is maintained. This phase is followed by an isotonic contraction of the agonists against the therapist's pressure until a new motion barrier is reached. There is no relaxation phase; the agonists are working all the time. The length of hold is typically 10–15 seconds and repetitions are typically 3–6.
- Stretch reflex (repeated stretch) – this may be used to enhance the contraction of the agonists. As the instruction is given to move into new range the therapist applies a short sharp stretch to the agonists. The spinal reflex kicks in and the agonist contraction is stronger due to greater recruitment of the motor units.
- To strengthen muscle – this technique is applied from the full length of the muscle to fully shortened.

Combining repeated contractions with soft tissue techniques

During the hold, palpation of the antagonist muscle may identify deep scarring. This then may respond to specific soft tissue mobilisations (SSTM). The reasoning therapist will apply a combination of active work for the contractile elements and passive holds to allow creep and viscoelastic changes in the non-contractile elements of muscle tissue.

Slow reversals (SR)

This involves continuous activity from one direction of movement to the opposite in a diagonal pattern. Greater motor recruitment leads to stronger contraction, increasing range of movement and co-ordination.

Stabilisations

The patient is positioned in a functional position and manual pressure is applied to the muscles until they are all working. This facilitates stability and co-ordination.

Reflexology

Reflexology originates from ancient traditions of working on the hands and feet for health. This concept is based on the hypothesis that the whole body is reflected in miniature on the hands and feet. Reflex points correspond to specific areas of the body. When pressure is applied to these points there is a change in the corresponding area of the body, helping to enhance the healing process. This approach works with whole body systems rather than a separate body part, influencing both body and mind.

Reflextherapy is an umbrella term that includes reflexology, incorporating a subtle, gentle touch, to include the head and the ear, and works holistically relating to the needs of the individual.

Areas of experienced clinical benefits include: musculoskeletal, respiratory, digestive, reproductive, neurological and endocrine disorders as well as relaxation, pain reduction, improved mobility, palliative care and chronic illness.

Rolfing (structural integration)

Ida Rolf developed a protocol of series of hands-on soft tissue techniques, giving a fundamental framework for unraveling and stretching the myofascial system. This allows patients to become aware of and therefore change their inhibiting movement patterns, which are manifested structurally in their body, and functionally as realignment alongside the forces of gravity.

Health benefits include improved mobility and function in musculoskeletal conditions, feelings of fitness and a reduction of tension patterns.

Segment massage

The practitioner targets the fascia under the skin. Small movements are made according to the segmental pattern of skin innervation. This East German technique gently stimulates the autonomic nervous system and is therefore used for a range of disorders

Shiatsu

Shiatsu literally means 'finger pressure' when translated from Japanese. It is the manual part of acupuncture and part of Japanese traditional medicine. Mainly fingers, thumbs and palms of the hands apply different depths of pressure over all the body, stimulating acupuncture points known as tsubos in Japanese. It is more than a mechanical stimulation of the points – it is an oriental healing art based on an energetic medical model.

Shiatsu is based on Chinese medicine and uses Eastern philosophy as its theoretical framework. Traditionally treatment is carried out on a cotton layer mat (futon) at floor level, with the body remaining fully and comfortably clothed. Nowadays some practitioners use a wide table, which is height adjustable. Shiatsu aims to maintain wellbeing and health, as well as treat specific conditions such as musculoskeletal disorders, pain, psychosomatic problems and stress-related symptoms, among others. (See Chapter 16.)

Soft tissue release (STR)

STR is a hybrid technique, combining movement and manipulation of soft tissues, particularly fascia and muscle, with elements of neuromuscular therapy (NMT) as well as connective tissue massage frictions and stretch. The technique is administered by applying and maintaining pressure or 'locking' into the relevant tissues, whilst simultaneously stretching away aligned fibres, through passive or active movement of the associated joint. This can produce a quick and effective 'release' in local areas of soft tissue tension. It is often used as a form of sports massage.

Specific soft tissue mobilisations (SSTMs)

These are oscillatory manual techniques applied to soft tissue. The techniques are graded. Pressure is applied to the structure at right angles to the longitudinal axis of the structure to be treated, in such a way as to create a bowing and therefore lengthening effect.

These techniques are very effective for lengthening and releasing scar-type collagen in healed, tight or adherent structures such as muscles, tendons and ligaments. Effectiveness is dependent on thorough examination to identify the problem structure, requiring the therapist to have a sound in-depth knowledge of applied anatomy and sensitivity in palpation.

Specific stretch

Specific stretch is similar to STR in that pressure is applied at the same time that a muscle is stretched. Variations of active and passive stretch are introduced and the pressure applied must be graded to influence/affect muscle and connective tissues at various depths.

Sports massage

The massage manipulations used in sports massage are as described in Chapter 6 and also involve acupressure, trigger pointing and ice massage. Sports massage can be divided into:

- Specific sports massage.
- Non-specific sports massage.

Any therapist involved in sports massage must know and understand the principles of the sport (see Chapter 14).

Swedish massage

Per Henrik Ling (1776–1839) of Sweden is credited with the development of Swedish massage. He explored massage techniques from different sources and co-ordinated some of them into a rationalised method, now termed Swedish massage. He founded the Royal Gymnastic Central Institute, where for the treatment of disease he advocated active and passive movements and massage. By the time of his death in 1839 his system had become recognised worldwide. Classical massage is based on Swedish massage but is more expansive in its manipulation techniques (see Chapter 6).

Thai massage (Thai yoga massage)

This technique is a combination of acupressure, gentle stretches and applied yoga, to assist energy flows around the body, and thus help the body's self-healing properties. The therapist uses hands, thumbs, elbows, knees or feet to apply pressure to energy lines along the body, using gentle stretches and applied yoga to enhance the benefits. The patient remains fully clothed, and the massage takes place on a mattress on the floor. A typical massage lasts at least 90 minutes and always treats the whole body, though specific attention can be paid to problem areas.

Therapeutic touch

Therapeutic touch is a contemporary approach to an ancient and traditional form of healing practice. Although there is a loose structural and philosophical framework to the clinical practice, therapeutic touch is not part of any religious doctrine, but is seen more as a natural human potential. In practical terms the therapist's hands may be working on the skin, through clothes or in the space around the subject's body. The therapist's mind intention and 'centering' (a form of focusing and meditation) are pivotal to the technique. The technique has been shown to reduce anxiety, improve mood, reduce pain (including phantom limb pain after amputation) and facilitate wound healing, and potentially could be of benefit in improving wellbeing and relaxation across all health care and patient groups.

Trager

This technique was developed and trademarked by Milton Trager in the USA. He describes it as psychophysical integration, as it involves a combination of 'tablework', which includes large passive movements, and rocking and mentastics, active movements performed after treatment. Trager therapy is said to induce a feeling of relaxation, ease of movement and reduced physical tension.

Transcadence massage

Properly called Linn transcadence massage (LTC) because it was devised by Denise Linn (of Cherokee Indian heritage), transcadence massage is a complete body system that blends the most potent aspects of Native American healing philosophy with altered states of conscious, through percussion massage movements. It is useful for dealing with deep-seated tension associated with old trauma, both physical and psychological.

Trigger point release

A feature common to many, if not all chronic pain conditions, is the presence of localised areas of soft tissue dysfunction which promote pain and distress in distant structures. These localised areas are known as trigger points.

The phenomenon of trigger points (commonly abbreviated as TrPs) is often overlooked in medical diagnosis and treatment of painful conditions. A sufferer may have been presented with an X-ray diagnosis of 'normal wear and tear' in a dysfunctional joint, and it is the bones, joints, bursae and nerves where physicians usually concentrate their attention. It is thought that TrPs are caused by dysfunction at the site of the motor endplates of skeletal muscle fibres.

The author's personal approach when assessing a patient with painful symptoms is to always include questions in the subjective assessment that enquire about a history of sudden contraction or stretch of muscles such as in a heavy fall or a history of prolonged overuse of a group of muscles such as in a heavy task or activity. The author has also found that TrPs are present in related muscle tissue following joint replacement surgery.

The patient is assessed objectively using palpation of suspected muscle areas as well as testing for joint range and muscle strength. Widely recognised diagnostic criteria for identification of TrPs include a taut palpable band; exquisite spot tenderness of a nodule within the taut band; a recognisable (familiar to the patient) referred pattern of pain on pressure of the tender nodule; and full stretch of the affected muscle being limited by pain.

Careful treatment of TrPs using a variety of approaches often brings about relief of painful symptoms – some conditions requiring an extremely light touch and some responding to firmer treatment. Comparative research has listed the following methods as being amongst the most effective for producing immediate benefits from the treatment of identified TrPs: ice spray and stretch; application of superficial local heat; and deep inhibitory pressure soft tissue massage.

Tuina/tui na (pronounced tweena)

Tuina is the ancient art of Chinese massage, using the operator's fingers, hands, arms, elbows and knees. It is based on the traditional Chinese medicine theory of balancing the flow of Qi (energy) throughout the body along certain lines called meridians. The methods used include the hand techniques of massage for the soft tissues of the body, acupuncture points to directly increase the flow of Qi, and manipulation to help realign the tissues.

Conditions for use are similar to some of those where classical massage may be utilised, e.g. alleviating chronic pain, particularly in the musculoskeletal system. The techniques are practised either on a couch or on a mat on the floor.

The Chinese tradition is not to take the clothes off, but they are loosened, and the shoes are removed. It is one of the three main components of Chinese medicine, the other two being acupuncture and herbal medicine.

Vibrational therapy (VT)

This is also called vibrational medicine and energy medicine. It is based on the scientific principles that all matter vibrates to a precise frequency, and that by using resonant vibration, balance of matter can be restored. Trauma may disrupt the normal rhythmic movements of tissue molecules and VT is directed at restoring the natural rhythm. All the senses may be stimulated to try to achieve this, including touch.

Zero balancing

The person's energy field is accessed by taking up the slack from the physical body (often with gentle traction and stretch), so that the hand acts as a fulcrum or balance point. Any additional pressure will then allow movement to orient around the hand and be felt as an energetic change at the interface of the 'physical and energetic'. The internal perceptions of elongation may take the person onto deeper states of relaxation and awareness. The normal flow of energy that permeates the bones is restored and realigned with the physical structure to optimise function. Energy balancing effects are of a holistic nature, reducing pain and stress, dealing with past trauma and enabling the person to develop his or her life potential.

References

Adler, S., Beckers, D. and Buck, M. (2008) *PNF in Practice: An Illustrated Guide*, 3rd edn. Springer, Heidelberg.

Holey, L.A. (1995) Connective tissue massage: towards a scientific rationale. *Physiotherapy*, **81**(12), 730–39.

Further reading

Cash, M. (1996) *Sport and Remedial Massage Therapy*. Ebury Press, London.

Chaitow, L. and DeLany, J. (2000) *Clinical Application of Neuromuscular Techniques*. Churchill Livingstone, Edinburgh.

Holey, E.A. and Cook, E.M. (1997) *Evidence Based Therapeutic Massage*. Churchill Livingstone, Edinburgh.

Oschman, J.L. (2002) Energy medicine: the new paradigm. In: *Complementary Therapies for Physical Therapists* (ed. R.A. Charman), pp. 2–33. Butterworth-Heinemann, Oxford.

Pert, C.B. (1999) *Molecules of Emotion. Why You Feel the Way You Feel*. Simon and Schuster, New York.

Simons, D.G., Travell, J.G., Simons, L.S. and Cummings, B.D. (1999) *Travell & Simons' Myofascial Pain and Disfunction: The Trigger Point Manual*, Vol 2, 2nd edn. Lippincott Williams and Wilkins, Philadelphia.

Watt, J. (1999) *Massage for Sport*. Crowood Press, Marlborough.

Useful websites

http://www.activerelease.com/about.asp
http://www.bowen-technique.co.uk
http://www.energysearch.us
http://www.hellerwork.com/
http://www.luminati.com/vibration.html
http://www.massagetoday.com/aboutmt
http://www.mic.ki.se/diseases/alphalist.html
http://www.noetic.org
http://www.reflexologyforum.org
http://www.reflextherapy.org.uk
http://www.rolfing.org/indexuk/htm
http://www.thaiyogamassage.co.uk
http://www.touch.org.uk/
http://www.zerobalancinguk.org

14 Massage in sport

Joan M. Watt

Massage has been used in sport from time immemorial. Athletes have resorted to massage since the days of the first Olympic Games, and the ancient athletes developed a special tool, the strygil, to scrape the masseur's oil from the skin (Williams 1974).

Sports massage can be divided into:

- Specific sports massage
- Non-specific sports massage

Basic rules of sports massage

Before embarking on any sports massage, the basic rules of such a regime must be addressed:

- Diagnosis
- History
- Contraindications
- Aims of treatment
- Position
- Materials
- Skin preparation
- Joint position
- Technique
- Check with the participant
- Clean up
- Warn the participant

Diagnosis

Diagnosis will only apply if massage is being used to treat a sports injury. Many sports massages are classified as specific, i.e. not only to treat a particular problem but also to help prepare prior to activity, between bouts of activity or after activity. Non-specific sports massage is also used to help keep the body in tune.

History

It is always good practice to gain a full history, either relevant to a particular problem or concerning previous experience of and reaction to massage.

Contraindications

Contraindications are listed in Chapter 3. It is vitally important when dealing with sports people to remember the great risk of recent injury being present.

Aims of treatment

Is the massage to be stimulating or sedative? The aim of treatment will depend on when massage is to be administered, e.g. pre or post event.

Position

It cannot be guaranteed that there will always be a treatment couch available when using massage in sport. Always ensure that the therapist is going to be able to perform all the necessary techniques with the greatest ease and that the recipient is at all times warm and comfortable.

Materials

Various oils may be used, most commonly vegetable based, ice, non-steroidal anti-inflammatory gel, towels, ranging from small to very large, and inflatable pillows.

Skin preparation

Many sports people shave their legs before competition and small nicks are not unusual. Aseptic conditions should apply, with absolute cleanliness essential.

Joint position

In the treatment rooms, positioning as described in previous chapters should be adhered to. At track or pitch side be prepared to be innovative and use whatever is available and suitable to obtain the best joint position.

Technique

This will be addressed later in the chapter.

Check with the participant

Always ask the participant if the massage is deep enough, too deep or as he/she wants it.

Clean up

Participants cannot enter the competition arena covered in oil. A basketball player with oil on his thighs can get this onto his hands with disastrous results. Soap and water are available in the treatment room but not necessarily at pitch side. In that situation wet-wipes or an astringent lotion should be available for use.

Warn the participant

Even if the participant has frequent massages, always warn what to expect as a result of this session, e.g. pre-competition stimulating massage may induce a feeling of warmth but the rules of warm-up must still be observed.

Massage manipulations in sports massage

The massage manipulations used in sports massage are as described in Chapter 6, plus acupressure, trigger pointing and ice massage.

Acupressure

Acupressure/acupuncture ('acu' is Chinese for needle) points are stimulated by finger or thumb pressure. There is a complete therapy using the 'tsubos'-specific sensitive points used in acupressure and also shiatsu (in Japanese 'shi' is finger, 'atsu' is pressure) where whole hands, elbows, feet and knees may be used to massage the body (Jarmey and Tindall 1991).

In sports massage acupressure tends to be to specific trigger points. These points are identified as tense, sometimes hard, and always producing pain in the muscle/connective tissue.

Once the point to be treated has been identified, the finger or thumb is used to apply pressure to that specific point. The technique is similar to that used in circular frictions but only one finger or the thumb tip is used. There are many different opinions as to the length of time the pressure should be held. A firm pressure accompanied by a slight circular motion applied for a maximum of 1 minute, relaxed and reapplied three or four times, gives good results. The object is to try to get muscle relaxation in as short a time as possible, thus making this technique very useful immediately prior to activity by removing particular spots of muscle/tissue tension. The use of both acupressure and shiatsu in sport is growing and there are many varying theories on the subjects, from basic applications to reduced muscle tensions right up to the complete science of the full holistic concept of Oriental medicine (Downer 1992).

Trigger pointing

Trigger pointing as first addressed by Travell and Simons in *Travell & Simons' Myofascial Pain and Dysfunction: The Trigger Point Manual* is an extremely efficient method of treatment in sport. This is particularly good pre and inter competition, when specific tight spots and tension are identified. As always with this technique it is vital to treat all areas and ensure you do not leave the point too soon.

Ice massage

The most convenient method of application of ice massage is to use a polystyrene cup which has been filled with water and then frozen. Cut a 1.25-cm ring from the top edge of the cup and then massage the injured area with the ice until an erythema is achieved. If dealing with tendinous or small areas an ice cube held in a tissue is best.

Specific sports massage

Specific sports massage is given for a particular reason and can be used in six different situations:

- Massage in conditioning
- Massage as treatment
- Pre-competition massage
- Inter-competition massage
- Post-competition massage
- Post-travel massage

These six specific sports massages may have to be carried out at pitch or track side and it may not always be possible to follow to the letter the manipulations, routines and methods suggested. The therapist must be prepared to be adaptable and use the manipulations and skills at his/her command in the most advantageous way to aid the participant in his/her chosen event.

Massage in conditioning

The conditioning time of year for any sports person will depend entirely on what his or her goals are for that particular year. The actual time of year will vary from sport to sport, dependent on the competitive season and major event(s). The object involves the SAID principle: specific adaptation imposed demands (Wallis and Logan 1964). This principle puts the body through safe and intense development, to achieve peak condition at the time of major competition. There may have to be more than one time of 'peaking' in each year, e.g. to qualify for Olympic selection in June and then to compete in the Olympic Games in September. Massage at the time of conditioning plays a very important part in the training regime.

Objects

- **To promote recovery from a hard training session.** It is to be expected after a hard bout of exercise that the sports person will experience various aches, pains and a feeling of tired and heavy limbs. Massage can be invaluable in speeding up recovery at this time.
- **To aid cool-down.** The object of cool-down is to return the body to its pre-exercise state as quickly and painlessly as possible. Massage at this time can be used to aid circulation, assist in the removal of waste products and enable the participant to perform his or her cool-down regimes more effectively.
- **To prevent delayed onset muscle soreness (DOMS).** It is widely appreciated that intense bouts of exercise will produce varying degrees of muscle soreness after the event. This soreness may not be noticed for up to 24 hours after cessation of the activity. Many learned sources will insist that there is no specific proof that massage will, in any way, prevent the occurrence of DOMS. On the other hand observation and anecdotal evidence lead those who are actively engaged in the field of sport massage to feel DOMS can be, and is, influenced positively by the application of the correct massage techniques.

- **Psychological effect.** The importance of the psychological effect of touch has never been fully quantified. At this hard time of training for the sports person a massage performed by a good knowledgeable practitioner can make a vast difference to his or her continued wellbeing and can enhance the benefits of the conditioning period.

Contact materials

Oils and mild warming rubs.

Routine and manipulations used

- Light effleurage to accustom the person to touch; also to test to see if there has been any micro trauma to soft tissue as a result of hard training.
- Deep effleurage to promote venous and lymphatic drainage.
- Petrissage to mobilise the soft tissues.
- Deep effleurage as above.
- Acupressure to address any specific tension or trigger spots identified.
- Stroking to provide relaxation and aid venous return.
- Tapôtement/shaking/vibrations to stimulate and give a feeling of wellbeing.
- Effleurage to aid venous and lymphatic return, and to assess the final state of the tissues.

Method

Start with the back, then the limbs, concentrating on the muscles most used in the training session. Often finish with a foot massage.

Duration

Whole body: 1–1.5 hours; half body: 30–45 minutes. This massage can be given on a daily basis throughout the conditioning period, with the first massage being given the day before the first day of hard training.

Contraindications

Contraindications are as described in Chapter 3, paying particular attention to identifying and avoiding any micro trauma that may have been occasioned by a particularly hard training session.

Massage as a treatment

Massage as a treatment for sports injuries can be used after 48 hours if all bleeding and tissue swelling has ceased, or, in the case of haematoma, after 4 days or dependent on the patient's tolerance.

Objects

- **To stimulate circulation.** Forty eight hours after trauma it is important to clear away the debris of the incident and remove the excess tissue fluid. Massage can play a useful part in reaching these goals.
- **To promote recovery from injury.** As stated above, to stimulate circulation and also to ensure the continued good state of surrounding tissues.
- **To break down adhesions.** The most important result after injury in sport must be that the individual has not been left with a tight shortened scar in any soft tissue. Adhesions and scar tissue are sources of trouble and can result in further trauma producing bigger and thicker areas of adherent tissue. Massage can play a very important part in the recovery.
- **To promote flexibility.** It is essential that all participants have returned at least to their previous level of flexibility after injury. Massage can provide a useful adjunct to the essential stretch routines performed by the patient.
- **To improve the range of movement.** Most types of injury, both soft tissue and bony, may well necessitate periods of strapping and/or immobilisation. A return to full range movement is necessary prior to return to full training and competition. Massage is used extensively to facilitate achieving a full range of movement.

Contact materials

Oil, cream, heat rub, ice, anti-inflammatory gel or cream.

Routine and manipulations used

- Stroking to accustom the sports person to touch and discover any areas of sensitivity.
- Effleurage to promote venous and lymphatic return; depth will depend on injury.
- Petrissage to mobilise soft tissue and induce slight stretch on those tissues; also to reduce muscle spasm.
- Effleurage as above.
- Frictions – to produce a counter-irritant effect as described in Chapter 6, to mobilise and break down scar tissue.
- Tapôtement to produce an excitation effect as described in Chapter 6, plus a feeling of wellbeing.
- Effleurage as above.
- Shaking applied both locally and to a total limb to aid relaxation and relief of muscle tension and cramp.
- Acupressure – by stimulating trigger points it is possible to gain muscle relaxation or an increase in muscle tone, dependent on depth and length of pressure applied.
- Connective tissue massage to mobilise the deep reticular layers of the dermis.
- Rolling as described in Chapter 6.
- Effleurage as above and to assess the final state of the tissues.

Method

Always massage proximal and then distal areas of the body before concentrating on the treatment area proper.

Duration

Dependent on area and sensitivity of the area to be treated the duration of massage may be 10–30 minutes. The treatment can be used daily depending on the patient's level of discomfort and training/competition schedule.

Contraindications

Contraindications are as described in Chapter 3. Also it is advisable not to massage within 3 days of training or competition if the methods are used to treat scar tissue or adhesions, and never if the patient cannot tolerate treatment.

Pre-competition massage

Massage prior to competition is to many sports people part of the ritual carried out before their sporting endeavour. The time of this massage as part of the adjunct to performance must be carefully planned. If dealing with a team sport and all players require a massage, there must be adequate staff so that massages are not carried out many hours before the actual physical warm-up. In the case of individual performance, the report time and/or start time will decide the time of the pre-competition massage: for example, start time 10.30 a.m., report time 10.10 a.m., warm-up 1 hour, therefore the pre-competition massage must start at 8.40 a.m. at the latest.

Warm-up is the preparation of the body for physical activity. It is divided into three components:

- Raising body temperature and increasing cardiovascular activity.
- Putting all joints through a full range of movement and all muscles into their greatest length of flexibility.
- Sport-specific warm-up by practising the activities to be carried out.

Thus, a rugby player will end his/her warm-up with ball skills, passing and tackling; a hurdler will hurdle; and a discus thrower will practise the movements required to throw the discus.

This massage cannot be used instead of the participant's own physical warm-up but definitely can be used to enhance the preparation.

Objects

- **To prepare muscles for exertion.** By increasing the circulation to specific areas and mobilising soft tissues. Massage prior to activity will make it easier to carry out the specific stretches needed for any performance.
- **To aid warm-up effect.** As the term implies, warm-up is about warming the body prior to activity. The vasodilatation caused by massage will enhance this phase of physical preparation.
- **Psychological effect.** The time spent on the massage couch is often used by participants to prepare mentally for the forthcoming action. This may be done in conversation with the therapist or may be inward and silent. There is

a great advantage if the therapist knows the competitor well and knows whether or not he/she likes to talk at this stage. It is also a good time to reinforce positive messages and allay fears about injury worries and the state of the opposition.

Contact materials

These must be carefully selected dependent on the activity about to take place and great care must be taken to clean the area well after the massage. Oils, creams and talcum powder are all appropriate, but do not use any heating agent. All rubefacients will cause vasodilatation of the skin and this will prove to be detrimental to the warm-up. The vasodilatation needs to be greatest below the dermis to aid warm-up.

Routine and manipulations used

- Stroking to accustom the person to touch.
- Effleurage to promote venous and lymphatic return, and discover any area that is particularly tight, tense or giving pain.
- Petrissage to increase mobility of the soft tissues and stimulate circulation.
- Tapôtement/shaking/vibration – all or one or two to promote a feeling of wellbeing and give relief from muscle tension.
- Effleurage to finish massage and ascertain that the desired effects have been produced.
- Trigger point and acupressure may be needed if there are specific areas of muscle spasm, tension or increased tone.

Method

Massage as requested by the participant. Many sports people only want/need massage to a particular area, e.g. hamstrings or calf, while others request a full body massage.

Duration

Duration of the massage is dependent on the area to be covered and length of time to achieve the desired effect of stimulation and to decrease any spasm or increase tone. Usually 20–30 minutes to a maximum time of 1 hour is best. As a last-minute attempt to decrease specific muscle tension, 5 minutes of acupressure can be used. It is best performed immediately prior to warm-up and it may well be followed by particular muscle stretch techniques such as contract/relax or stretch/relax as used in progressive neuromuscular facilitation techniques. **Do not use hot rubs.**

Contraindications

Contraindications are as stated in Chapter 3. Also it is advisable not to massage if the competitor has not used massage prior to competition on previous occasions.

Inter-competition massage

When there is prolonged competition it will be necessary to provide inter-competition massage. During a competition that has several rounds such as qualifying, quarter-final, semi-final and perhaps even finals on the same day, there are periods of rest in between. This is when massage can be very useful to the participant; also in multi-events at track and field, when the men do ten events over 2 days and the women seven. In this circumstance, if the athletes spent their normal time before and after each discipline doing warm-up and cool-down, they would be too tired to compete. Cool-down is the time immediately after training or competition when the participant will jog and perform specific exercises all aimed at returning the body to its resting state. Massage is extremely useful to complement a shortened warm-up and cool-down, but again cannot replace these essential activities. The only time massage can replace cool-down is if the participant is too exhausted to perform an active cool-down or if injury precludes activity. **Massage can never replace active warm-up.**

Objects

- **To promote recovery.** After a bout of exercise there will be waste products in the tissues. Massage, by stimulating venous and lymphatic return, aids the process of elimination of such products.
- **To refresh the competitor.** In a prolonged competition it is not unusual to experience muscle fatigue and general tiredness. Stimulating massage can be advantageous to combat both feelings.

- **To work out niggles.** After hard exercise there may well be a feeling of tightness in certain muscle groups, which will not respond to the competitor's normal series of stretching exercises. Massage can be used to help physically and also to reassure the participant that there is no major problem developing.
- **To prevent muscle cramps and spasms.** It is not unusual, especially if the competition is taking place in a situation where dehydration can occur, to be presented with cramps. While the competitor rehydrates with the correct fluids, massage can be used to help increase the circulation to the affected part.

Contact materials

Be careful to select the correct medium. If the area is sweaty or has sand or chalk on it, it must first be cleansed. The pores will be open and you do not want to clog these with any medium which will impede heat loss. A very light oil or soapy water is best. Never use any hot rubs at this stage. It may be necessary to use ice massage if there is an area where there could be actual tissue damage.

Routine and manipulations used

- Stroking to accustom the person to touch and to assess the temperature and state of the area to be massaged.
- Effleurage to promote venous and lymphatic return and discover any particularly tense spot(s).
- Petrissage to help remove the waste products and mobilise the soft tissues. The rolling manipulations described in Chapter 6 are particularly useful here.
- Acupressure to any area that is excessively tense or tending to cramp.
- Vibrations and shaking – whole-limb shaking and vibration are very good towards the end of this massage to ensure the limb is ready for the next bout of exercise and unlikely to go into cramp.
- Trigger pointing and acupressure – always be sure there is no underlying soft tissue damage.
- Effleurage to complete the session and prepare the competitor for warm-up.

Method

Massage as needed by the competitor. Early on in the day the request may be to address one specific area that is bothering the competitor. However, as the competition continues and usually before and/or after the last event of the day, it may be necessary to cover the full body.

Duration

Massage as time allows; this may be for only several minutes or up to an hour. It is best to perform inter-competition massage immediately after cool-down and/or prior to the next warm-up.

Contraindications

Contraindications are as stated in Chapter 3. Also any area of recent trauma must be avoided.

Post-competition massage

At the cessation of activity the competitor will do cool-down. Massage can be used to enhance the effects of this procedure. On certain occasions it may be necessary to replace active cool-down with massage and passive movements, e.g. after a marathon, long-distance event, or when the competitor has sustained an injury that precludes active cool-down.

Objects

- **To carry away waste products** (see 'Inter-competition massage' above).
- **To allow body functions to return to normal.** At the end of any period of physical activity the cardiovascular system may be working excessively hard, or as a result of the cessation of activity the blood pressure can suddenly drop. Massage, especially centripetal effleurage, is very useful in restoring normality.
- **To prevent post-exercise pain** (as previously described in 'Massage in conditioning').
- **To work out niggles.** Frequently after activity the participant may complain of certain specific areas of pain or tension. If any tissue damage is suspected, ice massage can be

applied. If the cause is purely exercise induced, then massage is beneficial to remove the tightness.

- **Psychological effect.** As previously described this can be very important if the competitor is either on a 'high' after competing successfully or, conversely, 'down' after a poor performance.

Contact materials

Ice, soapy water or light oil, but not any hot rubs or talcum powder.

Routine and manipulations used

All manipulations should be slow and rhythmic.

- Stroking to assess the area and accustom the sports person to touch.
- Effleurage – at first light and centripetal, then deeper if there is no tension or pain. It can be performed in all directions, to increase circulation and remove waste products.
- Petrissage – starting fairly light and deepening to a level the participant can tolerate.
- Effleurage interspersed between all other strokes and for at least 5 minutes at the end of the massage to enhance tissue drainage.

Method

Massage as requested by the competitor. This may be to one specific area only or to the whole body area and in some instances may be used in place of active cool-down.

Duration

Duration is dependent on the area to be covered; it may last 15–30 minutes or may take a full hour. This massage is best performed after the active cool-down and preceded by a tepid shower. When taking the place of an active cool-down it is essential to ensure that the participant is adequately rehydrating as well as receiving massage.

Contraindications

Again contraindications are as described in Chapter 3. Also be very circumspect around painful areas which might well be caused by micro trauma, in which case only ice massage should be applied.

Post-travel massage

It is very common for all types of sports people to have to travel varying distances to participate in competition all over the world. Wherever possible sufficient time should be allowed to permit adequate acclimatisation both to time change and climatic conditions. In reality the competitors may not be able to allow this time to adjust. The length of time spent travelling and the frequency of this travel can adversely affect performance. Travel problems highlighted in sport are:

- A general feeling of stiffness.
- A feeling of lassitude.
- Aches, especially in the lower back, neck and shoulders.
- Swelling of lower legs and feet.

Solutions are:

- Light exercise
- Shower
- Jacuzzi
- Massage

Objects

- **To increase venous and lymphatic flow, thus removing swelling and stiffness.**
- **To remove aches and increase flexibility** by gently and deeply stretching the soft tissues.
- **To remove any residual stiffness** without tiring the competitor with exercise.
- **To restore normal balance of the body.**
- **To create a feeling of wellbeing.**

Contact materials

Oil or creams. Do not use talcum powder or hot rubs as there may well be some dehydration present.

Routine and manipulations used

- Stroking to assess the condition of the skin and accustom the participant to touch.

- Effleurage – first centripetal to aid tissue drainage and increase venous and lymphatic return, then multidirectional to promote tissue stretching.
- Petrissage – especially kneading, wringing, picking up and rolling techniques to assist drainage and stretch the soft tissues.
- Effleurage should be interspersed regularly with all other strokes.
- Tapôtement, vibration and shaking to aid venous and lymphatic return and to promote a feeling of wellbeing.

Method

Start with the back and neck, then the legs and if necessary the arms as well. Finish with assisted stretches to the major muscle groups used in the participant's activity.

Duration

Duration is dependent on the areas to be covered but should be a minimum of 30 minutes and may last over an hour. Best results are gained if the participant has already carried out some gentle activity, such as a jog and gentle stretches, and then had a tepid shower prior to massage.

Contraindications

Contraindications are as described in Chapter 3, paying particular attention to the effects of dehydration.

Non-specific sports massage

There are times in the competitor's year when there is no competition or conditioning taking place. At those times the athlete will still be maintaining his/her body in a state of preparedness for the activities of the future. Massage can play a very important and helpful part at those times and is referred to as non-specific massage. This term also applies to massage given when the competitor has arrived at the competition site ahead of the event by at least 2 days, or finished competition and is still present at the competition site, waiting for the rest of the team to complete competition and return home. Basically we are referring to a massage that is given for no specific treatment purpose, and is not before, between or after competition or travel. Non-specific sports massage can be divided into two applications:

- General body massage
- Specific areas of massage

General body massage

Sports people spend a large part of their lives conditioning and preparing their bodies for the rigours of their particular sport. Many of them firmly believe that regular full body massage will aid them in their pursuit of excellence.

Objects

- **To enhance a general feeling of wellbeing.**
- **To promote relaxation**, if this is desired by the participant.
- **To stimulate**, if requested by the participant.
- **To monitor condition of the musculature and soft tissues.**
- **To highlight and deal with any area that could develop into a problem.**

Contact materials

Oils. If knowledgeable, aromatherapy can be used (see Chapter 15), creams, mild warming rub or talcum powder.

Routine and manipulations used

For objects 1 and 2:

- Stroking to accustom to touch.
- Effleurage – long slow manipulations used continuously.
- Kneading deep enough not to tickle, slow and rhythmical.
- Effleurage – slow to end the session.

For objects 1 and 3:

- As described in 'Pre-competition massage'.

For object 4:

- Deep effleurage.

For object 5:

- Trigger pointing and friction may be added and in this case the non-specific massage will change to a treatment massage if specific problem areas are highlighted.

Method

- For objects 1 and 2, as described in Chapter 2, starting with the back and neck, then each limb in turn, foot massage as opposed to facial massage and, if deemed necessary, finish by returning to the back.
- For objects 1 and 3, as described in 'Pre-competition massage'.
- For object 4, extra effleurage at the start and finish of the session.
- For object 5, as described in 'Massage as a treatment'.

Duration

For objects 1 and 2, massage as long as is needed to gain the desired relaxation, usually 1–1.5 hours. It is important that the competitor can lie and relax for at least half an hour after completion of the massage.

For objects 1 and 3, it is as described in 'Pre-competition massage'.

For object 4, a few extra moments at the end of each session are required.

For object 5, duration is as your findings necessitate.

Contraindications

Contraindications are as described in Chapter 3.

Specific areas of massage

Dependent on the muscle groups most used in a particular event, the competitor may request an area of body to receive massage, rather than a full body massage, e.g. a thrower's back and/or shoulders; a sprinter's hamstrings, quadriceps and calf muscles; a distance eventer's and soccer player's calf muscles.

Objects, contact materials and manipulations

These are as described in 'General body massage'.

Method

Concentrate on the area highlighted by the participant, but do not forget to clear the surrounding area.

Duration

Massage for as long as is needed to gain the desired effects.

Contraindications

Contraindications are as described in Chapter 3.

Summary

- Never give a first massage to a participant within 48 hours of competition.
- Arrange for the first massage to take place when there is plenty of time for any adverse effects to be worked off.
- Adverse effects may be:
  - producing too much relaxation;
  - stirring up old problems such as scar tissue.

Sports massage may be sport specific and any therapist involved must know and understand the principles of that sport. Most importantly, the rules and call-up times of the sport must be understood. As already stated, there will not always be time to perform the beginning, middle and end of a massage as you might wish. The most important issue in a situation where time is of the essence is to be absolutely clear about the main object of this massage. It may be to eliminate a particular point of tension or increase range of movement. Having identified the object, choose which of the techniques can best deliver the desired effect and use them. If the sport is an outdoor activity it may not even be possible to remove clothing, e.g. skiing, orienteering, distance running – participants frequently wear tights or jogging bottoms to protect their legs. In instances like these whole limb shaking, vibration or trigger pointing through the clothing will be the best massage techniques to use.

Case study

This case study by Joan M. Watt originally appeared in *Sportex Dynamics* and is reproduced with permission of Centaur Publishing.

What is sports massage? Sports massage is applying massage modalities for the specific benefit of sports and exercise participants and can be applied to any active person. It covers the manipulation and management of the soft tissues of the body. Sports massage can address specific muscle, ligament, tendon or fascia problems or be used to enhance the activity of healthy tissue. This type of massage should be administered to positively enhance each person's ability to move, exercise and compete.

Event information: decathlon is a track and field athletics event and is only for male competitors. There are ten events in all which take place over 2 days. Day one consists of 100 m, long jump, shot put, high jump and 400 m. On day two the events are 110 m hurdles, discus, pole vault, javelin and 1500 m.

Scenario: a 20-year-old student who is about to compete in the decathlon for his university team presents with limited range of movement in his right hamstring 30 minutes prior to his first event.

General health: excellent, very fit, no known illnesses, current injuries or allergies.

Previous history: originally tore his right hamstring at age 17 and has had no problems since.

Previous treatment: physiotherapy at time of injury, ice strapping, exercise and stretching. No follow-up or advice.

Medication: none.

Surgery: none.

Assessment:

- Questioning – this revealed previous injury history, a dislike of doing flexibility exercises and only paying lip service to warm-up and cool-down.
- Observation and movement – very fit, well-muscled young man but exhibits slightly stiff movement patterns. Right hip flexion was 20 degrees less than left and lower musculotendinous junction of the right biceps femoris was scarred and showing evidence of loss of elasticity. All other ranges of movement could be improved by stretching. Medial rotation of both hip joints was reduced by 20%.
- Palpation – sensation was normal, no lower back problems, skin temperature normal, no evidence of skin abrasions, cuts or rashes.

Treatment plan and outcome:

- Considerations – this young man did not stay in the area of the competition and was only going to be present for the 2 days of competition.
- Aims and objectives – it was agreed that we should try to get enough relaxation into the affected muscle tissue to allow safe participation. It was explained that long term the damaged area would need to receive intensive care with correct soft tissue mobilisation, passive and active stretching and conditioning. The competitor was advised to seek professional help at home, and contact details of a practitioner in his home area were supplied.
- Treatment pre-event – general massage to posterior aspect of right thigh and calf using stroking, effleurage, grades 1 to 2, petrissage, specific kneading, picking up, wringing and rolling grades 1 to 3. This was then followed by trigger pointing and acupressure grades 1 to 2 on specific areas, and ended with myofascial release and proprioceptive neuromuscular facilitation.

Range increased following treatment to allow a good pattern of movement with no pain.

Massage was administered before each of the events on day one, with ice massage being introduced between events four and five.

Post-event massage concentrated on gently loosening the tightest area and consisted mainly of effleurage, myofascial release, rolling, wringing and muscle energy technique. Ice was applied for 10 minutes at the end of massage and the athlete was advised to do gentle non-weight-bearing stretches for 5–10 minutes every hour awake and stretching to be held for 30–40 seconds.

Day two started with slightly increased range, but pain was experienced from mid to end of range of movement.

Massage as on day one was administered before each event and post competition, with ice being used on each occasion.

By the end of day two the musculotendinous junction was slightly slacker but showing active trigger points with very noticeable attachment to good tissue. Range of movement was almost full and the athlete experienced slight tightness and occasional twinging.

Since this event the competitor has received treatment from a sports-specific physiotherapist and sports massage practitioner in his home area. He now has equal pain-free range of movement in right and left hamstrings, strength is equal and he is training and competing fully. On palpation of the original problem area there is a small but mobile area of scar tissue. Ongoing it is vital that the athlete continues all stretching and strength work and attends for regular assessment of the scar tissue.

References

Downer, J. (1992) *Shiatsu (Headway Lifeguides)*. Hodder and Stoughton, London.

Jarmey, C. and Tindall, J. (1991) *Acupressure for Common Ailments*. Gaia Books, London.

Wallis, E.L. and Logan, G.A. (1964) *Figure Improvement and Body Conditioning Through Exercise*. Prentice Hall, New York.

Williams, J. (1974) *Massage and Sport*. Bayer, Switzerland.

Further reading

Andrade, C.K. and Clifford, P. (2001) *Outcome Based Massage*. Lippincott Williams and Wilkins, Philadelphia.

Cafarelli, E. and Flint, F. (1992) The role of massage in preparation for and recovery from exercise. *Sports Medicine*, **14**(1), 1–9.

Hilbert, J.E., Sforzo, G.A. and Swensen, T. (2003) The effects of massage on delayed onset muscle soreness. *British Journal of Sports Medicine*, **37**, 72–5.

Holey, E.A. and Cook, E.M. (2003) *Evidence-Based Therapeutic Massage*. Churchill Livingstone, Edinburgh.

Robertson, A. Watt, J.M. and Galloway, S.D.R. (2004) Effects of leg massage on recovery from high intensity cycling exercise. *British Journal of Sports Medicine*, **38**, 173–6.

Simons, D.G., Travell, J.G., Simons, L.S. and Cummings, B.D. (1999) *Travell & Simons' Myofascial Pain and Dysfunction: The Trigger Point Manual*, Vol **2**, 2nd edn. Lippincott Williams and Wilkins, Philadelphia.

Watt, J. (1999) *Massage for Sport*. Crowood Press, Marlborough.

Weerapong, P., Hume, P.A. and Kolt, G.S. (2005) The mechanisms of massage and effects on performance, muscle recovery and injury. *Sports Medicine*, **35**(3), 235–56.

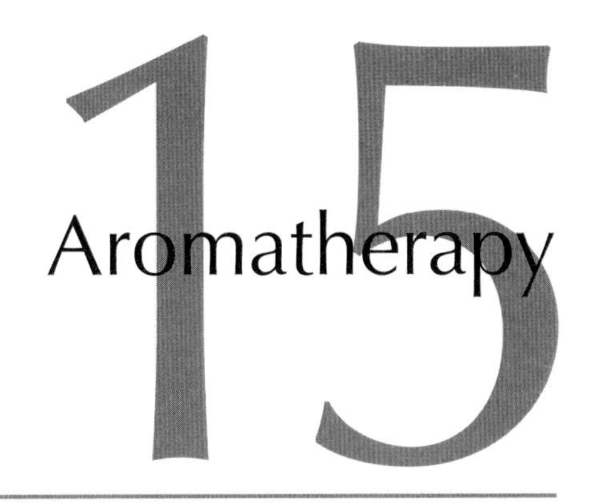

15 Aromatherapy

Elisabeth Jones

Introduction

Aromatherapy may be defined as a therapeutic treatment that utilises the fragrant components extracted from aromatic plants. The aromatic substances generally used by aromatherapists are the essential oils of these plants. Aromatherapy massage must only be practised by those therapists who have nationally recognised qualifications.

Historical uses of essential oils

Since time immemorial aromatic plants and their extracts have been used for religious, medicinal and cosmetic purposes.

Egyptians: 3000–1500 BC

The ancient Egyptians used them not only for religious rites (embalming of bodies, using in particular cedarwood oil), but also for their therapeutic effects (scented unguents on sun-baked skin to soothe and maintain elasticity). A famous perfume, 'Kyphi', was made of a mixture of fragrant herbs and resins. Plutarch said that the aromatic substances included in the perfume Kyphi 'lulled one to sleep, allayed anxieties and brightened dreams' (Genders 1972).

Greeks: 500–40 BC

The Greeks also used aromatics for medicinal as well as body-enhancing purposes. A famous Greek perfume 'Megaleion', named after its Greek creator Megallus, was used not only for its scent but also for healing wounds and reducing inflammation.

Europeans

Twelfth century

Many monasteries had their own aromatic herb gardens and used the plants and extracts to heal the sick who came to their doors. Abbess Hildegard of Bingen is known to have utilised both the plant and the essential oil of lavender.

Sixteenth century

To ward off the plague, according to a book written in French, *Les Secrets de Maître Alexis de Piedmont*, the house should be fumigated with all manner of fragrant substances including rosemary, cloves, nutmeg, sage, aloes and juniper wood (Genders 1972).

Seventeenth century

By the beginning of the 17th century approximately 60 oils were being used for their perfume and medicinal effects (Valnet 1980).

Nineteenth century

'The first research into the antiseptic powers of essential oils was undertaken by Chamberland in 1887 in his work on the anthrax bacillus. He noted the active properties of origanum, Chinese cinnamon, Singhalese cinnamon, angelica and Algerian geranium' (Valnet 1980).

Twentieth century

Cavel's research on microbial cultures in sewage has shown many essences to have the power to render inactive 1000 cc of culture at considerable dilutions (Valnet 1980). Cavel in fact researched 35 oils, finding thyme, origanum and sweet orange the most effective (Cavel 1918).

Gattefosse, a French chemist, was the first to coin the term 'aromatherapy', having during and after World War I made an extensive study of the uses of plants, and published a book termed '*Aromatherapy*' in 1937.

During World War II, Dr Jean Valnet, another Frenchman, inspired by Gattefosse's work, started to use essential oils in his clinical practice. His medication included both internal and external use of essential oils.

By the 1960s a small band of enthusiasts (the foremost being Madame Maury, a French biochemist) began to incorporate essential oils into massage treatments. This use of essential oils has grown steadily and aromatherapy massage, when given by properly qualified practitioners, is now widely used in hospitals, hospices and clinics.

Essential oils

An essential oil may be defined as an odorous, volatile substance, present within all aromatic plant matter. In many cases the amount is so minute that it is not practicable, or is too expensive, to isolate it. Essential oils are not confined to flowers. They may be found in leaves, grasses, seeds, roots, rhizomes and fruits as well as woods and resins.

When essential oils are produced in more than one part of a plant, the individual oils will differ in composition and fragrance, e.g. the bitter orange tree gives bitter orange oil from the rind of the orange, petitgrain oil from the leaves and the green twigs, and neroli oil from its freshly picked flowers.

Basic chemistry

A typical essential oil is a complex mixture of chemical compounds, each of which possesses its own individual properties (Williams 1989).

'All of the constituents of an essential oil are organic; that is, their molecular structures are based upon arrangements of carbon atoms blended into one another and to atoms of hydrogen. Oxygen atoms are present in many of the constituents of essential oils and sometimes atoms of nitrogen and/or sulphur' (Williams 1989).

The constituents that have molecules containing carbon and hydrogen only are called hydrocarbons. The number of constituents in an essential oil varies, and an oil may have 100 or more when analysed. The contribution of any one constituent to the unique scent of an essential oil depends on:

- The proportion of the constituent.
- The volatility of the constituent.
- The quality of the constituent.
- The strength of odour of the constituent.

The varying evaporation rates of the individual constituents will affect the fragrance of the essential oil over the passage of time. 'It is the odours of the oxygenated constituents and to a secondary degree the odours of their sesquiterpenes which determine the odours of almost all the essential oils' (Williams 1989).

Mind and body

A perfume uses natural and synthetic materials to combine odour and volatility to give the wearer maximum psychological pleasure from the fragrance that he/she has chosen. This pleasure results from the stimulation of the olfactory (smell) nerve endings in the nose. An aromatherapist combines psychological with physiological effects to gain maximum therapeutic value from the essential oils.

Aromatherapists remain firmly committed to using only natural essential oils from aromatic plants.

> 'It has been demonstrated that the anti-inflammatory and other medicinal properties of some natural oils, some of which have been used since Biblical times, are gentler and less toxic than the pure active drugs isolated from the oil' (van Toller and Dodd 1988).

These essential oils offer a state of wellbeing not only for the mind but also for the body.

Extraction methods

Figure 15.1 describes methods of extraction and the aromatic derivatives from plants. Essential oils used in aromatherapy may be extracted from plant materials in the following ways:

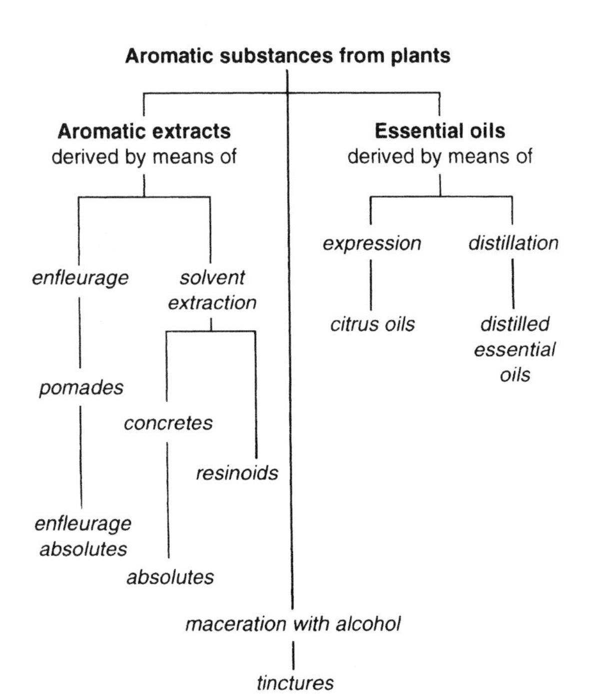

Figure 15.1 Aromatic derivatives from plants.

- Distillation: this is the method usually employed for extracting the essential oil from a plant. The plant material is heated either in boiling water or in steam and the essential oil molecules are released and are ultimately distilled.
- Expression: the expression technique is reserved for citrus oils because they are unable to withstand the rigours of distillation. Hand or mechanical pressure is applied to the rinds of citrus fruits, thereby expressing their essential oils.
- Solvent extraction: aromatic extracts such as concretes and absolutes and resinoids contain considerable amounts of non-volatile matter and cannot therefore be truly termed essential oils. They are removed by chemical solvents from the plant matter that stores them. They are sometimes used by aromatherapists.
- Enfleurage: this method used to be used to extract absolutes for perfumery. Glass plates were covered with a film of cold fat on which fragrant flower petals were laid, their essential oils being absorbed by the fat.
- Hydrofusion/percolation: this is the newest method of extraction and though it uses steam as in distillation it is considered to be a faster process.
- Maceration: some essential oils are too difficult or too costly to distil and are therefore extracted by a method called maceration. Plants such as calendula, lime blossom and Melissa are cut up and placed in a vat of vegetable oil, e.g. almond or sunflower, and agitated for some days. The molecules of the essential oils are absorbed by the vegetable oil, and the liquid is filtered and then bottled.
- Carbon dioxide extraction: this method was introduced in the 1980s for the perfumery trade, but it remains an expensive method. The oils are supposed to be more like the 'natural' oil.

A working knowledge of essential oils

It is important that an aromatherapist has a working knowledge of the traditional uses of at least 40 different oils, and a list of the most commonly used is given below:

Basil (*Ocimum basilicum*)
Benzoin (*Styrax benzoin*)
Bergamot (*Citrus bergamia*)
Cajaput (*Melaleuca cajaputi*)
Cedarwood (*Cedrus virginia*)
Chamomile – Moroccan (*Ormenis multicaulis*)
Chamomile – Roman (*Chamaemelum nobile*)
Clary sage (*Salvia sclarea*)
Cypress (*Cupressus sempervirens*)
Eucalyptus (*Eucalyptus globulus*)
Fennel (sweet) (*Foeniculum vulgaris*)
Frankincense (*Boswellia carteri*)
Geranium (*Pelargonium graveolens*)
Ginger (*Zingiber officinalis*)
Grapefruit (*Citrus paradisi*)
Hyssop (*Hyssopus officinalis*)
Jasmine (*Jasminum officinale*)
Juniper (*Juniper communis*)
Lavender (*Lavender angustifolia*)
Lemon (*Citrus limon*)
Lemongrass (*Cymbopogon citratus*)
Mandarin (*Citrus reticulata*)
Marjoram (sweet) (*Origanum marjorana*)
Melissa (lemon balm) (*Melissa officinalis*)
Myrrh (*Commiphora myrrha*)
Neroli (*Citrus aurantium*)
Niaouli (*Melaleuca viridiflora*)
Palmarosa (*Cybopogon martinii*)
Patchouli (*Pogostemon cablin*)
Pepper (black) (*Piper nigrum*)
Peppermint (*Mentha piperita*)
Petitgrain (*Citrus aurantium bigaradia*)
Pine (*Pinus sylvestris*)
Rose (*Rosa centrifolia/Rosa damascena*)
Rosemary (*Rosmarinus officinalis*)
Sandalwood (Spanish) (*Santalum album*)
Sweet orange (*Citrus aurentium/Citrus vulgaris*)
Teatree (*Melaleuca alternifolia*)
Thyme (*Thymus vulgaris*)
Ylang ylang (*Cananga odorata*, var. *genuina*)

Methods of administering essential oils

Figure 15.2 illustrates methods of use and the passage of essential oils into the body.

Aromatherapists generally administer essential oils therapeutically via olfaction, inhalation or skin absorption.

Olfaction

Olfaction occurs when the sense of smell is interpreted by the olfactory apparatus. This starts in the nose where the olfactory receptors are situated, and spreads via impulses along the olfactory nerve (C1) to the olfactory bulbs on the underside of the brain. There are two groups of receptors of about 25 million cells each of which lie in a small area at the top of the nose.

Protruding from the cells are olfactory hairs which are so small as to be visible only when very highly magnified by the electron microscope; they lie immersed in the thin watery secretion of the mucus which covers the surfaces of the nasal cavities (Williams 1989).

Odour molecules from the essential oils are volatile and fat and water soluble.

'As a result when we breathe in these molecules they easily penetrate the mucus layer and come into contact with the olfactory cilia. The incoming molecules fit into the receptor sites and initiate an electrochemical reaction in a "lock and key" action' (Vickers 1996).

The olfactory apparatus is closely associated with the limbic system (hippocampus and amygdala), once known as the rhinencephalen or 'nose-brain'. The limbic system is that part of the brain that is concerned with feelings, emotions, moods and motivation. It influences eating, aggressive action and sexual activity and controls certain hormones and the autonomic nervous system. There is quite a lot of observational evidence that shows that odours influence mind and body, e.g.

(1) Menstrual synchrony in female humans is an example thought to be due to odour (Schwartz and Natyncuk 1990).
(2) Communication in the insect world by the volatile chemical pheromones is often cited in support of this theory.

The fragrance of essential oils transmitted via the olfactory system to specialised areas of the brain undoubtedly creates psychological effects which in turn may achieve physical effects of a therapeutic nature.

Inhalation

Inhalation occurs when we breathe air into the lungs. When the vapour from an essential oil con-

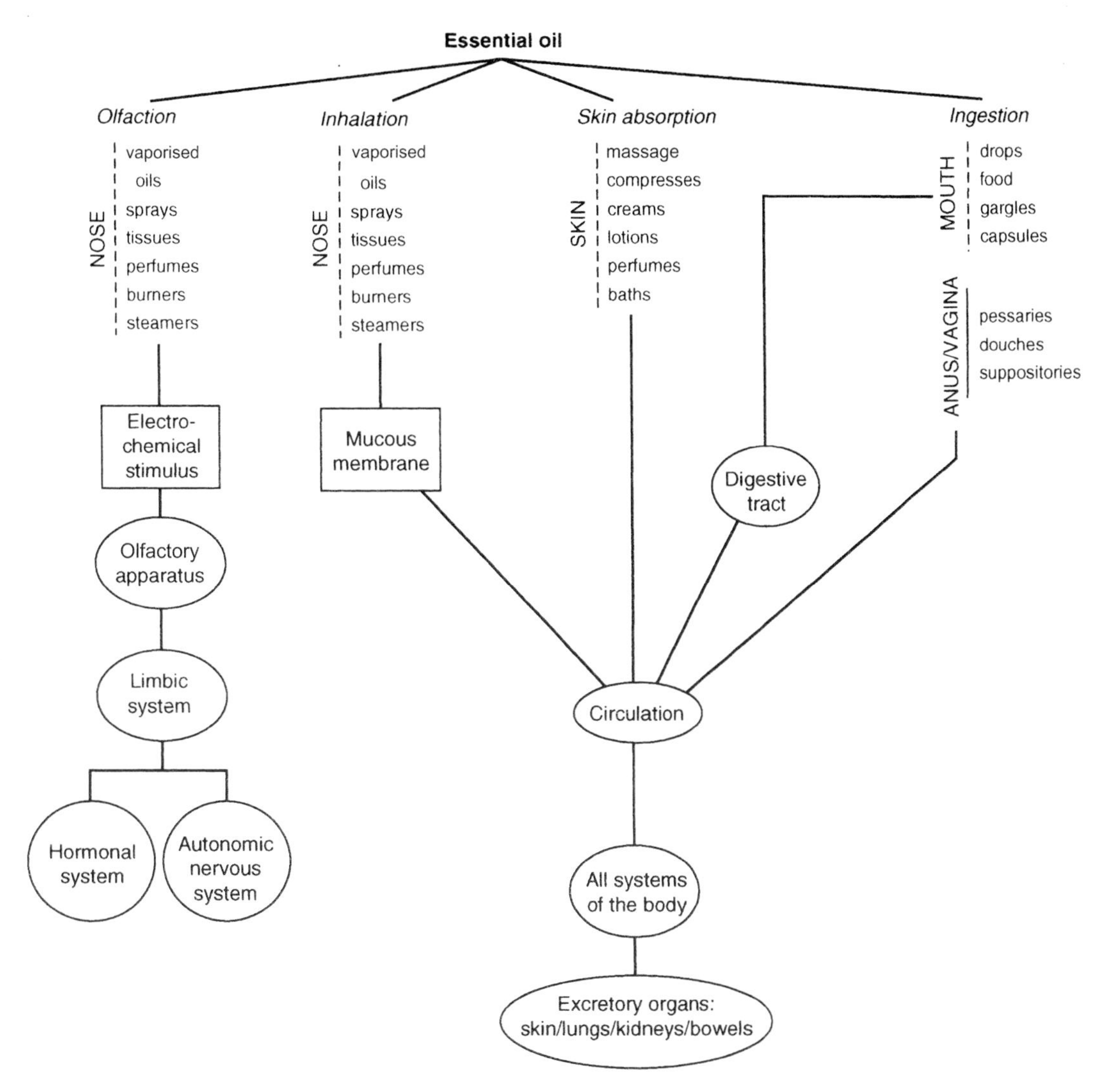

Figure 15.2 The practical application of essential oils: methods of use, and passage of essential oils in the body.

taining aromatic molecules passes into the respiratory system it can have an effect throughout the system. Many traditional remedies advocate the use of essential oils in boiling water and vaporising chest rubs to improve respiratory function. A number of clinical tests have been done that support the use of such inhalations (Berger *et al.* 1978; Saller *et al.* 1990).

The aromatic molecules also pass through the walls of the alveoli in the lungs and enter the bloodstream. Again, clinical research has shown this to happen (e.g. Kovar *et al.* 1987; Buchbauer *et al.* 1993; Falk-Filipsson *et al.* 1993).

Skin absorption

Until relatively recently it was thought that the skin was virtually impermeable, but it is now known that the skin and mucous membranes are able to absorb lipophilic substances (Brun 1952). Traditionally, the action of oils when they are absorbed through the skin is considered to be similar to when they are absorbed into the capillary network around the alveoli of the lungs. They enter the bloodstream and are transported round the body until naturally eliminated.

Whether absorbed by the lungs or the skin it is possible they influence the body processes. Some may stimulate the release of endorphins – the body's own chemicals which can have an analgesic or anti-depressant effect. Others appear to have a diuretic effect, whilst yet more may be able to help with hormonal balances of the body or support the immune system.

Just as the oils work on the respiratory tissue itself during inhalation, so essences can have an effect on the skin during skin absorption. Essential oils therefore not only provide pleasing fragrances, which have an effect on the mind, but also can have beneficial effects on the body.

Ingestion

Essential oils may be administered orally or via the anus or vagina. However, ingestion as a method of treatment should only be undertaken by those qualified, for instance in phytotherapy. The reason for this is that this method has the greatest risks of adverse effects. Though some doctors in France specialise in treatment by ingestion, it is rarely used in the UK or the USA.

Glossary of terms and properties of some essential oils

The terminology applied to the uses of essential oils has been borrowed from herbal medicine. Table 15.1 shows a list of such terms (with explanations), together with some essential oils that offer these properties.

The practical application of essential oils

Figure 15.2 illustrates the different methods by which essential oils may be utilised for therapeutic purposes, and their passage in the body.

Olfaction/inhalation

- Vaporised oils
- Sprays
- Tissues
- Perfumes
- Burners
- Steamers

Skin absorption

- Massage
- Compresses
- Creams
- Lotions
- Perfumes
- Baths

Ingestion

- Drops
- Food
- Gargles
- Capsules
- Pessaries
- Douches
- Suppositories

The holistic approach

There are various ways of viewing the cause and treatment of disease. It is held that conventional medicine locates all disease in the physical body, and even emotional distress is viewed as a biochemical disorder that requires biochemical intervention. Holistic medicine seeks the roots and treatment of disease not just in the individual's body but also in the mind, family, environment and community. In cancer, for instance, it has been claimed that an individual's temperament (Eysenck 1988) and social and family links (Reynolds *et al.* 1994) affect the onset cause of disease (Vickers 1996).

The practical application of essential oils for therapeutic purposes uses the holistic approach both during consultation and in treatment. Aromatherapy is considered to be one of the complementary therapies, but its usefulness in the treatment of many conditions is now widely appreciated by those working in orthodox medicine. Consequently an ever-increasing number of doctors, nurses, physiotherapists and other paramedical

Table 15.1 Glossary of terms and properties of some essential oils.

Term	Property	Essential oil
Analgesic	gives pain relief	basil, benzoin, bergamot, cajaput, chamomile, clary sage, coriander, cypress, eucalyptus, geranium, ginger, juniper, lavender, lemon, lemongrass, marjoram, melissa, orange, pepper (black), peppermint, pine, rosemary, thyme
Anticontusive	prevents bruises	geranium, ginger, hyssop
Antidepressant	counters low spirits	bergamot, chamomile, clary sage, coriander, geranium, jasmine, lavender, melissa, neroli, orange, patchouli, pine, rose, sandalwood, thyme, ylang ylang
Antifungal	inhibits growth of fungi	myrrh, tea-tree
Antiphlogistic	reduces inflammation and vasoconstricts	benzoin, chamomile, clary sage, cypress, geranium, jasmine, lavender, myrrh, neroli, niaouli, peppermint, rose, sandalwood
Antiseptic	inhibits growth of bacteria	almost all oils
Antispasmodic	relieves smooth muscle spasm	basil, bergamot, cajaput, chamomile, coriander, cypress, eucalyptus, fennel (sweet), frankincense, geranium, hyssop, jasmine, juniper, lavender, mandarin, marjoram, melissa, pepper (black), peppermint, rose, rosemary, sandalwood, thyme
Antiviral	inhibits replication of viruses	niaouli, tea-tree
Aphrodisiac	increases sexual desire	clary sage, jasmine, neroli, patchouli, pepper (black), rose, sandalwood, ylang ylang
Astringent	tightens tissues	bergamot, cedarwood, frankincense, geranium, grapefruit, juniper, lemon, patchouli, rose, rosemary, sandalwood
Carminative	eases bowel pain and expels wind	basil, bergamot, chamomile, coriander, fennel (sweet), ginger, hyssop, juniper, lavender, mandarin, melissa, myrrh, neroli, pepper (black), peppermint, rosemary, sandalwood, thyme
Cordial	acts as a tonic for the heart	benzoin, lavender, lemon, mandarin, rosemary
Cytophylactic	stimulates cell regeneration	almost all oils
Depurative	purifies the blood of toxins and waste	eucalyptus, hyssop, jasmine, juniper, rose
Digestive	aids digestion	basil, bergamot, cajaput, chamomile, geranium, ginger, hyssop, lemongrass, marjoram, myrrh, orange, thyme
Diuretic	removes fluid from the body through the kidneys	cedarwood, chamomile, cypress, eucalyptus, fennel (sweet), frankincense, geranium, juniper, lavender, lemon, marjoram, orange, patchouli, pepper (black), pine, rosemary, sandalwood, thyme
Emmenagogue	aids menstrual problems	basil, cajaput, chamomile, clary sage, cypress, fennel (sweet), ginger, hyssop, jasmine, juniper, lavender, marjoram, melissa, myrrh, peppermint, rose, rosemary, sandalwood, thyme, ylang ylang
Euphoric	uplifts into an excitory state	clary sage, ylang ylang
Expectorant	expels mucus from the chest	basil, benzoin, cedarwood, cypress, eucalyptus, frankincense, hyssop, lemon, myrrh, niaouli, peppermint, sandalwood, thyme
Febrifuge	reduces fever	chamomile, cypress, eucalyptus, hyssop, lemongrass, melissa, orange, pepper (black), peppermint

continued

Table 15.1 Glossary of terms and properties of some essential oils (*continued*).

Term	Property	Essential oil
Haemostatic	helps to arrest bleeding	geranium, rose
Hepatic	helps with liver problems	chamomile, mandarin, peppermint, rose, rosemary
Hyperpnoea	Reduce abnormally fast breathing	ylang ylang
Hypertensor	raises blood pressure	mandarin, rosemary, thyme
Hypotensor	Reduces blood pressure	clary sage, hyssop, lavender, lemon, marjoram, melissa, ylang ylang
Laxative	helps to evacuate bowels	camphor, fennel (sweet), ginger, hyssop, mandarin, orange, pepper (black), rose
Nervine	useful for nervous disorders in general	basil, cedarwood, chamomile, coriander, cypress, hyssop, juniper, lavender, lemon, lemongrass, mandarin, melissa, orange, peppermint, rosemary, thyme
Rubefacient	stimulates circulation	benzoin, coriander, eucalyptus, juniper, lemon, pepper (black), peppermint, pine, rosemary, thyme
Sedative	soothes the nervous system	benzoin, bergamot, cedarwood, chamomile, clary sage, cypress, frankincense, geranium, hyssop, jasmine, juniper, lavender, marjoram, melissa, neroli, patchouli, peppermint, rose, sandalwood, ylang ylang
Stimulant	has a tonic action on mind and body	coriander, eucalyptus, grapefruit, hyssop, lemon, niaouli, orange, pepper (black), pine, rosemary
Tonic	acts as a mild astringent	grapefruit, lemon, mandarin
Vulnerary	heals sores and wounds	benzoin, cajaput, chamomile, eucalyptus, frankincense, geranium, hyssop, jasmine, juniper, lavender, lemon, orange, patchouli, rosemary, sandalwood, thyme

workers are including aromatherapy as part of the 'care package' they offer in hospitals, hospices and clinics.

Aromatherapy massage

The combination of the therapeutic effects of essential oils with the therapeutic effects of the 'laying on' of hands, namely massage, provides a 'natural' treatment of considerable value. The oils are utilised not only by skin absorption but also by olfaction and inhalation when applied by massage.

Aromatherapy massage probably creates the most diffuse therapeutic effect if compared with other methods of use of essential oils. It is also a very safe treatment when practised by a competent and well-trained, qualified aromatherapist. The massage techniques described in this book that would be the most appropriate would be:

- Effleurage/stroking
- Petrissage/kneading

Many aromatherapists, myself included, use further techniques such as lymphatic drainage, neuromuscular massage and acupressure manipulations of the soft tissue.

Lymphatic drainage

These manipulations involve short or long, light or deep stroking movements which help move on excess fluids, waste matter and toxins, through the lymphatic system, towards the heart and into the general circulation, and thence to the excretory organs of the body.

Neuromuscular massage

The manipulations involve a knowledge of the relationship between the cutaneous sensory zones of the body, the autonomic nervous system and the internal organs. Movements include deep palmar kneadings and deep finger kneadings in the zones.

Acupressure

These manipulations include a knowledge of the philosophies of acupuncture and shiatsu. The movements include working with the thumbs on meridians (energy lines) and tsubo points (areas where energy blockages may be released) of the body.

Effects and uses of aromatherapy massage

My personal experience (and that reported by many aromatherapists) has shown me that aromatherapy massage is the most popular form of treatment with essential oils. There are a number of consistent themes in different patient groups' experience of and response to massage and aromatherapy. (Vickers, who has been a member of the Research Council for Complementary Medicine, in his book *Massage and Aromatherapy – A Guide for Healthy Professionals* (1996), supports these findings.)

Muscle tension

It is claimed that massage and aromatherapy can relieve muscle tension. This can sometimes lead to short-term improvements in mobility. Muscle tension and mobility is said to be a particular issue in physical disability, AIDS and primary care.

Blood circulation

Aromatherapists say that essential oils can also stimulate local blood flow. This is reportedly of value in physical disability, cancer care and where patients spend significant periods of time in bed or in a wheelchair, e.g. in intensive care units and AIDS in some cases.

Pain

Aromatherapy is reported to have a short-term effect on pain. This is of particular importance in physical disability, cancer care, hospice care, primary care and AIDS.

Fatigue

Certain essential oils are said to act as stimulants. Aromatherapy treatment of fatigue is reportedly of benefit in cancer, AIDS, mental health and primary care in particular.

Infection

Essential oils are known to be antimicrobial. More controversially, aromatherapy is claimed to stimulate the immune system. Complementary treatment of infection is an issue of particular interest in the treatment of disabled children and people with AIDS.

Relaxation

Aromatherapy can be a relaxing experience. Patients may also undertake self-help with essential oils, as inhalations or in baths. Relaxation is generally beneficial, especially where patients are anxious, such as in cancer care, disabled children, hospice care, mental health, HIV and AIDS.

One-to-one care

One-to-one care and attention associated with massage or aromatherapy treatment is not common in health care. This has been found to be important in physical disability, primary care, mental health, HIV, AIDS, hospice care and cancer care.

Support for staff and carers

Massage and aromatherapy can be an important means of providing support to staff and carers.

Sleep

Aromatherapy is reported to improve sleep.

General wellbeing

Most people report feeling generally better in themselves after massage or aromatherapy treatment (Vickers 1996). Aromatherapy is useful at all stages of life.

Pregnancy/childbirth/baby care

Aromatherapy massage can help pain and insomnia and give a sense of deep relaxation. It is therefore of considerable benefit to those who are pregnant, in labour or have post-natal depression.

Massage for babies is common in certain countries and the use of essential oils with massage for babies is becoming widespread in Western countries. It helps the 'bonding' process between parent and child, and may increase the child's resistance to infection, improve weight gain and help general mental and physical development.

The elderly

Aromatherapy massage is being used more widely in the care of the elderly. This is a time of life when people may feel especially alone, depressed and fearful. Aromatherapy massage to hands, feet, neck and shoulders can help to break the sense of isolation and inspire calm and peace.

Problems that may be helped are:

- Pain in the musculoskeletal system
- Constipation
- Dyspepsia
- Insomnia
- Pressure sores

Consultation procedures

As aromatherapy is an holistic therapy, the consultation procedure should take a full 25–30 minutes. Different aromatherapists will approach a consultation in a variety of ways, but all well-qualified professionals will seek to discover a complete picture of the events leading to the patient's condition. This will include such areas as the patient's medical, social and family background.

The patient consultation is a vital prelude to a session of treatments. It is this that leads to correct assessment of the patient, both physical and psychological, and therefore to correct treatment. My approach is shown below. A Consultation Card/Sheet is required and on which the results of three major techniques are recorded:

- Verbal
- Visual
- Tactile

Verbal

This is the first very important point of communication. The patient may make a booking by telephone or come to your clinic. Either way, it is very important that he/she is made to feel relaxed and at ease and that the person to whom he/she talks has a detailed knowledge of aromatherapy. If the patient decides to come for treatment then the consultation procedure will begin.

First, ensure that the treatment room is warm and quiet and gives the atmosphere of peace. The treatment couch needs to be firm and comfortable with suitable drapes.

Let the patient undress and lie down, well covered and warm. Sit beside the patient and begin quietly to discuss the points outlined on the Consultation Sheet. Take a name, address and telephone number, and also that of the patient's doctor.

One cannot, unfortunately, rely entirely on verbal communication alone, for a variety of reasons. First, a patient who has come for treatment for the first time might feel shy or even embarrassed and therefore be very non-committal in some areas. Second, the patient may genuinely have forgotten past problems which in fact may have a bearing on his or her present state of mental and physical health.

There are three areas that need to be covered:

- Medical
- Social
- Family history

The pattern of events leading up to the consultation session will have a profound influence on the patient's current wellbeing. Needless to say, problems that have a genuine medical significance must be referred to the GP before undertaking a treatment programme for such a condition.

Visual

This is a second technique that is vital for obtaining a correct assessment of the patient's condition. More often than not it is combined with another technique, namely tactile.

Tactile

Tactile adds a third dimension to assessment and is a final 'back up' to the information already gained. The areas examined by visual and tactile means are:

- The back
- The face
- The abdominal area
- The feet (reflexology)

The back

- Spinal alignment
- Colour
- Texture
- Connective tissue massage tension areas of fascia
- Pain
- Flare reaction by stimulation to circulation

The face

The following points need to be noted:

- Colour
- Skin type (sensitive, dry, oily, combination)
- Tone
- Expression

Abdominal

The following points need to be noted:

- Pain
- Tension

Foot reflexology

The following point needs to be noted:

- Reflex pain areas on either foot

Personality type

The temperament of the patient is taken into account and it is noted whether he/she is Yin (passive, lacking in energy, debilitated) or Yang (active, hypertensive, often irritable and nervous and certainly prone to stress symptoms). Depending on the personality type, the acupressure techniques are also varied, so it is important to know the temperamental characteristics of the patient.

Other information

- It is important to know whether the patient is on drugs, medicinal or otherwise, and to find out if there are any other items of medical information that have not been listed on the chart.
- Precautions – contraindications. It is vitally important to find out if there are problem areas before treatment. This way, the appropriate oils and massage can be given.
- The GP's name, telephone number and permission. Should there be a medical problem that should be referred to the doctor before treatment, ensure permission is given in writing.
- Facts, full and true. This ensures that the patient signs to say that he/she has given you full and true facts before you give treatment.
- Oil blends and home care. For each treatment, mark the date of treatment and fill in details of oil blends and home care advice and whenever this changes according to new patient needs.

Oils

Once all the previous facts have been correlated, an assessment may be made as to which essential oils and base oils are suitable for the patient's condition. Usually no more than three different oils are required to cope with most of the problems the therapist can deal with, and these are blended carefully to produce a therapeutic, individual blend suitable for that patient alone.

It is important to identify whether it is necessary to have a special facial blend as well as a body blend, so ensure that at the consultation, accurate formulae are given.

Contraindications

Aromatherapy massage is an extremely safe treatment when given by a competent, well-trained, qualified aromatherapist (Price and Price 1995; Tisserand and Balacs 1995). The very small percentage of essential oils in relation to the carrier oil when blended (i.e. a maximum of 0.5–2% essential oils, namely 3–12 drops, to a maximum of 30 ml of carrier oil) ensures this is the case.

Such a treatment means that there is a 'controlled' use of essential oils. Only 'gross misuse' would cause problems. However, because of the media attention focused on certain oils mentioned in some books on aromatherapy it is probably sensible for an aromatherapist generally to avoid certain oils for particular conditions, mainly because a perception has been created in the popular mind that there is 'something wrong' with them. This is particularly true of certain oils that some literature claims may have adverse effects in the first 3 months of pregnancy. Those aromatherapists who have gone on courses of a high standard of training will be fully aware of which oils are safe to use for different conditions.

Hazards

Certain hazards are associated with some oils, namely the possible problems of toxicity, irritation or sensitisation.

- Toxicity: this is commonly called poisoning and at a certain level becomes fatal whether applied to the skin or taken orally. Toxicity is dose dependent – the greater the amount of essential oil, the greater the hazard. The very small amounts of essential oil put into a carrier oil for an aromatherapy massage by a well-trained professional would not present a problem in any way.
- Irritation: here there is a localised inflammation affecting the skin or mucous membranes, depending on where the essential oil is applied. Respiratory conditions should be treated with care when using essential oils. The amount of oil(s) chosen, the medium in which it/they are carried and the length of time of inhalation must be safely controlled.
- Sensitisation: here there is an allergic response to an essential oil. Only small amounts are required to trigger a reaction. Photosensitisation occurs when the sun shines on the skin on which certain oils have been applied. A photochemical reaction takes place, causing pigmentation. Bergamot is one of the best known oils that can produce this effect.

Certain oils present risks either of toxicity, skin irritation or skin sensitisation and are not considered safe in general use. Below is a list of oils that should not be used in aromatherapy.

Oils not to be used at all in therapy

According to the International Federation of Aromatherapists (2008), the following oils should not be used:

Almond (bitter)	*Prunus amygdalus*
Boldo leaf	*Peumus boldus*
Calamus	*Acorus calmus*
Camphor (brown)	*Cinnamomum camphora*
Camphor (yellow)	*Cinnamomum camphora*
Cassia	*Cinnamomum cassia*
Cinnamon (bark)	*Cinnamomum zeylancium*
Costus	*Saussurea lappa*
Elecampane	*Inula helenium*
Fennel (bitter)	*Foeniculum vulgare*
Horseradish	*Amoracia rusticana*
Jaborandi (leaf)	*Pilocarpus jaborandi*
Mugwort (armoise)	*Artemisia vulgaris*
Mustard	*Brassica nigra*
Pine (dwarf)	*Pinus mugo*
Rue	*Ruta graveolens*
Sassafras	*Sassafras albidum*
Sassafras (Brazilian)	*Ocotea cymbarum*
Savine	*Juniperus sabina*
Southernwood	*Artemisia abrotanum*
Tansy	*Tanacetum vulgare*
Thuja (cedarleaf)	*Thuja occidentalis*
Thuja (Western red/Washington)	*Thuja plicata*

Wintergreen	*Gaultheria procumbens*
Wormseed	*Chenopodium anthelminticum*
Wormwood	*Artemisia absinthium*

Oils never to be used on the skin

Clove bud	*Eugenia caryophyllata*
Clove leaf	*Eugenia caryophyllata*
Clove stem	*Eugenia caryophyllata*
Origanum	*Origanum vulgare*
Origanum (Spanish)	*Thymus capitatus*

In the author's experience also sage, either Dalmation (*Salvia officinalis*) or Spanish (*Salvia lavandulifolia*) should not be used for aromatherapy treatments.

Oils not to be used with patients who have epilepsy

According to Epilepsy Action/British Epilepsy Association (2007) the following oils should not be used on patients who have epilepsy:

Fennel (sweet)	*Foeniculum vulgare*
Hyssop	*Hyssopus officinalis*
Rosemary	*Rosmarinus officinalis*
Sage	*Salvia officinalis* and *Salvia lavandulifolia*
Wormwood	*Artemisia absinthium*

Pregnancy

Regarding pregnancy, where there is controversy over which oils to use or not to use, particularly in the first trimester, it is vital that the therapist has a nationally recognised qualification in aromatherapy, from which he/she will obtain information to help make safe choices. A midwife needs to have up-to-date knowledge of the United Kingdom Central Council (UKCC) Rules for Midwives, the Standards for Administration of Medicines and the Code of Practice as applicable to aromatherapy as well as locally agreed protocols drawn up by various midwifery and gynecological services.

Only 1%, i.e. a small amount of essential oil, is the maximum one would use in a carrier oil for pregnancy. If there is a history of miscarriage, do not use at all.

Precautions

Apart from these contraindications, there are certain basic precautions to be taken when using essential oils:

- They should not be taken internally unless prescribed by a suitable qualified medical practitioner.
- Although the majority of essential oils do not harm the skin, if there is sensitisation or irritation, wash off with mild soap and water.
- If an essential oil gets into the eye it may cause pain and distilled water is best for washing it out.
- Essential oils in most circumstances should be diluted in some carrier medium (vegetable oil, water, cream).
- When making up a massage oil, the dilution is 0.5–2% (3–12 drops) per 30 ml of carrier oil. Sensitive skins should only have 3 drops of essential oil in 30 ml of carrier oil.
- Avoid giving essential oil massage to skin with acne as the passing of the hands may spread infection. Other useful methods utilising essential oils may be used instead, namely compresses and vaporisers.
- Essential oils that are rubifacient in effect should not be used on dry, sensitive or vasodilated skin.
- Essential oils should be kept away from flame as they are flammable.
- Babies and children need to have much less percentage essential oils to a carrier oil than an adult because of their relatively smaller body area. Usually this would be about 25% of the normal adult dose, and the treatments should be of less duration, and less frequent.
- Medical conditions, if presented on consultation, should be discussed (with the patient's permission) with his or her medical practitioner and a written letter of approval received from the medical practitioner before aromatherapy massage is given. In particular the treatment of a patient with cancer must only be carried out with the approval of the patient's

consultant. Some consultants are quite happy to give this approval, others are not, whether the patient is on chemotherapy/radiation therapy or whether without medication at all. As yet there is no complete knowledge of the effects of essential oils combined with massage when a patient is undergoing medical treatment involving drugs. It is imperative therefore that an aromatherapist has the agreement of the patient's medical practitioner before embarking on treatment.

Blending of oils and formulation

When the aromatherapist decides after consultation with the patient to make up a special blend for that patient's aromatherapy massage, two separate components are used:

- A vegetable carrier oil.
- An essential oil or oils incorporated in the carrier oil.

Many types of carrier oil are available, each useful and having its own properties; these include:

- Almond: softening, soothing to the skin, a light oil suitable for face and body.
- Avocado: deeply penetrating and very nourishing. Contains vitamins A and B and is good for dry, mature skin.
- Grapeseed: a light oil, good for body and face.
- Jojoba: a very nourishing oil, which is particularly recommended for dry, mature skins.
- Safflower: light and nourishing, recommended for body and face treatments.

Many hundreds of essential oils are available for use, but it is more practical to utilise the better known ones.

The decision on how to blend the oils depends on the information gained from the patient during the consultation. The important factors are:

- The problems discerned during the consultation, which can safely be treated by the aromatherapist.
- Fragrance appreciation by the patient of the essential oils that the therapist intends to put together in the special blend.

Basic formula

There can be anything from one to five oils in a blend with a carrier oil, but it is usual to have three. This is so that it is possible to cover most problems and at the same time be able to appreciate the subtlety of different essences without finding that they have been swamped. It is usual to put approximately 0.5–2% (3–12 drops) of essential oils (in total) to 1 oz (30 ml) of carrier oil. Fewer drops are required for strong-scented oils and more drops for the gentle fragrances. Each essential oil has many therapeutic values. In making up the special blend it is sensible to write down the problems that you want to treat, and against each write a list of the oils that can be helpful in each case. Often it will be seen that a number of oils will be helpful with each of the problems. Provided the fragrances appeal to the patient and blend well together it is sensible to aim for maximum benefit by choosing to put these together. Otherwise one can choose an oil suitable for each problem, ensuring that the patient likes each fragrance and that each will blend well, one with the other.

The blend needs to be built up carefully, a drop of each oil at a time. It is wise not to overpower gentle scents such as rose with, for instance, too much eucalyptus. If one wishes to 'fix' the blend it is sensible to incorporate a base note such as patchouli. Sometimes one is asked if there are essential oils that will not combine. The answer is that one can combine any essential oil with any other essential oil, but that some oils blend better with each other than others. It takes time and considerable practice to achieve blends that have a harmony of fragrance.

Finally it is important to remember that the patient's needs may change over successive treatments and that one may have to reformulate the blend accordingly.

Preparation of the patient

After consultation:

(1) The patient lies supine, warm, comfortable and well covered.
(2) A headband is placed on the head to protect hair from creams and oils.
(3) The face and neck are deep cleansed with herbal products.
(4) The aromatherapy oil is lightly massaged over the face for 1 minute, with stroking movements.
(5) The patient is then asked to move into the prone position, the head supported by the patient's own hands or a small roll of towelling, and a roll of towelling under the ankles.

Treatment by aromatherapy massage

As stated before, the effleurage (stroking) and petrissage (kneading) movements described earlier in this book are techniques often employed by aromatherapists during an aromatherapy massage treatment. In addition I use lymphatic drainage, neuromuscular massage and acupressure techniques.

I first work on the back; then the backs of the legs; then turn the patient into supine again and commence with the front of the legs, the arms, the abdomen and finish with the scalp, neck, face and shoulders. It must be emphasised that an aromatherapist adapts his/her massage techniques and the areas treated according to the patient's needs and any precautions noted in the consultation procedures.

Case study

A 55-year-old woman, recently divorced, came to have aromatherapy because she had been told it was very helpful in stress situations. She was suffering from severe tension headaches, pain in the neck and shoulders and bloating in her colon area. It was decided on her first session that she would like to have a full body treatment, with head, neck, shoulders and abdomen to be given extra attention.

Lavender was chosen to have an analgesic, sedative and uplifting effect. Bergamot was also chosen for the above effects and because of its usefulness in helping digestive upsets. Finally, sandalwood was added as it would aid the reduction of the visceral muscle spasm and because of its calming and uplifting effects. Total drops of essential oils were 12–30 ml of almond carrier oil (i.e. 2% essential oils to 100% carrier oil).

On the next session, a week later, she reported a reduction in pain in the head, neck and shoulders and in her abdominal area, but still felt anxious and low. Clary sage, a euphoric, was added, reducing the sandalwood amount so that the percentage of essential oils (2%), i.e. 12 drops, to 30 ml carrier oil (100%) remained the same.

This new combination turned out to be very successful and after four weekly sessions the patient reported that she felt very much better in every way. Thereafter she had monthly sessions for a total of 6 months and professed to feel well again at that time. Whenever she feels stressed she returns for treatment.

Purity of essential oils

Essential oils used by aromatherapists for therapeutic massage should be of the highest quality, and of natural and not synthetic origin. The quality of the oil will depend on the good reputation of a high-grade supplier.

Storage

Essential oils can deteriorate rapidly. It is very important therefore that they are stored under the following conditions:

- They should be in containers that will not interact with the oil. Glass is usual for small amounts. Over 10 kg, then internally lacquered steel drums are used. Plastic containers are no good as the plastic and oil interact.
- They should be sealed very well.
- They should be protected from light, particularly from strong sunlight, because it has a chemical catalytic effect (photocatalytic) which precipitates chemical changes in the oil. Artificial light is not so damaging.
- They should be kept in cool conditions. Almost all oils can be kept in a refrigerator at 5°C. Vetivert, sandalwood, cedarwood and patchouli

should be kept at a room temperature of 15°C. Rose oil, rose absolute and some other oils will solidify, but this is no problem as they will remelt at room temperature. Under no circumstances should they be heated.

- For the therapist running a clinic it is sensible to order only small quantities, to avoid deterioration.

Conclusion

It may be concluded that aromatherapy massage is a safe, useful and effective treatment for a wide variety of conditions, when given by a properly trained therapist. As a result its role in the health care setting, both in the UK and worldwide, has expanded enormously in recent years. It is therefore most welcome to see that the orthodox and complementary medicine practitioners can work harmoniously together in the further interest of patient care and treatment.

References

Berger, H., Jarosch, E. and Madreiter, W. (1978) Effects of Vapourub and petrolatum on frequency and amplitude of breathing in children with acute bronchitis. *Journal of International Medicine Research*, **6**, 483–6.

Buchbauer, G., Jirovitz, L., Jager, W., *et al.* (1993) Fragrance compounds and essential oils with sedative effects upon inhalation. *Journal of Pharmaceutical Science*, **82**(6), 660–64.

Brun, K. (1952) *Les essences vegetales en tant qu'agent de penetration tissulaire*. These Pharmacie, Strasbourg.

Cavel, L. (1918) Sur la valeur antiseptique de quelques huiles essentielles. *Comptes Rendus (Academie des Sciences)*, **166**, 827.

Epilepsy Action/British Epilepsy Association (2007) *Leaflet*, July 2007. Epilepsy Action/British Epilepsy Association, Leeds.

Eysenck, H.J. (1988) Personality, stress and cancer protection and prophylaxis. *British Journal of Medical Psychology*, **61**, 57–75.

Falk-Filipsson, A., Löf, A., Hagberg, M., Hjelm, E.W. and Wang, Z. (1993) d-limonene exposure to humans by inhalation; uptake, distribution, elimination and effects on the pulmonary function. *Journal of Toxicology and Environmental Health*, **38**(1), 77–88.

Gattefosse, R.M. (1937) *Aromatherapy (translated 1993)*. Daniel, Saffron Walden, p.87.

Genders, R. (1972) *A History of Scent*. Hamish Hamilton, London, pp. 20, 126.

International Federation of Aromatherapists (2008) *IFA Cautionary Essential Oils List*. IFA, London.

Kovar, K.A., Gropper, B., Freiss, D. and Ammon, H.P.T. (1987) Blood 1evels of 1,8 cineol and locomotor activity of mice after inhalation and oral administration of rosemary oil. *Planta Medica*, **53**(4), 315–18.

Price, S. and Price, L. (1995) *Aromatherapy for Health Professionals*. Churchill Livingstone, Edinburgh.

Reynolds, P., Boyd, P.T., Blacklow, R.S., *et al.* (1994) The relationship between social ties and survival among black and white breast cancer patients. National Cancer Institute Black/White Cancer Survival Study Group. *Cancer Epidemiology, Biomarkers and Prevention*, **3**(3), 253–9.

Saller, R., Beschomer, M., Hellenbrecht, D. and Buhrimg, M. (1990) Dose dependency of symptomatic relief of complaints by chamomile steam inhalation in patients with common cold. *European Journal of Pharmacology*, **183**, 728–9.

Schwartz, D. and Natyncuk, S. (eds) (1990) *Chemical Signals in Vertebrates*. Oxford University Press, Oxford.

Tisserand, R. and Balacs, T. (1995) *Essential Oil Safety, A Guide for Health Professionals*. Churchill Livingstone, Edinburgh.

Valnet, Dr. Jean (1980) *The Practise of Aromatherapy*. Daniel, Saffron Walden, pp. 28, 33, 34.

van Toller, S. and Dodd, G.H. (1988) *Perfumery, the Psychology and Biology of Fragrance*. Chapman and Hall, London, p. 29.

Vickers, A. (1996) *Massage and Aromatherapy – A Guide for Health Professionals*. Chapman and Hall, London, pp. 33, 174–6.

Williams, D. (1989) Lecture 1, p. 7. In: *Lecture Notes on Essential Oils*. Eve Taylor, London.

Further reading

Campbell, T. and Jones, E. (2000) Aromatherapy. In: *Complementary Therapies for Physical Therapists* (ed. R. A. Charman) pp. 231–46. Butterworth-Heineman, Oxford.

Davis, P. (2005) *Aromatherapy A–Z. Vermilion*. Ebury Publishing, London.

Useful websites

http://www.ifaroma.org – International Federation of Aromatherapists.

http://www.ifparoma.org – International Federation of Professional Aromatherapists.

16

Shiatsu – the Japanese healing art of touch

Andrea Battermann

Introduction

This chapter opens with a description of the history, theory and practice of shiatsu. The photography demonstrates some of the basic shiatsu techniques and principles and an example of self-shiatsu massage shows the manual stimulation of acupuncture points for relieving headaches. The chapter ends with an outline of the professional development of shiatsu practitioners. It is beyond the scope of this chapter to explain shiatsu theory and terminology in detail; interested readers are referred to the Further reading.

What is shiatsu?

Shiatsu literally translated means 'finger pressure'. It is the manual therapy of acupuncture and part of traditional Japanese medicine. Mainly fingers, thumbs and palms of the hands apply different depths of pressure over the whole body, stimulating acupuncture points known as tsubos in Japanese. It is more than a mechanical stimulation of points – it is an oriental healing art based on an energetic medical model. Shiatsu is based on Chinese medicine and uses Eastern philosophy as its theoretical framework. Chinese medicine incorporates acupuncture and moxibustion (application of heat), acupressure, herbalism, diet and therapeutic exercises known as T'ai Chi and Ch'i-Kung (breathing exercises).

Traditionally, treatment is carried out on a cotton layer mat (futon) at floor level with the body remaining fully and comfortably clothed. Nowadays, some practitioners use a wide table, which is height adjustable. Shiatsu aims to maintain good health and wellbeing, as well as to treat specific conditions.

History

Shiatsu has its roots in Chinese medicine and developed about 5000 years ago. It evolved over centuries and was practised by people who developed a high sensitivity of touch and body awareness. They were able to localise points and areas on the body that relieved pain and stiffness, locally and distally. Simultaneously, shiatsu influenced the function of internal organs; headaches, for example, are relieved by pressing specific points on the hands and feet. Manual techniques like pressing and rubbing (Anmo) were used long before stimulating acupuncture points with fish bones, stones and later needles. Massage techniques remained an important prerequisite of the physician's training before he/she was allowed to progress to needles (Beresford-Cooke 1996). Chinese doctors observed the effects on the body and categorised the points that treat certain conditions, as well as developing an holistic diagnostic medical model and treatment.

Chinese medicine started to appear in Japan in the 5th century AD, in fragmented form, in the hands of Japanese warlords returning from incursions in Korea. It was not until the 8th century AD when a Buddhist monk named Jian Zhen brought a systematic corpus of written texts into Japan. The materials introduced by Jian Zhen mostly derived from the Han dynasty, dating to about 200 AD, and contained many herbal prescriptions of 'Han Fang' which is pronounced 'Kam Po' (also Kan Po) in Japanese. Over the following centuries in Japan, various schools of Japanese acupuncture arose, and variations in diagnostic approaches appeared. For example, whereas in China more emphasis was placed upon diagnosis from the pulse in the wrists, in Japan more emphasis was accorded to diagnosis by palpation of the abdomen, or 'Hara' in Japanese. This process of evolution of Kam Po and Japanese acupuncture continued. At the beginning of the 20th century acupressure massage developed into a medical form of treatment, changed its name to shiatsu and was legally recognised in 1950 in Japan. A well-known shiatsu practitioner, Shizuto Masunaga, created a unique system incorporating four paradigms into shiatsu: Chinese medicine, Western physiology, psychology and oriental philosophy (Daoism and Zen). His style and approach are now used worldwide. Masunaga developed the abdominal (Hara) diagnosis and extended the length and location of the traditional energy pathways, known as meridians, throughout the whole body. He also developed techniques to work with one meridian in the entire body.

Introduction to oriental medicine

Shiatsu is based on an energetic concept of Ki (the body's vital energy, known as Qi in Chinese). It is essential to understand this concept in order to grasp Chinese medicine theory and its practical application. Chinese medicine, as well as shiatsu, aims to stimulate a free flow of Ki in the meridians in the body and at the same time strengthen the body's general constitution. In disease and illness, Ki energy becomes deficient or excessive in the meridians and moves into a state of imbalance (Masunaga and Ohashi 1977).

Diagnostic methods

A detailed examination of all physical, emotional and mental expressions and symptoms is carried out by the practitioner using different forms of diagnostic methods in Chinese medicine.

Four forms of diagnosis

- **Asking questions:** present and past medical and social history, appetite and digestion, stools and urination, taste and thirst, body temperature and perspiration, eyes and ears, menstruation.
- **Observing:** noting posture, colours of clothes and facial skin, and condition of hair and nails.
- **Hearing and smelling:** listening to the tone of the voice and noting any body smell.
- **Touching:** this is the most important diagnostic and treatment method in shiatsu. The practitioner feels the quality of Ki with the fingers in defined zones in the abdomen, meridians and tsubos of the patient's body. Each zone in the Hara, as well as the diagnostic Bo and Yu points (in the front and back of the body), mirror the state of Ki in the associated meridian. The Hara diagnosis is used before and after the treatment (see Fig. 16.1). The Hara is defined in zones that are related to individual meridians. Figure 16.2 shows Hara diagnostic zones in the abdomen (after Masunaga and Ohashi 1977). The quality of each zone indicates how the Ki circulates in the meridian. The palpation of the Hara, Yu and Bo points, together with all the other diagnostic signs and symptoms, determines which meridian and points are treated. The practitioner diagnoses states and patterns of disharmonies in the Ki, Blood, Yin and Yang long before they manifest physically in the body or develop into a disease; for that reason traditional Chinese medicine (TCM) plays a major role in

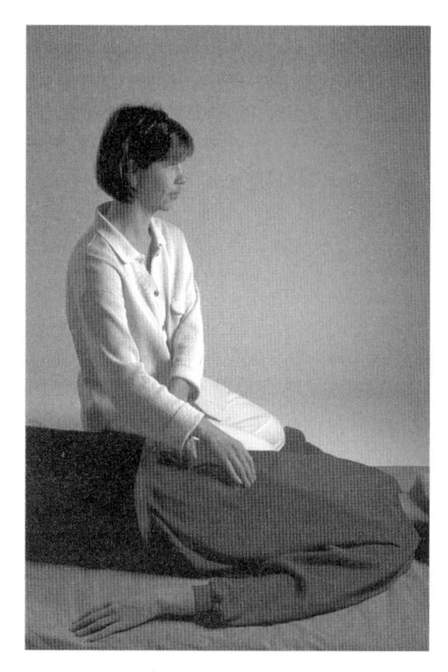

Figure 16.1 Hara palpation.

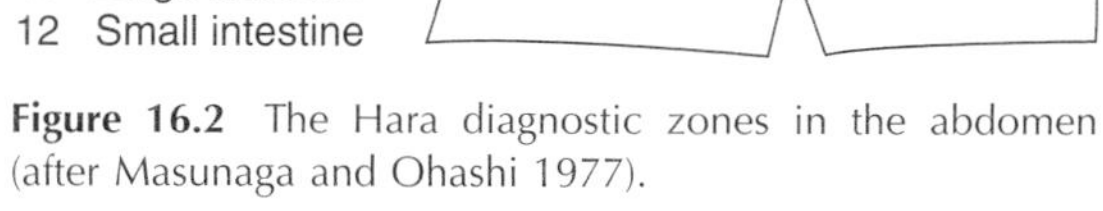

Figure 16.2 The Hara diagnostic zones in the abdomen (after Masunaga and Ohashi 1977).

preventative medicine and complements the Western medical model. A treatment method is chosen according to the results of all diagnostic rnethods and follows a phenomenological approach.

Shiatsu theory

There are several models in Chinese medicine explaining the Ki circulation throughout the body: Yin and Yang, the five phases or elements, the eight principles and the kyo–jitsu theory. Kyo and jitsu are interdependent and cannot be separated. Kyo is the condition of deficient energy which manifests itself as weakness or stiffness. The shiatsu technique for treating a kyo condition is called tonification, which requires a holding touch to encourage Ki flow. Jitsu is the condition of most concentrated energy (excess) which manifests in hard but elastic and more resistant body tissue. The jitsu is worked with a sedating technique and requires a more active technique to disperse the excess energy. Either one meridian, part of a meridian or any body part or Hara zone can be described as having a degree of kyo or jitsu quality. Throughout the shiatsu treatment the practitioner diagnoses and treats kyo and jitsu areas either in the meridian, tsubos or body parts and aims to balance the Ki in the whole body.

Basic principles and techniques of shiatsu

The following principles are relevant in giving a treatment:

- Controlled body weight and relaxation are used when pressure is applied; no muscular power is used. Figure 16.3 shows controlled body weight.
- Stationary and perpendicular pressure is applied in order to access and sense the Ki in the meridians and points. Figure 16.4 shows stationary and perpendicular pressure.
- Two-hand connection is maintained in which there is a stationary, listening hand called a 'mother hand', which gives support, stability and stillness, as well as an active hand, called a 'child hand', which works with a penetrative technique. The practitioner holds awareness in both hands as well as the interaction between them. Figure 16.5 shows the two-handed technique.
- Meridian continuity is used, in which the practitioner works along the whole length of any chosen meridian to find points of deepest penetration in order to access the Ki and manipulate it.

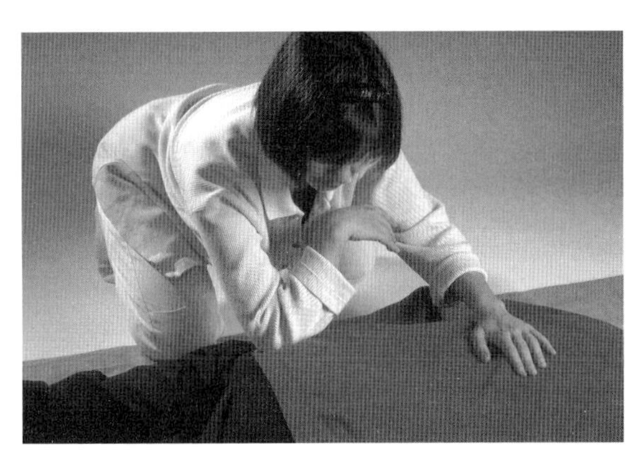

Figure 16.3 Elbow technique. Photograph ©ALIKI SAPOUNTZI www.aliki.co.uk.

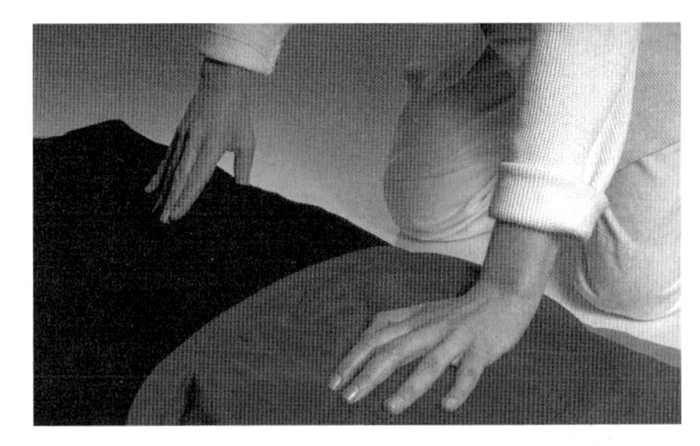

Figure 16.5 Two-hand technique. Photograph ©ALIKI SAPOUNTZI www.aliki.co.uk.

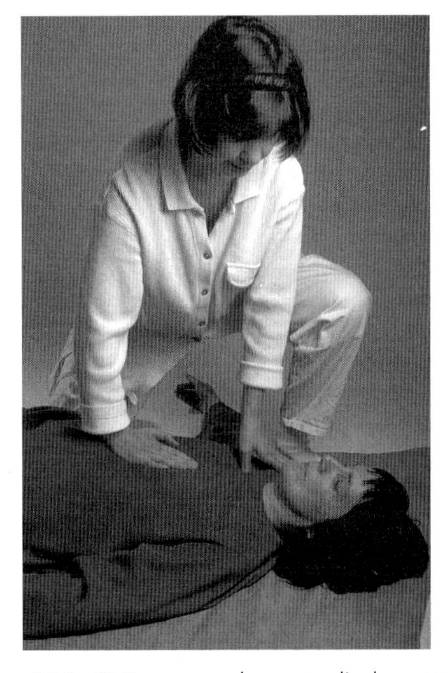

Figure 16.4 Stationary and perpendicular pressure. Photograph ©ALIKI SAPOUNTZI www.aliki.co.uk.

- An holistic approach of treatment is followed, in which the client's emotional, mental, spiritual and physical states are considered.
- Use of a steady rhythm throughout the treatment enhances the patient's deep relaxation, physically and mentally.
- A relaxed manner of the therapist is important as he/she needs to work in the most comfortable position with an aligned and open posture.
- There is a reciprocity of process, involving a constant inner listening and responding to the patient's needs and expressions. It is like a non-verbal dialogue through touch between therapist and patient, affecting the patient's whole wellbeing. Each shiatsu treatment is unique and cannot be precisely repeated. The external techniques can be reproduced, but the internal dialogue as well as the proprioception-sense is unique and personal to that moment between patient and therapist.

Clinical indications

Shiatsu can be used for many conditions. It is especially effective for musculoskeletal disorders, arthritis, respiratory conditions, immunodeficiency problems, psychosomatic conditions, hormonal imbalances, digestive problems, headaches and migraine, childbirth and pregnancy, anxiety and depression, as well as stress-related symptoms. A national survey carried out by Harris and Pooley (1998) discovered that musculoskeletal and psychological disorders are the most common conditions treated by shiatsu practitioners. Most treatments are given for neck/shoulder problems, followed by lower back problems and arthritis (see Fig. 16.6). The main psychological disorder treated is depression, followed by stress and anxiety.

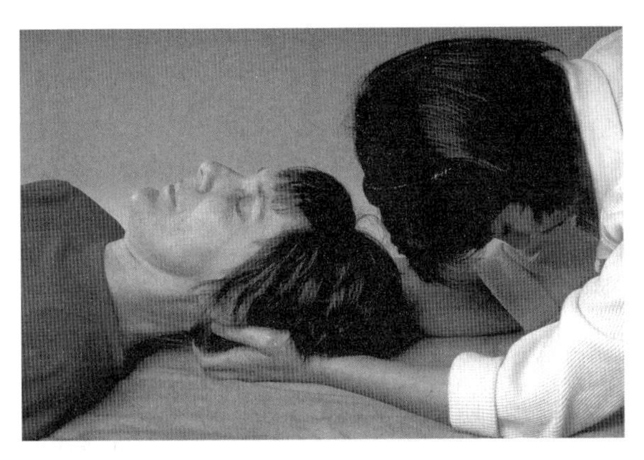

Figure 16.6 Neck release. Photograph ©ALIKI SAPOUNTZI www.aliki.co.uk.

Contraindications

Shiatsu is contraindicated in the following conditions:

- Cerebrovascular accident (not yet stabilised).
- Fever.
- Systemic/contagious infections.
- Any acute inflammations.
- Thrombosis.
- Haemophiliac patients or patients on anticoagulant medication.
- Varicose veins.

Cautions

- Light touch should be used on lymphatic areas below the ears, throat area and groin.
- Treatment of the abdominal area should be careful, with a light touch and for a short time.
- Ulcerous conditions and open wounds or serious burns should not be worked upon.
- New scar tissue or skin rashes should not be worked on directly.
- A patient who is very hungry and weak should not be worked on, because he/she may faint after the treatment.
- Special care should be taken in pregnancy in the first 3 months. Gentle work is recommended avoiding the following points: GB-21, SP-6, BL-60, Li-4 and LiV-3.
- Light touch should be used for patients with hypertension.

Physiological effects associated with shiatsu

- Drowsiness. Some patients relax very deeply and it can take some time until they sit up and their reaction response can be delayed, e.g. driving or walking in traffic. It is advisable to sit for some time after the treatment.
- Low muscle tone and sweating can appear in areas of hypertonicity.
- Stress response: hyperventilation, dry mouth and light headedness.
- Temporary aggravation of symptoms and increased pain for a maximum of 2 days following the treatment. Clients should be informed about this possible effect and reassured that this is a normal response.
- Improvement of lymphatic and general circulation of body fluids.
- Strong analgesia due to an increase of opioid-like hormones and other neurohormones, which is noticeable after a short treatment time. The patient tolerates a much stronger and more penetrative touch towards the end of the treatment.
- Increased peristaltic sounds, which can be noticeably loud, with embarrassment for the patient. Reassurance of the patient is needed that the autonomic nervous system is strongly activated.
- Reduced heartbeat.
- Strong stimulation of the autonomic nervous system.
- Stimulation of the neuropathways from muscles to the brain, e.g. flaccid muscles increase in muscle power and tone.
- Increase of sensation of areas that were numb due to scars or neurological causes.
- Improvement of proprioception sense.

Case study: self-shiatsu massage

The following case study describes a treatment that can be applied to oneself to relieve headaches and migraines. It is easy to use and to teach to patients as a self-help method. The author has given this treatment to many patients and students.

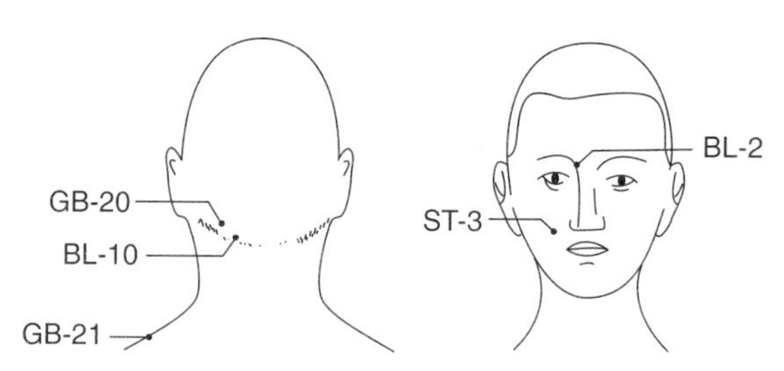

Figure 16.7 Acupuncture points for relief of headaches.

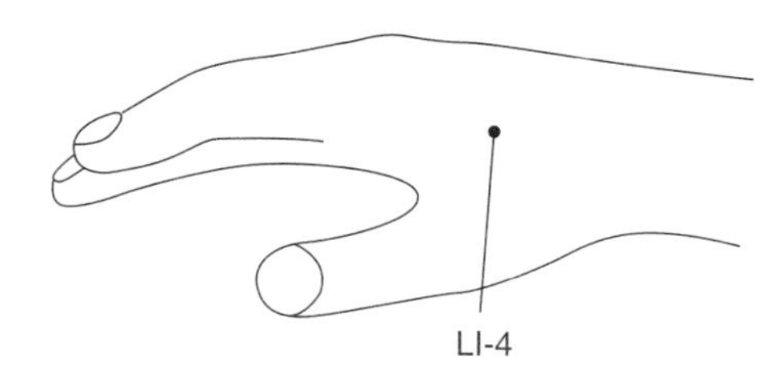

Figure 16.8 Point LI-4.

A neurological consultant once referred a patient with persistent unilateral headaches which could not be clearly diagnosed and no treatment had been effective. The patient's signs and symptoms were assessed with Chinese medicine methods. The location and symptoms of his headaches corresponded precisely with the bladder meridian and its pathway on the skull. He was taught the following treatment and advised to practise twice daily and write a pain diary. His second session focused on supervision of point locations and treatment techniques. After the third session, the patient reported relief from headaches after each self-shiatsu massage.

The following point locations were taught (see Fig. 16.7):

- BL2 Zanzhu (Gathered Bamboo): in a depression on the medial end of the eyebrows.
- M-HN-3 Yintang (Hall of Impression): at the midpoint between the medial ends of the eyebrows.
- GB-20 Fengchi (Windpond): below the occiput, in the hollow between the origins of the sternomastoid and trapezius muscles.
- BL-10 Tianzhu (Celestial Pillar): on the midline of the neck, in a depression directly below the occipital protuberance, on the lateral side of the trapezius muscles.
- GB-21 Jianjing (Shoulder Well): midway between the occiput of the neck and the tip of the acromion, at the highest point of the shoulder.
- ST-3 Juliao (Great Crevice): eyes look straight forwards, below the pupil, level with the border of the ala nasi, on the lateral side of the nasolabial groove.
- LI-4 Hegu (Joining Valley): on the dorsum of the hand, between the thumb and index finger, at the midpoint of the second metacarpal bone, close to its radial side (Fig. 16.8).

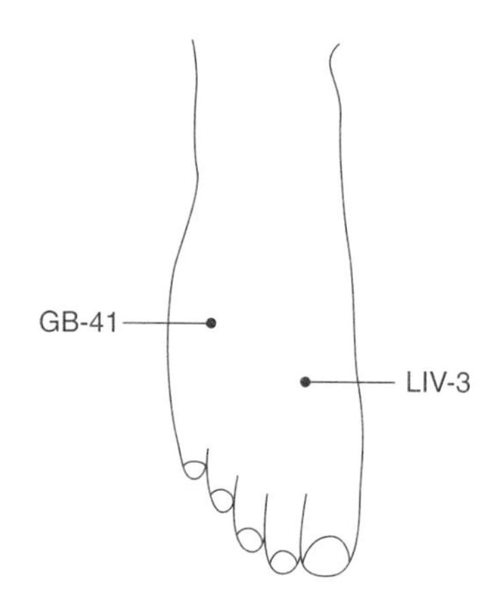

Figure 16.9 Points LIV-3 and GB-41.

- LIV-3 (Taichong Great Rushing): on the dorsum of the foot, in the hollow distal to the junction of the first and second toe (Fig. 16.9).
- GB-41 Zulinqi (Foot Governor of Tears): in the depression distal to the junction of the 4th and 5th metatarsal bones, on the lateral side of the tendon muscle extensor digitorum longus (Fig. 16.9).

The self-shiatsu routine

Self-shiatsu massage can be practised sitting comfortably in an upright position.

Press the inside corners of each eye. You will find the points if you pinch the bridge of the nose (Fig. 16.10).

Press the points under the eyebrows. Rest your head heavy and relaxed on your fingertips (Fig. 16.11).

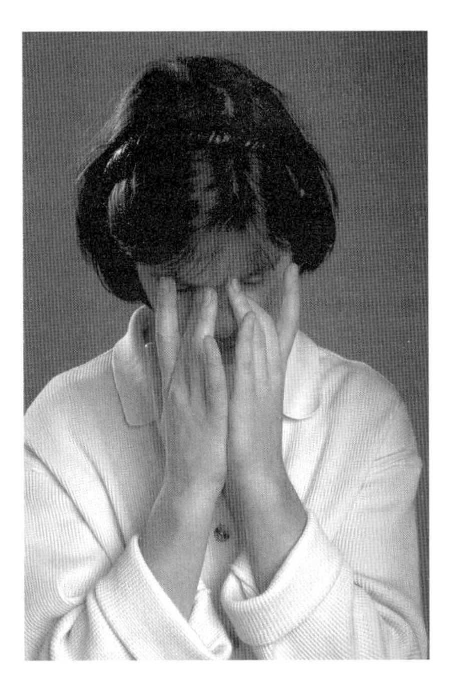

Figure 16.10 Working on BL-2. Photograph ©ALIKI SAPOUNTZI www.aliki.co.uk.

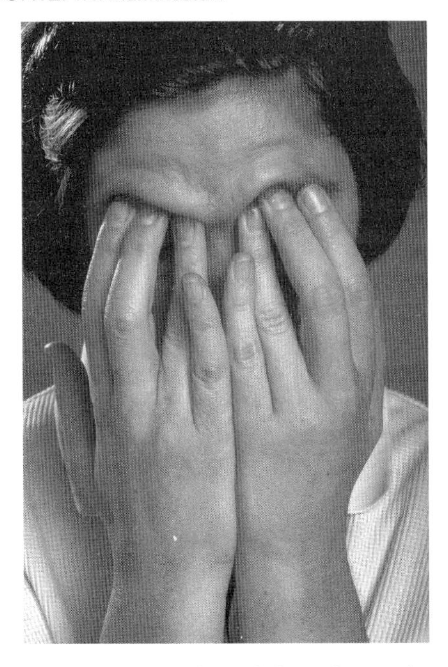

Figure 16.11 Pressure underneath the eyebrows. Photograph ©ALIKI SAPOUNTZI www.aliki.co.uk.

Lightly press the point M-HN-3 with the palm of the hands together. Let your head tilt forwards and position your middle fingers in between the eyebrows. Hold the point for 2 minutes as you relax and breathe deeply (Fig. 16.12).

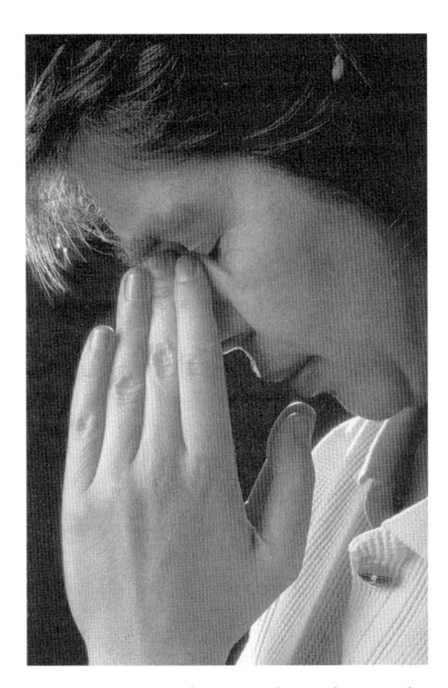

Figure 16.12 Pressure in between the eyebrows. Photograph ©ALIKI SAPOUNTZI www.aliki.co.uk.

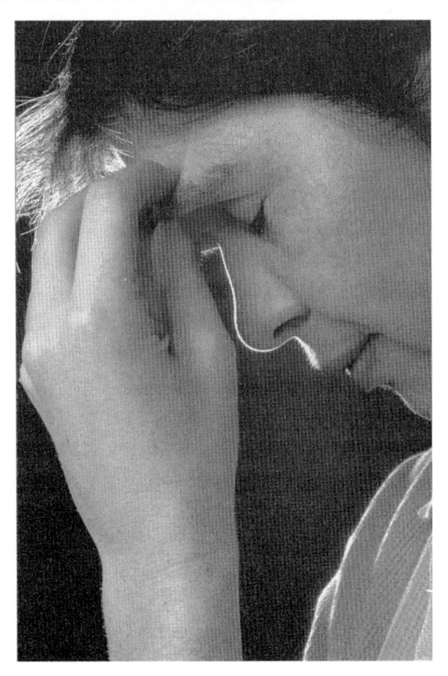

Figure 16.13 Massage of the eyebrows. Photograph ©ALIKI SAPOUNTZI www.aliki.co.uk.

Pinch and massage your eyebrows from the inside to the lateral ends several times (Fig. 16.13).

Grip your head with fingers apart.

Work along parallel lines extending over the top of your head towards your neck. Then circle around

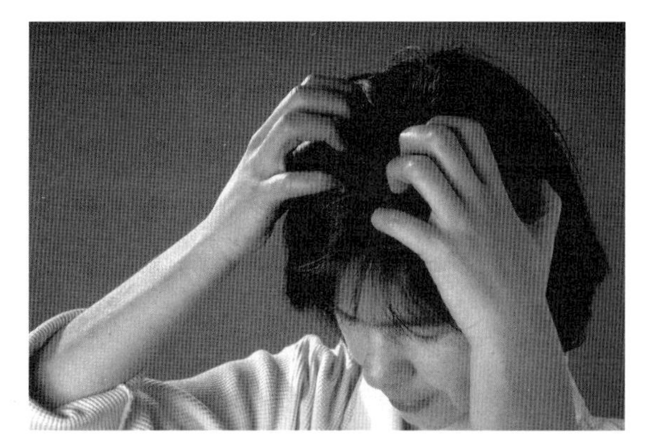

Figure 16.14 Working on the meridian on the head. Photograph ©ALIKI SAPOUNTZI www.aliki.co.uk.

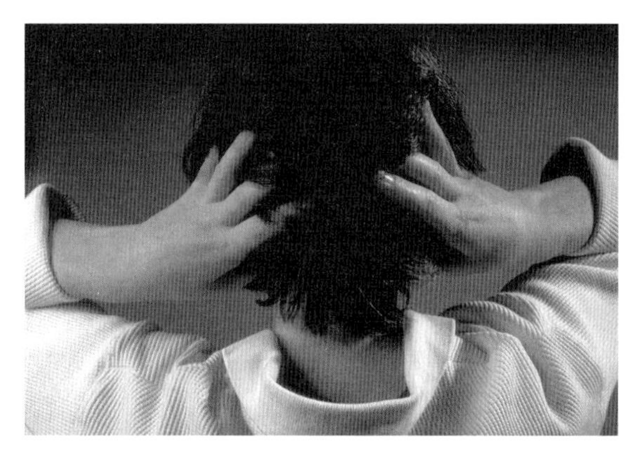

Figure 16.15 Working on BL-10 underneath the occipital line. Photograph ©ALIKI SAPOUNTZI www.aliki.co.uk.

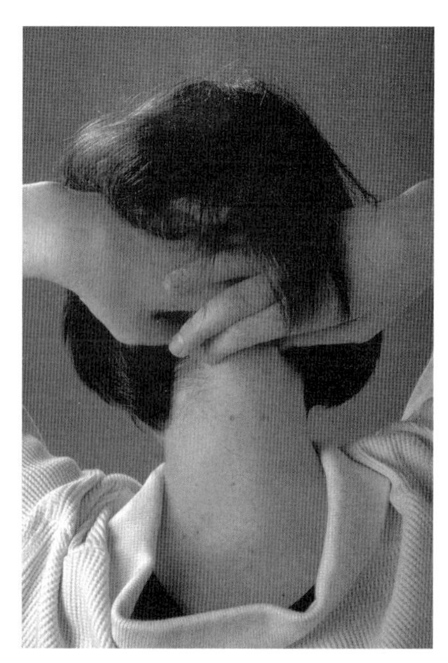

Figure 16.16 Self-massage technique on the neck. Photograph ©ALIKI SAPOUNTZI www.aliki.co.uk.

your ears and temples with the palm of your hands, pressing towards the centre of your head (Fig. 16.14).

Firmly press the point GB-20: place your thumbs underneath the base of your skull in the hollows between the origins of the sternomastoid and trapezius muscles. Apply the pressure gradually underneath the base of your skull as you slowly tilt your head backwards. Take a deep breath and hold the point for 1 minute. Then work the point BL-10 as you direct the pressure towards the opposite eye. You can work other tight points under the occipital ridge on the hairline (Fig. 16.15).

Press the back of your neck with both thumbs lateral to the cervical spine from the top to the base of the neck (Fig. 16.16).

Curl your fingers and place them on the highest point of your shoulder muscles at GB-21 close to the neck on the left side. Simply relax the weight of your arm in front of your chest. Keep your fingers curled like a hook. Sink deeper into the muscles as they soften and relax. Hold for 1 minute and take a few, long, deep breaths. Repeat on the other side (Fig. 16.17).

Press the point ST-3: use your thumbs to gently press upwards underneath the cheekbones directly below the centre of your eyes. Tilt your head forwards and relax, taking a couple of deep breaths (Fig. 16.18).

Firmly press the point LI-4: relax your left arm and hand on your thigh. Place your right thumb on the webbing between your thumb and index finger of your left hand. The pressure is directed towards the base of the left index finger at the highest point of the bulge of the muscle. Repeat on the other hand. You will feel a dull ache if you are on the point (Fig. 16.19).

Stimulate the points LIV-3 and GB-41: take off your shoes and sit comfortably. Place your left heel on top of your right foot between the first and second toe for 1 minute. You can also rub this area gently.

Stimulate the point GB-41: place your heel between your fourth and fifth toe and work as above. Repeat on the other foot (Fig. 16.20).

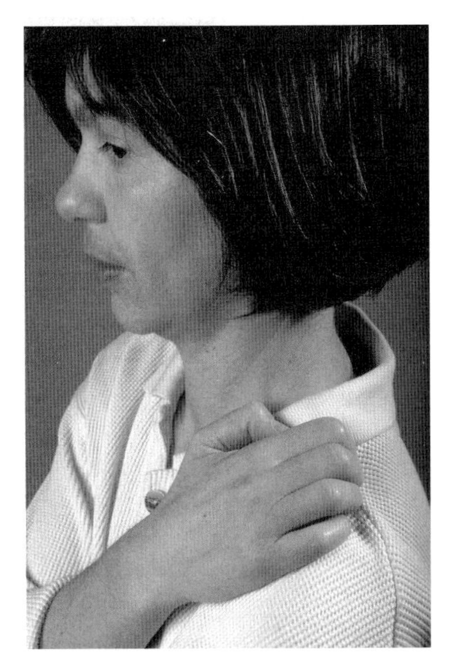

Figure 16.17 Working on GB-21. Photograph ©ALIKI SAPOUNTZI www.aliki.co.uk.

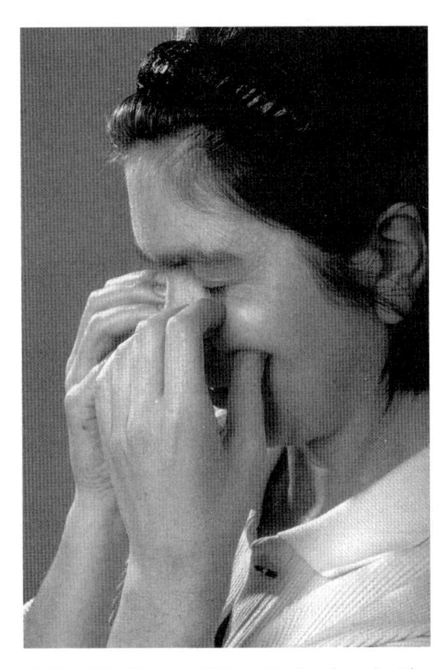

Figure 16.18 Working on ST-3 with the thumb. Photograph ©ALIKI SAPOUNTZI www.aliki.co.uk.

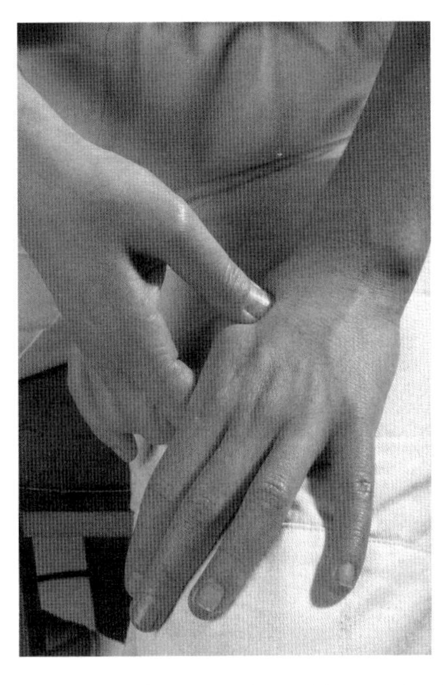

Figure 16.19 Working on LI-4. Photograph ©ALIKI SAPOUNTZI www.aliki.co.uk.

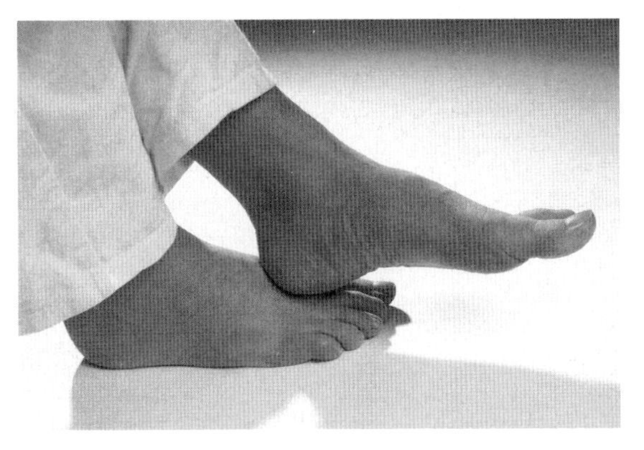

Figure 16.20 Working on LIV-3. Photograph ©ALIKI SAPOUNTZI www.aliki.co.uk.

How to apply pressure

- Use your body weight to lean into the tsubo.
- Apply finger pressure gradually and then hold the tsubo deeply with a firm and steady penetration for up to 3 minutes.
- Never press a tsubo with an abrupt, forceful or jarring technique.
- Most tsubos and meridians appear bilateral on the body. The tsubos are like coin-size areas.

You may feel a dull ache or pleasant tingling if you are on the tsubo with the right angle and depth of penetration. The anatomical location of the acupuncture points will describe only the area where you have to touch in order to find the location of the tsubo.

- If you feel increasing pain or discomfort by pressing a tsubo, gradually decrease the pressure until you find a more tolerable sensation, which is called 'sweet pain' in shiatsu.
- Do not continue to press a tsubo that is excruciatingly painful.
- Approximately 2 minutes should decrease pain of the tsubo with firm pressure; if not, stop pressing this tsubo.
- If you feel pain in another part of your body (referred pain), press the points in these related areas as well. Each tsubo belongs to a meridian. Sometimes the next point or more distant points on the same meridian are activated.
- Avoid self-shiatsu during pregnancy unless an experienced practitioner has supervised your treatment.

Professional development of the therapist

Shiatsu requires long and complex training over a period of years involving an immense amount of practice and theoretical study in order to master this skill and gain an understanding of it. The perception of Ki in the patient's body and our own is developed by practising Qi-Gong and meditation, receiving treatments and working on the teacher's body.

In a tutorial lesson, the teacher will give direct feedback on how to sense and direct Ki in the body while the student is working. In shiatsu the emphasis in training is on the development of Hara, from which all movements originate and physical stamina and relaxation are gained. A practitioner with a strong Hara is able to sense, transmit and manipulate Ki more effectively and keeps the awareness in the Hara throughout the whole treatment.

Makko-Ho meridian stretches (similar to yoga) are taught to students; this is a simple workout for the whole body and meridian system.

Do-In (literally 'leading and guiding') Ki throughout the body is a system of working on the whole body with self-shiatsu techniques or exercises. Specific Makkho-Ho stretches are recommended by practitioners to support the outcome effects between treatments. The student is taught how to keep a healthy lifestyle using the principles of a Chinese medicine diet, general exercise to keep flexibility and strength, and maintaining the balance between rest and activity.

Conclusions

This chapter has provided an introduction to shiatsu with some practical applications. Due to the popularity of complementary therapies (CT) in the UK and patients frequently using CT beside or instead of Western medicine, it is important that health care professionals know what most CT entail in order to converse with patients. Nowadays CT is more integrated within the medical system. Acupuncture is one of the most frequently used CT by doctors and physiotherapists. Shiatsu is recognised as the manual treatment of acupuncture by the Acupuncture Association of Chartered Physiotherapists (AACP) and the Chartered Society of Physiotherapy in the UK.

Physiotherapists can use shiatsu as it is a recognised practice. There is no doubt about the clinical effectiveness of shiatsu. The problem is more how it can be integrated partially and effectively into physiotherapy treatments. It is unrealistic due to the constraints of time to aim to carry out a full-length shiatsu treatment. Over many years the author has used physiotherapy techniques with an energetic awareness of Ki movement and has achieved very good clinical outcomes with long-lasting effects.

Glossary

Anmo: a traditional form of Chinese massage, literally translated as 'pressing and rubbing'.

Blood: with a capital 'B' indicates Blood in the sense of Oriental medicine, which represents more than it does in Western medicine. For example, in Oriental medicine, poor memory indicates deficient Heart Blood and the lustre of the head hair depends upon the Liver Blood. Where Ki goes, Blood goes and Ki also follows Blood. The function is to moisten, nourish and relax on the physical and psychological level.

Bo and Yu points: diagnostic acupuncture points in the front and back of the body.

Ch'i or Qi: Chinese word for energy (Ki in Japanese).

Do-In: self-shiatsu includes percussion or tapping techniques, meridian stretching and breathing exercises for guiding and leading the Ki throughout the body. For clarification the terminology self-shiatsu is used in the text when massage techniques are described to work on oneself.

Eight principles: ways of categorising various symptoms into recognisable patterns to determine the extent and seriousness of the illness and which points to use, e.g. cold and hot, interior or exterior causes of disease.

Five elements or five phases: used in Chinese medicine and shiatsu. Organs are characterized by the elements metal, water, wood, fire and earth and the relationship between them.

Hara: Japanese word for the abdomen, acknowledged as the centre of physical and spiritual strength.

Hara diagnosis: zones on the abdomen where the practitioner feels the state of Ki in the meridian and the body.

Ki: Japanese word for energy.

Kyo: a deficient or empty meridian, which responds slowly to treatment.

Kyo–jitsu: the theory used in Zen shiatsu describing the dynamic relationship between a more kyo and a jitsu meridian (full or overactive) and their physical manifestations.

Makko-Ho: meridian stretches (similar to yoga), a simple workout for the whole body and each meridian.

Meridian: an energy pathway in the body where Ki flows more strongly.

Moxa: a treatment warming the body by burning the herb Mugwort (*Artemisia vulgaris* leaf) on or over specific acupuncture points.

Qi (or Ch'i): Chinese word for energy.

T'ai Chi and Ch'i Kung: Chinese therapeutic exercises for building and circulating the Qi in the body using the breath.

Tsubo: Japanese word for acupuncture point.

Yin Yang: the dynamic relationship of all forms in which complementary and opposing forces interact in a never-ending flow. This theory is used to categorise various symptoms of the body and mental states.

Zen: an Eastern philosophy, a form of Buddhism, which encourages spontaneity and living in the present moment. It is used in shiatsu to still the mind and create an atmosphere of heightened awareness.

Acknowledgements

I would like to thank Aliki Sapountzi for the photography, Mark Wright, Clifford Andrews, Sensei Akinobu Kishi and many other teachers, colleagues, students and patients for their encouragement and inspiration.

References

Beresford-Cooke, C. (1996) *Shiatsu Theory and Practice.* Churchill Livingstone, Edinburgh.

Harris, P.E. and Pooley, N. (1998) What do shiatsu practitioners treat? A nationwide survey. *Complementary Therapies in Medicine*, **6**(1), 30–35.

Masunaga, S. and Ohashi, W. (1977) *Zen Shiatsu.* Japan Publications, Tokyo.

Further reading

Charman, R.A. (2000) *Complementary Therapies for Physical Therapists.* Butterworth-Heinemann, Oxford.

Deadman, P., Mazin, A. and Baker, K.(1998) *A Manual of Acupuncture Point Cards.* Journal of Chinese Medicine Publications, Hove.

Ferguson, P. (1995) *Self-Shiatsu Handbook.* New Leaf Publishing, Houston.

Kaptchuk, T.J. (1983) *Chinese Medicine.* Rider, London.

Liechti, E. (1998) *The Complete Illustrated Guide to Shiatsu.* Element Books, Shaftesbury.

Lundberg, P. (2002) *The Book of Shiatsu.* Gala Books, London.

Masunaga, S. (1987) *Zen Imager! Exercises.* Japan Publications, Tokyo.

Useful websites

http://www.holisticphysiotherapy.org.

http://www.shiatsu.org.

17 Myofascial release and beyond

Ann Childs and Stuart Robertson

Introduction to the fascial matrix

There are many types of massage/bodywork techniques focusing more specifically on the fascial component of tissues (rather than muscle or bone) to effect a global, whole body response, for example connective tissue massage, structural integration, rolfing, trager, shiatsu, positional release and craniosacral therapy. Rather than become embroiled in semantics, or in the classification of techniques identified by goals of treatment or clinical effects (Sherman *et al.* 2006), this chapter broadly looks at the underlying approach widely termed myofascial release (MFR) currently gaining much popularity in both traditional and complementary medicine. Although muscle is implicated, the salient feature that loosely distinguishes this approach from 'traditional' massage is the interconnectivity of the fascial system, subtlety of palpation and a gentle (low load) sustained stretch. The approach is driven more by perception, palpation and the patient's tissue response rather than following a structured framework based on symptom-driven techniques.

There has been a tendency to identify muscles in terms of anatomical structure and functional isolation, yet other body systems are identified in relation to their total anatomical and functional continuity through connective tissue, for example the vascular, lymphatic, osseous, respiratory and neural systems. The term connective tissue and fascia for the purposes of this chapter are interchangeable. Fascia is composed of the proteins collagen, providing strength, and elastin, providing flexibility, and the ground substance, a polysaccharide gel complex surrounding every cell (Gray and Williams 1995; LeMoon 2008).

The fascia surrounds, supports and give structural integrity and interconnectivity to all the systems of the body (Stecco *et al.* 2008), down to cellular and nuclear level (Chaitow 2006).

The muscular and fascial systems are both derived from the mesoderm and known together as the myofascial system. On a gross level, individual muscles are enveloped in a fascial matrix, the endo-, peri- and epimysium, interconnecting not only muscles, but also all the functional body systems (Juhan 1987; Gray and Williams 1995). Body movements either tension or slacken some part of this three-dimensional fascial matrix providing a key component to movement and structure. The nervous system receives the greatest amount of afferent sensory nerves from the muscles and related fascia, potentially forming the largest sensory organ (Schleip 2003, part 1).

Aims of the MFR approach

- Identify and palpate subtle, discrete areas of restriction within the fascial matrix.

- Apply a *gentle* sustained three-dimensional stretch for approximately 90–120 s.
- Facilitating with hands, follow and allow this restriction to elongate and 'unwind' as a spontaneous (not preconceived) release of the myofascial tissue.
- Acknowledge and encourage changed awareness of any somatic, postural, emotional or mental changes in a supportive, trusting environment.
- Maintain improved range of movement and resulting new ways of moving with home exercises.

Palpation philosophy and possible barriers to effectiveness

In order to locate these fascial restrictions, the practitioner needs to relax, let go of expectation and pay attention to the tactile and proprioceptive information received through the hands. During MFR teaching sessions students tend to focus on what they think they are supposed to be feeling, rather than what they are actually feeling in their hands. This has led to the following response:

- *'This is a waste of time, how can palpating so lightly tell us anything?'* – the more effort required the more out of touch you seem to be (Blackburn 2004, part 3).
- *'I'm never going to get this.'* – this may become a self-fulfilling prophecy.
- *'What exactly is it I'm supposed to be feeling?'* – needing to fulfill an expectation.
- *'I really, really, really, want to be able to do this.'* – the practitioner is trying too hard and is too tense to feel any subtle tensions in the body.

As these undermining thoughts, beliefs and attitudes arise in our mind, palpating at a subtle level becomes more difficult to the point where the analytical, right-brained thinking process may inhibit the more left-brained palpatory sensitivity (Payne 2000).

The mind needs to be free to explore, in a non-judgemental way, an appreciation of incoming information, rather than analysing and referencing each thought. Imagine our hands working as radio receivers; if they only tune into one frequency they will only receive one radio station, but if free to scan all the different frequencies then potentially all radio stations may be received. If some of those stations are in a foreign language, to filter them out would diminish the bigger picture. If the mind intention is to feel solely for myofascial restrictions (tuning into the myofascial station), this will be the station received. As this becomes more accomplished other stations can be received at the same time; for instance, tuning into emotions that may be related to the palpated area.

Exercises to enhance palpatory skills

The space apportioned here to palpatory skill description is indicative of the importance and relevance to the MFR technique.

Exercise 1: Attuning whole and bilateral hand sensitivity

During palpation we may become aware of being able to feel more easily with the right or left hand or with only part of that hand. The following exercise helps to develop feeling with the whole of one hand and then bilateral sensitivity.

- Place your flat hands palm down on a table surface as lightly as possible. Become aware of which areas you can feel in contact with the surface. Do both hands feel equally relaxed?
- Allow the hands to rest fully on the surface of the table. Does one hand melt and mould (meld) into the table surface more than the other? Bring awareness into each finger, thumb and palm of the hand. Avoid pushing the hands into the surface; simply allow the weight of just the hands to sink into the table.
- Notice what has to shift in you, for your sensitivity and awareness to develop more fully throughout the whole hand.
- Then notice what has to change in order for you to be able to feel more equally with both left and right hand.
- Identify in your own body areas of tension and how that may affect your ability to palpate.

Exercise 2: Enhancing palpatory sensitivity

- Repeat the above exercise with your hands lightly resting on your thighs.
- Having paid attention to what is happening in your hands start to notice what is actually underneath your hands. Does one hand sink into the tissues more freely? Develop a sense of density of the thigh tissue.
- Change hands in order to feel the left leg with the right hand and right leg with the left hand. How deeply into the tissues can you feel with either hand? Is there a difference? Change over hands to see if the difference is consistent.
- Return the right hand to the right leg and left hand to the left leg. If there is asymmetry in perception between your hands, what needs to shift in you or where do you need to release tension in order for the hands to feel more equal?
- Repeat the above with hands on the right and left side of the abdomen and thorax to develop this symmetry in hand perception.

Exercise 3: Palpating fascial glide

- Placing your hands on your thighs, imagine that your hands are part of the thighs (light touch as in Exercise 2).
- Now traction away from the hip (south), then away from the knee (north), then back to the starting position, then to the left and the right. Describe how the tissues felt in each leg and the amount of excursion from the starting position.
- Repeat this whilst extending your awareness beyond the surface to engage all the tissues of the thigh.
- Repeat with the hands placed on the abdomen and thorax.

Exercise 4: Influence of palpation and body tension

- Now you have greater awareness in your hands, notice how your palpatory sensitivity is influenced by your own body tension and posture.
- If unsure continue to practise Exercises 1–3.

Exercise 5: Palpation changes with different states of mind

- Ask a consenting colleague/friend to bring to mind one negative and one positive thought they have on a regular or daily basis, then forget the thoughts and focus on the present.
- Place your hands over the person's diaphragmatic area (anterior hand over the xiphoid process, posterior hand over the T10 area). Observe the feelings in your hands and then beyond into the tissues.
- Once you have a clear feeling of the tissues, ask the person to take a deep breath in, and when he/she breathes out, to bring the positive thought to the forefront of his/her mind. Notice what happens at the interface of your hands and beyond into the person's body.
- After approximately 20 s, ask the person to take another deep breath in, and on breathing out to bring his/her focus into the negative thought and notice changes.
- Notice how with the different mind states there may be a change in feeling between your hands.

Exercise 6: Identification and documentation of fascial restrictions

- A body chart may document the hand placement for assessing the whole of the fascial matrix. With light touch learnt from the palpation exercises previously, glide the tissues in the north, south, east and west directions as in Exercise 3.
- Mark on a body chart areas of tissue restriction, i.e. where you feel the tissues move freely and where they are restricted.

Exercise 7: Identification of the dominant holding pattern in the body

- Having assessed areas of tension/restriction throughout the body, each of these restrictions are prioritised (explained on training courses) in a similar manner to prioritising primary over secondary trigger points.

Myofascial release techniques

There are many ways of releasing perceived myofascial restrictions. The two most basic techniques are recoil stretch (direct technique) and positional release (indirect technique). The recoil stretch takes tension up in the tissues and the positional release relaxes tension in the tissues. For the purpose of this text, focus will be on the direct stretch technique as it is the safest to learn from text.

A sustained stretch technique

Conventionally, tissue has been stretched from a two-dimensional perspective in many therapeutic interventions; however, the body functions three dimensionally, and hence assessment, treatment and functional change is three dimensional.

- Place your hands either side of the restriction, and engage the fascia by taking up the slack in the tissues.
- Gently stretch (a few grams) by increasing the tension three dimensionally until you feel the tissues 'lock' under your hands and hold. Imagine you have an elastic cord between your hands and wind the tension up. This tension is developed between the hands without pushing down into the body excessively; more a sense of pulling the tissues apart three dimensionally.
- Hold this gentle stretch (sustained low load pressure) for a minimum of 90–120 s (Barnes 1997). As the restriction eases, warmth, motion and softening of the tissues is often palpated.
- Follow this release, holding the gentle pressure against any new restriction/barrier. Repeat until the tissues are softened and pliable.

Often there is no clear distinction between assessment and treatment as the gentle kinaesthetic perception of a fascial restriction initiates a physiological stretch (unwinding).

Contraindications

The same subjective and objective assessment preceding treatment and clinical judgement is applied as in all massage therapy. The following are absolute contraindications (J. Annan, teaching material 2006; see 'Course information'):

- Malignancy.
- Aneurysm.
- Acute circulatory conditions.
- Acute rheumatoid arthritis.
- Cellulitis.
- Febrile state.
- Advanced osteoporosis.
- Obstructive oedema.
- Anticoagulants.
- Severe hyperalgesia.
- Advanced diabetes.
- Systemic infection.
- Healing fracture sites, haematoma and open wounds (use clinical judgement).

Beyond the anatomy

Involving the mind and feelings

It is of great importance for the therapist and patient to be equally 'present', that is to have a shared awareness of the physical and mental experience of the patient to facilitate the patient's therapeutic process (Blackburn 2004; Blackburn and Price 2006). King (2002) suggests a deeper interactive tissue engagement is facilitated between patient and therapist by the patient focusing his/her breathing into the fascial restriction.

The concept of the mind and body being inextricably linked is now taken as a given. The growing integration of mind, body and feelings demonstrated in cognitive behavioural therapy (CBT), psychoneuroimmunology (PNI) and mindfulness in the practice of manual therapy are testament to the growing interest and significance of mental and emotional stresses in relation to the presentation of symptoms. Our posture can be seen as a reflection of our mental and emotional states becoming habitual over time. Latey (1996) describes in depth how the somatic body encapsulates mind and feelings at different levels, enabling exploration, understanding and the potential for therapeutic change. Therapeutic rapport facilitates personal meaning of these bodily responses to stress, enabling the patient's insight and motivation to change previous habitual physical and mental responses to stress.

An exploration of suggested rationale and their clinical implications

Responsive biomechanical model

Fascia has tended to be considered as an inert container and passive contributor to biomechanics. However, immunohistological analysis has demonstrated the presence of contractile smooth muscle-type features in cells called myofibroblasts, in normal fascia occurring particularly in the fascia lata, plantar and lumbar fascia (Schleip *et al.* 2005). An increasing body of evidence is demonstrating how physical manipulation may potentially influence profound and rapid structural, functional and mechanical interactions between fibroblasts and the extracellular matrix, resulting in fascial changes (Grinnell 2008). These fascial contraction properties may be actively influencing biomechanical behaviour, enabling an active temporary adjustment of passive muscle stiffness in response to increased mechanical and/or emotional tensional demands (Schleip *et al.* 2006). This may have an impact on fascial proprioception where an alteration of fascial tone may contribute to sacro-iliac instability and spinal segmental instability (Schleip *et al.* 2005) in a similar way that stiffness in plantar fascia contributes to stability of the foot (Cheung *et al.* 2004).

Neural-mechanoreceptor model

Schleip (2003, part 2) discuses how Ruffini sensory mechanoreceptors in the broad fascial sheaths give sensory and proprioceptive feedback to the central nervous system when stimulated by slow deep steady manual pressure involving lateral stretch. The Ruffini mechanoreceptors and other interstitial fascial mechanoreceptors (types III and IV) when stimulated can also affect autonomic function by increasing vagal activity (increased parasympathetic response), promoting global muscle relaxation and less emotional arousal. Increased vagal activity also changes local fluid dynamics and tissue metabolism (Schleip 2003, part 2). A diminished number of mechanoreceptors in the thoracolumbar fascia may relate to chronic low back ache and be possibly implicated in the ageing process (Schleip *et al.* 2005). Considering the possibility that MFR's specific sensory input might activate the central nervous system, thus eliciting neural reactions, Bertolucci (2008) suggests that EMG activity could objectively measure simultaneous subjective palpatory phenomena.

Gel-to-sol model

Thixotrophy is the gel-to-sol (dense to more fluid state) transformation confirmed to occur after mechanical pressure to connective tissue (Twomey and Taylor 1982).

The extracellular ground substance of fascia is a viscous colloidal semi-liquid in the immediate environment of every cell in the body, bathing the collagen fibres and composed of water-binding complex sugar mucopolysaccharides. As a general process, stress, disuse and lack of movement cause the gel to dehydrate, contract and harden. Dehydrated tissue feels gnarled and stringy (King 2002).

The application of pressure or stretch brings about a rapid rehydration and change to sol, yet removal of pressure allows the system to rapidly re-gel. However, during the 'sol' phase, the ground substance becomes more porous, providing an improved medium for the diffusing entry and exit of nutrients, oxygen, waste products of metabolism and enzymes. If the stretch is gentle and sustained (less is more) and the following rest period sufficiently long enough, more water soaks into the ground substance than before the stretch. This water content then increases to a higher level than before the stretch. This increased hydration could account for the palpable tissue changes after long-duration MFR but not below 2 minutes (Barnes 1997; Oschman 1997, part 5; Schleip 2003, part 1). However, this still does not account for the therapist's experience of tissue change after a few seconds.

Piezo-electric model

The structure and architecture of each cell consists of connective tissue, called the cytoskeleton, having the ability to communicate and process electromechanical and electrochemical signals. On a more subtle scale, fascia may act as a liquid crystal. When fibroblasts are distorted by movement, pressure, compression or tension, piezo-electrical fields spread throughout the body. The strength of these fields depends on the angle with which the pressure is applied (Oschman 1997, part 5; Schleip 2003, part 1).

Oschman (2005) discusses how the reliable detection of extremely low-frequency, non-thermal and non-ionising energy fields, as experienced in gentle sensitive manual touch, can potentially have important biological effects which optimise rapid cellular communication. These may be partially explained by emerging concepts of semiconduction, quantum mechanics, liquid crystals and biological coherence. In practical terms, this may be explained as less input producing greater clinical outcomes with the possibility of a physical intervention being directed some distance from the presenting symptoms, yet still clinically affecting the symptoms. Clinical evidence is discussed in Oschman (1997, part 5) and Schleip (2003, part 1).

Trauma release model

In a positive context, just as myofascial tissue appears to be therapeutically responsive to manual therapy, equally, within a negative context, for example, physical trauma or poor posture, the myofascial tissue change may appear to support dysfunction, as seen in adhesions and scar tissue. Oschman (2006) hypothesises how the fascial matrix extending into every cell and nucleus in the body senses and absorbs the physical and emotional impact in traumatic experiences. As these 'structural memories' are laid down in the fascia at an unconscious, non-verbal level, it is suggested that the non-verbal subtle MFR may release and resolve this 'tissue–held' trauma (Blackburn 2003; Oschman 2006).

Evidence of effectiveness in clinical practice

There is much positive anecdotal evidence arising from MFR ranging from objective specific musculoskeletal improvements in mobility, pain and dysfunction to wider holistic mind–body responses. The individualised nature and diverse responsiveness of MFR together with the varied outcomes poses complex methodological issues for research design, resulting in few rigorous studies. However, the following descriptions give a flavour of clinical potential:

- Barnes *et al.* (1997) demonstrated the effect of a myofascial release treatment technique on obtaining pelvic symmetry. Acknowledging the small sample size ($n = 10$), the results indicated that the treatment had the potential to be effective in facilitating a change in asymmetric pelvic position toward symmetry. Limitations of the study described subjects already undergoing MFR and the questionable reliability of measurements.
- Davis *et al.* (2005) compared MFR and exercise to exercise alone in two case studies involving two older people with severe kyphoscoliosis from osteoporosis and pain that necessitated walking with a rolling walker. Subjective and objective measures were taken pre and post MFR/exercise compared with exercise alone. After MFR, both cases reported improved feelings of energy, improved posture and greater ease in reaching and walking. Objectively there was improved balance, height, walking speed (timed-up-and-go or function) and pain reduction compared with exercise only.
- A single case study describing MFR in the treatment of a chronic thoracic outlet syndrome with nerve root irritation and gross postural asymmetry fully explained the treatment rational. The successful outcome of 2 weeks of intensive daily treatment described clinically significant changes in function, ROM, pain and postural symmetry (Barnes 1996).
- A single case study of amyotrophic lateral sclerosis showed improvements in range of movement, vagal tone, self report and timed-up-and-go at 12 weeks follow-up (Cottingham and Maitland 2000).

The following suggest potential clinical applications:

- Myofibroblast-facilitated contraction in the intramuscular perimysium fascia will influence passive muscle stiffness in conditions such as

torticollis, Parkinson's rigor, ankylosing spondylitis, shortened soleus in muscular dystrophy and chronic muscle tension, e.g. of the upper trapezius. It is suggested that very slow, sensitive manual deep tissue techniques may target and release these particular restrictions (Schleip *et al.* 2006).
- Increased alkalinity of blood in hyperventilation may cause contraction of intrafascial smooth muscle, increasing overall fascial tension. This may have implications in fibromyalgia and chronic fatigue syndrome (Schleip 2003, part 2).
- Post mastectomy and reconstruction, fibrous scar tissue and adhesions are eased and function improved (Hobden 2006).

So what do we feel with our hands?

If MFR affects local blood supply and local tissue viscosity, it is conceivable that these tissue changes could be rapid and significant enough to be felt by the 'listening' hand of the practitioner (Schleip 2003, part 2). The tissue responses our hands experience could be related to the sponge-like squeezing and refilling in the semi-liquid ground substance. Manual stimulation of fascia leads to tonus changes in the motor units which are mechanically linked to the tissue under the therapist's hand, enabling the hand to feel local specific changes in tone (Schleip 2003, part 1). It would seem that our understanding of the traditionally passive containing role of fascia is moving towards an adaptable and sensitive organ, responsive to the human hand.

Future implications

In the past, many therapies without an acceptable biomedical explanation were seen as alternative to the orthodox health care system of that time. Ongoing research and emerging concepts briefly addressed in this chapter are beginning to give some explanation of how the gentle sustained touch and global clinical changes observed in MFR may change the perception of this 'alternative therapy' towards an accepted integrated clinical practice.

The work of Myers (2004, part 13) in metaphorically describing the functional, articulated chains of myofascial structures as train lines dovetails well into Langevin *et al.*'s (2001) parallel concept of how the interconnected myofascial network appears to relate to the acupuncture meridian network, acupuncture points and myofascial trigger points. The propagation and amplification of cellular signals, from mechanical pressure/stretch, through the fascial network, may potentially further our understanding of the integrative communication and function of the whole body.

This described ability to sensitively palpate and therapeutically respond to changes in the myofascial tissues to affect the whole body may enhance (and change) our clinical practice, regardless of the specific manual therapy technique or discipline of the therapist (Myers 2004, part 1; Bertolucci 2008).

References

Barnes, J. (1996) Myofascial release in treatment of thoracic outlet syndrome. *Journal of Bodywork and Movement Therapies*, **1**(1), 53–7.

Barnes, M.F. (1997) The basic science of myofascial release: morphological changes in connective tissue. *Journal of Bodywork and Movement Therapies*, **1**(4), 231–8.

Barnes, M.F., Gronlund, R.T., Little, M.F. and Personius, W.J. (1997) Efficacy study of the effect of a myofascial release treatment technique on obtaining pelvic symmetry. *Journal of Bodywork and Movement Therapies*, **1**(5), 289–96.

Bertolucci, L.F. (2008) Muscle repositioning: a new verifiable approach to neuro-myofascial release. *Journal of Bodywork and Movement Therapies*, **12**, 213–24.

Blackburn, J. (2003) Trager: psychophysical integration – an overview. *Journal of Bodywork and Movement Therapies*, **7**(4), 233–9.

Blackburn, J. (2004) Trager part 2, 3, 4: Hooking up: the power of presence in bodywork. *Journal of Bodywork and Movement Therapies*, **8**, 114–21, 171–88, 265–77.

Blackburn, J. and Price, C. (2006) Implications of presence in manual therapy. *Journal of Bodywork and Movement Therapies*, **2**(1), 68–77.

Chaitow, L. (2006) Fascia 2007 Congress. *Journal of Bodywork and Movement Therapies*, doi:10.1016/j.jbmt.2006.07.004.

Cheung, J.T.K., Zhang, M. and An, K.N. (2004) Effects of plantar fascia stiffness on the biomechanical responses of

the ankle–foot complex. *Journal of Clinical Biomechanics*, **19**, 839–46.
Cottingham, J. and Maitland, J. (2000) Integrating manual and movement therapy with philosophical counselling for treatment of a patient with amytropic lateral sclerosis: a case study that explores the principles of holistic intervention. *Alternative Therapies*, **6**(2), 120–28.
Davis, C.M., Doerger, C., Rowland, J., Sauber, C. and Enton, T. (2005) Myofascial release as complementary to exercise in physical therapy for two elderly patients with osteoporosis and kyphoscoliosis: two case studies. *Australian Journal of Physiotherapy*, **51**(Suppl 4), S15.
Gray, H. and Williams, P.L. (1995) *Gray's Anatomy*, 38th edn. Churchill Livingstone, Edinburgh.
Grinnell, F. (2008) Fibroblasts mechanics in 3-dimensional collagen matrices. *Journal of Bodywork and Movement Therapies*, **12**, 191–3.
Hobden, J. (2006) Ties that bind. Frontline, January, p. 31.
Juhan, D. (1987) *Handbook for bodyworkers: Job's body*. Station Hill Press, Barrytown, New Jersey.
King, K. (2002) Myofascial breathwork: a regenerative bodywork approach. *Journal of Bodywork and Movement Therapies*, **6**(4), 224–5.
Langevin, H.M., Churchill, D.L. and Cipolla, M.J. (2001) Mechanical signalling through connective tissue: a mechanism for the therapeutic effect of acupuncture. *FASEB Journal*, **15**, 2275–81.
Latey, P. (1996) Feelings, muscles and movement. *Journal of Bodywork and Movement Therapies*, **1**(1), 44–52.
LeMoon, K. (2008) Terminology used in fascial research. *Journal of Bodywork and Movement Therapies*, **12**, 204–212.
Myers, T.W. (2004) Structural integration – developments in Ida Rolf's recipe. *Journal of Bodywork and Movement Therapies*, **8**; Part 1, 131–42; Part 2, 189–98; Part 3, 249–64.
Oschman, J.L. (1997) What is healing energy? *Journal of Bodywork and Movement Therapies*, **1**(2–5). Part 2, 117–22; Part 3, 179–94; Part 4, 239–47; Part 5, 179–94.
Oschman, J.L. (2005) Energy and the healing response. *Journal of Bodywork and Movement Therapies*, **9**, 3–15.
Oschman, J.L. (2006) Hypothesis: trauma energetics. *Journal of Bodywork and Movement Therapies*, **10**, 21–34.
Payne, R. (2000) *Relaxation Techniques – A Practical Handbook for the Health Care Professional*, 2nd edn. Churchill Livingstone, London.
Schleip, R. (2003) Fascial plasticity – a new neurobiological explanation. *Journal of Bodywork and Movement Therapies*, **7**(1–2), Part1, 11–19; Part 2, 104–16.
Schleip, R., Klinger, W. and Lehmann-Horn, F. (2005) Active fascial contractility: fascia may be able to contract in a smooth muscle-like manner and thereby influence musculoskeletal dynamics. *Medical Hypotheses*, **65**, 273–7.
Schleip, R., Naylor, I., Ursu, D., *et al.* (2006) Passive muscle stiffness may be influenced by active contractility of intramuscular connective tissue. *Medical Hypotheses*, **66**, 66–71.
Sherman, K., Dixon, M., Thompson, D. and Cherkin, D. (2006) Development of taxonomy to describe massage treatments for musculoskeletal pain. *BMC Complementary and Alternative Medicine*, 6, 24. Available from http://www.biomedcentral.com/1472-6882/6/24 (open access article).
Stecco, A., Masiero, S., Macchi, V., Stecco, C., Porzionato, A. and De Caro, R. (2008) The pectoral fascia: anatomical and histological study. *Journal of Bodywork and Movement Therapies*, **12**, doi:10.1016/j.jbmt.2008.04.036.
Twomey, L. and Taylor, J. (1982) Flexion, creep, dysfunction and hysteresis in the lumbar vertebral column. *Spine*, **7**(2), 116–22.

Further reading

Andrade, C.K. and Clifford, P. (2001) Outcome-based massage, In: *Connective Tissue Techniques*. Lippincott Williams and Wilkins, Philadelphia, pp. 244–74.
Barnes, J.F. (2004) Myofascial release: the missing link in traditional treatment. In: *Complementary Therapies in Rehabilitation* (ed. C.M. Davis). Slack Incorporated, Thorofare, New Jersey, pp. 59–81.
Oschman, J. (2003) *Energy Medicine in Therapeutics and Human Performance*. Butterworth Heinemann, Oxford.

Useful websites

http://www.fasciaresearch.com.
http://www.i-sis.org/brainde.shtm (articles by M.W. Ho).
http://www.johnlatz.com/keyelements_article.html.
http://www.rolf.org/about/research.htm.
http://www.sciencedirect.com/science/journal/13608592.
http://www.softtissuetherapy.com.au.
http://www.somatics.de/fasciaresearch/innervation.htm.

Course information

http://www.dmbem.com/mfrb.htm (Stuart Robertson).
http://www.physiouk.co.uk/html/courses/fascial.htm (John Annan). Acknowledgements to John Annan for kindly providing information regarding contraindications, as taught in his courses.

Index